FOODS *for* HEALTH

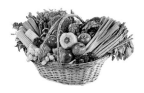

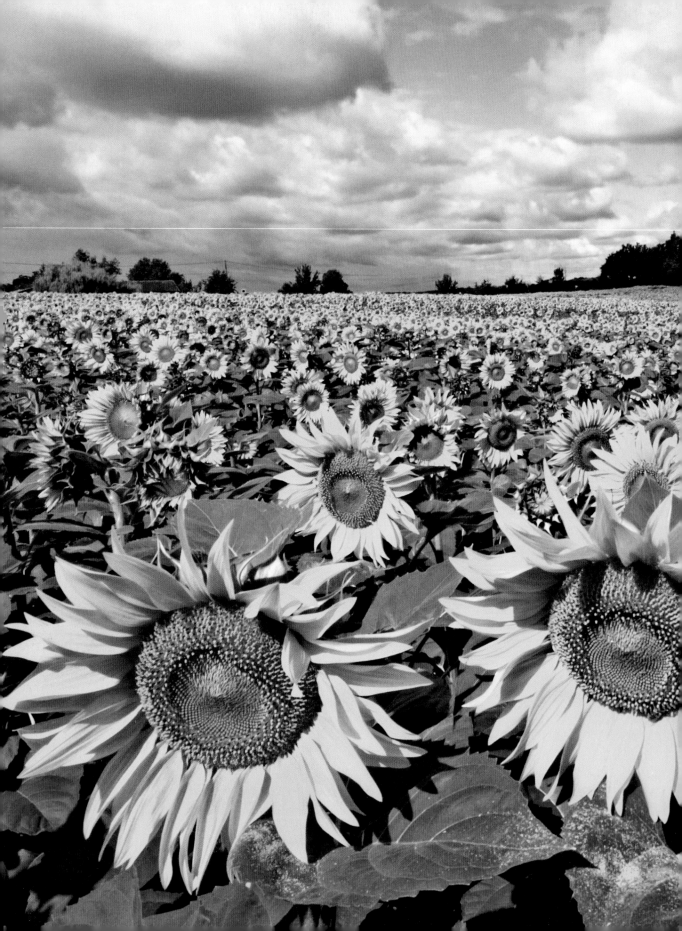

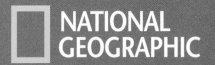

FOODS
for
HEALTH

Choose and Use the Very Best Foods
for Your Family and Our Planet

Barton Seaver
P. K. Newby, Sc.D., M.P.H.

NATIONAL GEOGRAPHIC
WASHINGTON, D.C.

CONTENTS

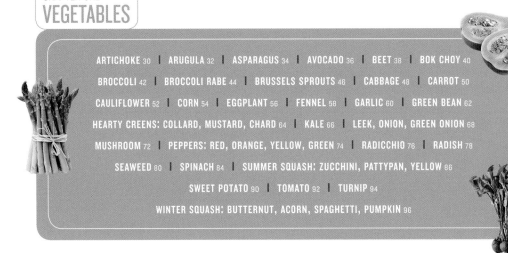
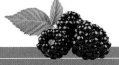

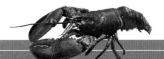

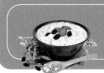

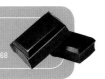

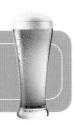

TOWARD A COMMUNION OF THE COMMONS:
EATING JOYFULLY AND RESPONSIBLY

✢ ✢ ✢

BARTON SEAVER

I grew up in a multicultural neighborhood in Washington, D.C. While the majority of the neighborhood hailed from El Salvador, there were large populations of Ethiopians, Guatemalans, Hondurans, Koreans, Chinese, Thai, and African Americans.

It was a Noah's Ark of people. Each of these groups had little bodegas that served their needs, importing to their new world a taste of home. I vividly remember exploring the aisles of these shops and being blown away by the heady, seductive spices, the exotic fruits and vegetables, and the variety of meats available, not to mention the cuts of meat not easily found in our regular stores. I warmly remember answering the dinner bell's clang and saying goodbye to my friends after an intense afternoon of street soccer. Arriving home I would find my father, tie off, apron donned, at work at the stove. My father was an excellent cook and was not shy to use new ingredients. Some nights the aroma of an East Indian curry filled the house. Other nights I would be put to work pressing out the moistened masa harina dough to form the tortillas, dry-fried, and then stuffed with fresh ingredients for taco night.

Muliticultural Food

Food was always an exploration for me. A window onto a world of new flavors, textures, aromas, experiences. But as much as dinner brought some new corner of the world into our house, these ingredients, dishes, and flavors also represented the cultures of the boys and girls with whom I spent my days. Just as these new ingredients and dishes helped me to better know the physical world, they also allowed me to better know the people who populated my life. I realized early on that food is an exploration of geography, of physical senses, of history, of culture, and is an expression of the needs that we all share as neighbors on this planet.

I was fortunate to spend a few weeks every summer on the shores of the Patuxent River in Maryland, a tributary of the Chesapeake Bay. There, every morning at the crack of dawn I would wake and begin my search for food. Walking down the dock I would deftly scoop up the blue crabs that had anchored on the pilings. I would cast my line into the deep water and with every third toss reel in a striped bass, bluefish, perch, croaker, spot, or mackerel. There was bounty in these waters, and our dinners were a reflection of whatever we were blessed to have received from the bay that day.

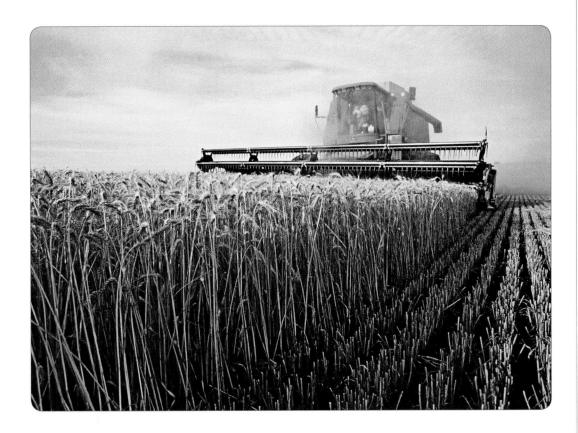

Respecting Earth's Resources

Years later I was offered my first executive chef position. As I created my menu, I asked myself what I wanted to communicate to my guests? I went back to those summer memories and hoped to share that same joy with my clientele. I phoned my fish purveyor and said, "Send me striped bass, crab, oysters. I want bluefish. I want mackerel." He gave a brief chuckle and dryly stated, "Sorry kid, we ate all of those. What else do you want?"

I was speechless. How could something that was part of my identity be gone? It turned out my fish supplier was right. Our demand for those species had been so great that they were effectively gone. Efforts were in place to restore the health of the bay, but for the time being I had to look elsewhere for my menu.

I realized at that moment that the guiding hand of natural selection in this world is quite firmly holding a fork. What we choose to eat describes how we choose to use the world. And in this case, we had used it all up.

I began to talk to friends in the conservation community and learned a great deal about how marine ecosystems work, how fishing pressure can diminish the health of our oceans, and how most people were unaware of the crisis. I looked back into the cannon of environmental literature and found out about the "tragedy of the commons." This idea, put forth beautifully in an essay by Dr. Garret Hardin, has become a cornerstone of modern environmentalism, and states that men and women acting in rational self-interest will ultimately bring ruin to our shared common. And this has given rise to a style of environmentalism that focuses on how humans negatively impact ecosystems.

People Create Solutions

Now I was a chef selling hospitality in a restaurant. I needed to come up with another perspective on the common story—describe how humans have a positive role to play in our relationship with nature. If humans can bring destruction to ecosystems through their quest for food, if humans can then use that food to give rise to unprecedented rates of diabetes, heart disease, obesity; if humans can make the earth and themselves sick by the choices that they make for dinner, then the opposite was also true—they could make the very same choices in order to heal. Heal their bodies and their planet.

In other words, we are the problem, and that means that we are also the solution. I began to call this perspective the communion of the commons. It's a narrative of how humans are impacted by ecosystems, a consideration of our role in nature that is more hopeful, useful, and human.

Sustainability

One of my favorite authors, E. B. White wrote, "I wake each morning torn, not knowing whether to save the earth or to savor it." Fortunately we don't have to make that choice, we cannot create more food, bulldoze more rainforests, find more fish in the sea. But we can learn how to balance our relationship with what nature provides. Sustainability and human health are about nourishing ourselves and our communities with the foods that we already produce.

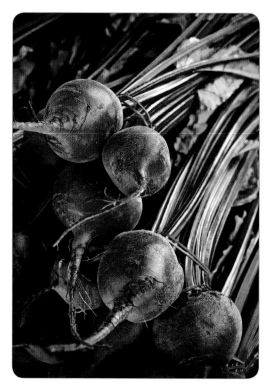

Sustainable food production is a continuously advancing effort. But it alone is not enough. We must also achieve a simultaneous behavioral shift that encourages and teaches us to use food sustainably. It's all about balance, finding the best products and then using them wisely. The same principles apply to sustaining environments and sustaining humans.

We eat to sustain ourselves, and food is the basis of all health. We eat for calories, nutrients, vitamins, and a host of biological interactions to serve our physiological needs, some known, others not. Nutrition allows for us to understand how foods impact the body, and why some are good and others less so. This biological approach to food is the science of nutrition, which is a science of discovery, revealing the inner workings of the human body's biochemistry. Understanding nutrition gives us an opportunity to gain wisdom on how best to use food to sustain our bodies.

SPRING

An Early Spring Celebration
THE RETURN OF THE VEGETABLES

Spring heralds the return of tender young vegetables.
Farmer's markets sprout up as eagerly as do the first shoots
of asparagus after a long winter's hiatus. This menu celebrates
the new flavors and crisp textures of the season

BEVERAGE
These heady-scented lemons, a holdover from the winter, make for a beguiling treat. Sweeten the lemon juice with maple syrup and add soda or flat water to your taste.

MEYER LEMONADE

ROASTED ASPARAGUS WITH POACHED EGG, TOASTED BARLEY, AND PARMESAN

VEGETABLE
Asparagus is easily combined with many flavors. Here the crisp stalks are paired with the creamy egg, the salty bite of shaved Parmesan, and the sweet crunch of toasted barley.

ENTRÉE
Fisheries begin anew in the warming spring weather. Halibut is one of the markers of the season and its snowy, white flesh is a perfect match to the sweet and delicate flavors of roasted carrots and crisp snap peas tossed in vinaigrette with pea shoots.

ROASTED ALASKAN HALIBUT, PEAS AND CARROTS SALAD WITH TENDER PEA SHOOTS

PANNACOTTA WITH MACERATED STRAWBERRIES

DESSERT
Pannacotta is the wonderfully simple thickened cream dessert of Italy. Similar to a crème brulée in texture, this creamy dessert is a perfect foil to the aromatic burst of the first of season strawberries.

CRISP CALIFORNIA SAUVIGNON BLANC

WINE
A crisp California sauvignon blanc pairs easily with many of the foods of spring dessert.

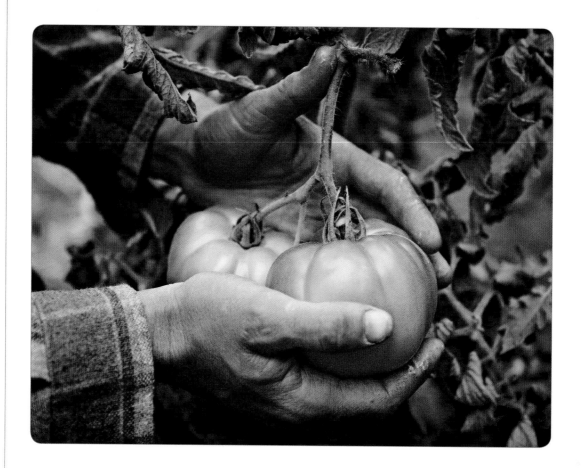

Fads versus Prudent Choices

Too often in the past, nutrition has been perceived incorrectly as a science of invention. People have looked to nutrition to alleviate their ills that have resulted from mismanagement of everyday health habits. Instead of changing our habits, we prefer to believe that doctors will invent a miracle cure or a magic pill that allows us to continue in our poor dietary habits that have hurt our health.

Invention is a part of human behavior and culture and responds to the cycles of popular preferences and trends. We see this often in the ever-recurring "new diet" that will radically change our appearance and life. Such promises offer more than an instant cure; they support the notion that our health can be guaranteed by science and not by our own prudent choices throughout our lives.

We do not need to reinvent the human diet. We have been getting along acceptably for the past 10,000 years, and the human relationship to food has been one of immense reward, allowing our diverse societies to succeed in magnificent ways. However, a part of the modern food industry has largely convinced us of the need to reinvent food, not for reasons of better health, but for their profit. What we need and fortunately are moving towards is a return to a more rational relationship with the foods that have sustained us throughout history.

◆ SUMMER ◆

A Midsummer's Feast
THE PLAYFUL DELIGHTS OF SUMMER

Summer is when cooking gets really easy.
The straightforward flavors of ripe fruit and produce
are best when left to speak for themselves.
The cook's role here is to buy great ingredients
and then let them shine.

BEVERAGE
Blackberries are a sweet-sour treat. Muddle a few berries with mint and sugar then stir into soda water or sparkling wine.

BLACKBERRY SODA

✛

SHAVED ZUCCHINI AND FENNEL SALAD WITH MUSTARD VINAIGRETTE

SALAD
Raw zucchini makes for a delicious dish when shaved thin with a peeler into long, thin ribbons. The aromatic crunch of fennel and the cool tang of mustard rounds this dish out.

✛

ENTRÉE
Fresh sockeye salmon takes to smoke like a fish to water. Spike your grill with woodchips and cook slowly. Romesco is a classic Catalan sauce of roasted then puréed vegetables.

GRILL-SMOKED SALMON WITH ROMESCO

✛

SPELT AND ALMOND PILAF

SIDE DISH
Spelt is delightful when paired with nutty sweetness of almonds. Start by toasting the spelt in olive oil with garlic then add almonds and water. Simmer till the spelt is soft.

✛

GRILLED PEACHES WITH BALSAMIC VINEGAR AND ICE CREAM

DESSERT
Grilling peaches couldn't be simpler. Pair the smoky, sweet fruit with the tang of balsamic for a balanced dessert.

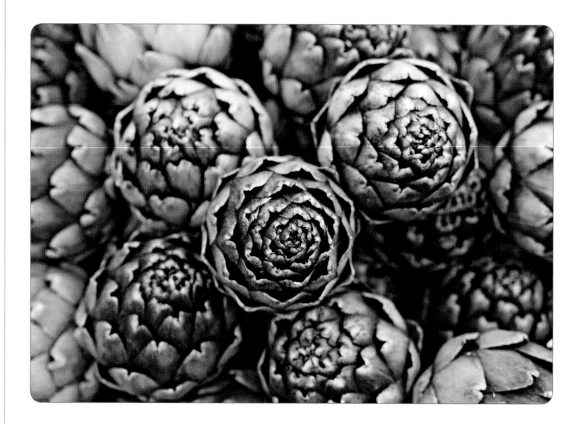

Craft Your Own Diet

This is not a plea that we all return to a farm to charm from the soil our daily bread. We do not need to cast aside our culinary preferences and cultural identities to adhere to a strict dietary prescription. The offerings in this book aim to encourage people to make food—its preparation, culture, and enjoyment—a pleasurable priority in our everyday life.

Good nutrition is not the result of denying ourselves the foods we love. It is not an all or nothing proposition. A hamburger now and then is not going to kill you. *Foods for Health* shares that it's not so much the unhealthy food we choose, but how much of it we consume.

So much of healthy eating is about behavior—setting expectations of what we hope food to accomplish in our lives and realigning our consumption behaviors to match our goals. Good nutrition is the result of eating a diverse range of foods within the framework of dietary guidelines, and delicious taste must always be of primary importance. You have to enjoy food in order to want to eat it again. And food is an incredibly personal topic. It represents the most intimate relationship we have with anything in our natural world, second only to our families and partners.

There is no right answer, no one answer, for how we eat. *Foods for Health* presents information and our own passions for fresh, natural ingredients to help you to understand the amazing opportunity available in every meal you craft.

Enjoying Delicious Food

To help you discover and experiment more, we offer many of our favorite ingredients

◆ AUTUMN ◆

Autumn's Splendor
A HARVEST CELEBRATION

There is much to celebrate in the Fall,
and this meal invites you to do just that.
Gather your friends and family and give a culinary
tip-of-the-hat to the seasons as they change.

APERITIF
A glass of warmed apple cider begs for a dash of brandy!

Spice-Mulled Apple Cider

⊹

Roasted Squash Panzanella with Pear and Walnut

SALAD
Panzanella is a salad of croutons and vegetables that combine for a well-textured dish.

⊹

Quinoa Cakes, Roasted Sweet Potatoes with Cilantro-Almond Pesto, and Braised Broccoli with Raisins and Almonds

ENTRÉE
A bevy of vegetables to celebrate the harvest is a perfect send-off to the bounty of the year.

DESSERT
Peel, core, and bake your favorite heirloom apple with a dash of cider in a covered pan. When soft, fill with cool plain yogurt sweetened with maple syrup and top with crunchy granola.

⊹

Baked Apples Stuffed with Yogurt and Granola

⊹

A Vibrant Oregon Pinot Noir

WINE
A refreshing yet luscious pinot noir is an excellent pairing for the earthy flavors of autumn.

and suggestions on how to approach these foods. Here you can find the groundwork to create or expand your relationship with food in a way that enables you to feel satisfaction and well-being.

When we eat we nourish more than just our bodies—we nourish our spirits. Through food we extend hospitality to ourselves and to others. We create bonds that transcend nationality, age, race, and beliefs. We nourish a complicated hunger in that we use food to connect to each other, to our past. Through food we also participate in tradition and acknowledge our place in the natural systems of this world. Ultimately, what and how we eat defines our health, and the myriad ways food comes into our lives defines the health of our planet.

Nutrition helps us to understand our biological needs, and sustainability helps us to understand what we can rationally expect our world to provide for us. When we combine these two efforts we find that we have a rare opportunity to acknowledge our dependence upon nature for our wellbeing and as a result embrace our relationship with nature and honor its ecosystems. Health and sustainability are social constructs with a singular purpose: to both savor and save the blessing of our time here on earth, one delicious bite at a time.

Our goal is for *Foods for Health* to inspire you to think about what you eat and how it can optimize your health and improve the environment. We hope that you use this book to increase the joy of eating and of eating together, so that we might all be reminded of what unites us on this beautiful, remarkable planet.

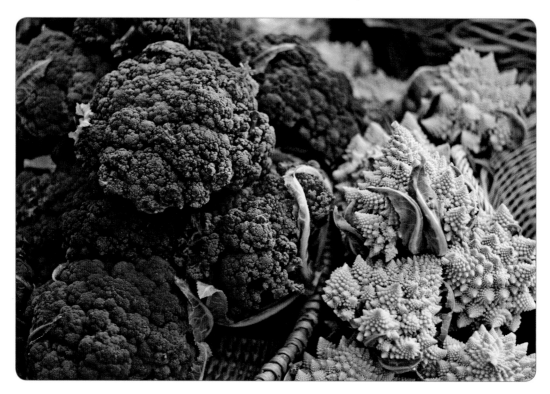

◆ **WINTER** ◆

Winter's Comfort
A MEAL TO BRING PEOPLE TOGETHER

In the winter months we want to snuggle
into the comfort of our homes
and gather around the warming fires of the kitchen.
The foods we crave are rich and filing.
The ingredients at market yield nothing new
as we settle into the dormant months on a farm.

SALAD
Spinach gives us a burst of fresh flavor, especially when this slightly bitter green is paired with the sweet, creamy taste of caramelized onion.

Spinach and Caremelized Onion Salad

VEGETABLE
Cauliflower has a beautiful flavor and is well suited to a long-simmered dish like this. Cut into florets and simmer with canned, diced tomatoes, onions, and slivered almonds. Finish with fresh mint and olive oil.

✛

Braised Cauliflower with Mint and Almond

ENTRÉE
Lots and lots of vegetables are what make this stew. Turnips, parsnips, carrots, potatoes, kohlrabi all add a unique twist to this balanced stew of flavors. You'll find yourself picking around the beef just to get to the vegetables!.

✛

Vegetable and Beef Stew

WINE
The rich foods of winter are well matched with fuller bodied red wines.

✛

Rich California Cabernet

✛

Hot Chocolate

BEVERAGE
Rich cocoa stirred into warmed milk is a perfect foil for the evening's chill. Carry a mug with you to the fire and snuggle in for the night.

FROM FARM TO FORK:
WHY WHAT WE EAT MATTERS

✤ ✤ ✤

P. K. NEWBY, Sc.D., M.P.H.

When you get right down to it, food is practically the whole story every time, wrote Kurt Vonnegut in his 1985 novel, *Galápagos*. Wise words indeed, for food is as fundamental to human life as it is to for the development of civilization itself.

A source of pleasure, a celebration of culture, and a foundation of health, food practically is the whole story every time.

Vonnegut's words certainly ring true in my own life. My love affair with food began as a child, baking and gardening at my mother's side. I began working in restaurants as a teenager and worked as a part-time cook in a local vegetarian restaurant in college. Despite my love of the culinary arts, I became increasingly fascinated with the larger role food plays in our lives, farm to fork, spoon to society. From examining the effects of food on health and disease to studying why we eat what we do and the impacts of our choices on the environment, I have dedicated my scientific career to understanding why what we eat matters. These days, I spend more time in the kitchen than the laboratory, where I work to communicate what we know about food—and we know a lot—to people like you. My goal is simple: to help individuals translate principles of sound science and sustainable eating to their plates in delectable ways. After all, if food doesn't taste good, no one's going to eat it, no matter how good it is for you.

As one of life's purest joys, there are plenty of occasions for indulgence when it comes to food and drink: moderation is a key facet of a healthful diet. Even so, some foods are better for our bodies and the environment than others. The foods we eat regularly that form our everyday diet have the power and potential to help us reduce our risk of disease, maintain a healthy body weight, and maybe, just maybe, save the planet in so doing. It is to this life- and planet-saving topic—foods for health—that this book is dedicated.

Eating "Whole"

I envision this book sitting on a kitchen shelf or coffee table, providing you with at-a-glance information to help guide your individual body and our planetary home toward better health. Our goal is to provide you with a compendium that brings together key elements of what we grow and eat in easy-to-use fashion. Each section includes

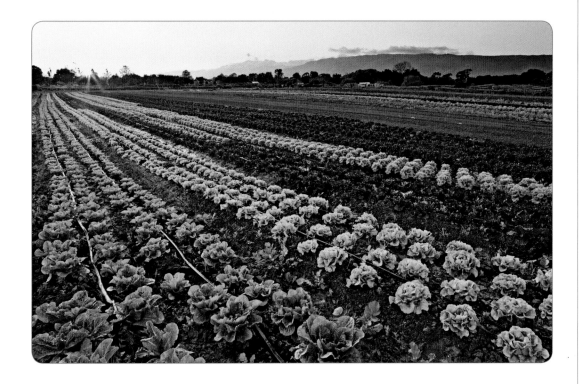

historical and agricultural food facts as well as science-based nutritional information, health benefits, and environmental considerations. We've also included a few of our favorite methods, techniques, and tips for selecting and preparing foods in ways you and your family will enjoy. Through its pages, I hope you will gain an increased appreciation for why what you eat matters, farm to fork.

The book is arranged alphabetically within each food category: vegetables, fruits, proteins, whole grains, fats, and oils, and beverages. Organizing the book one food at a time makes logical sense when it comes to reading, but less so when it comes to eating. For while we might snack on a handful of juicy blueberries or crunchy almonds, our diet includes a mixture of foods and drinks that, together, create an indelible impact on our health and the planet. In other words, when it comes to diet, the whole is greater than the sum of its parts.

Combining Foods

This is certainly obvious from a taste perspective: combining foods in delectable ways creates memorable meals, and we all have our favorite examples of things that just "go together." Eating foods in mixtures also provides a major health benefit, as nutrients often interact with each other in the body. Fat-soluble vitamins, for example, are better absorbed if consumed alongside fat, as their name implies. Thus, not only is our salad more flavorful with a zesty vinaigrette, it also helps us gain the maximum nutritional value from all of those nutrient-rich vegetables—more so than if we had eaten the salad without any dressing at all.

The whole is also greater than the sum of its parts when it comes to individual foods, as foods are complex packages that include vitamins, minerals, and phytonutrients (powerful chemicals found in plants), many of which work in concert to impact our health. Scientific studies have shown that whole foods evoke a greater benefit to our bodies than consuming any one particular nutrient. Moreover, foods undoubtedly include a host of beneficial elements that scientists have not yet discovered: what we don't know about an individual food may turn out to be just as important to our health as what we know now.

For these reasons, it's best to fill your diet with whole foods that have been minimally processed so as to preserve and maximize their health benefits. Stripping away the germ and bran from grains, for instance, results in a far less nutritious food than consuming its "whole" counterpart. (Think: bread or pasta made from the whole wheat kernel rather than the "white" version.) And eating the whole fruit rather than just extracting the sweet juice will deliver more nutrients and less sugar than simply drinking the liquid. While it's necessary to wash produce to remove unwanted dirt and chemical residues, consuming the fiber- and (phyto)nutrient-rich peels alongside the flesh delivers more nutrients than removing the skins. By consuming all the different parts of foods, root to leaf, we also reduce our methane-producing, climate-warming food waste that gets dumped into landfills—much of it perfectly edible.

Your Personal Plate

While most people eat pretty much everything, it is the degree to which we do so that defines our overall dietary pattern, our whole diet. There are obvious examples of how we might classify the way we eat, like omnivore or vegetarian. Yet even within those groups exists considerable variation in what we cook, colored by geography

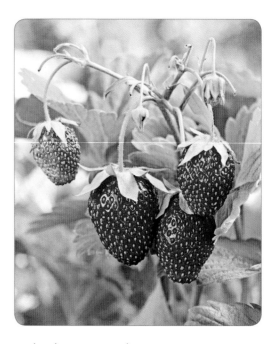

and culture as much as taste, cost, convenience, and healthfulness. Are you a meat-and-potatoes person who enjoys traditional comfort foods, or do you enjoy global cuisine? Do you have a penchant for sweet or salty foods, or do you consume alcohol? Is your diet filled with fast-food favorites like burgers, fries, and pizza or does it burst with whole grains, fruits, and vegetables? More so than the consumption of any one particular food, it is the combination of all the foods you eat regularly (alongside other genetic and lifestyle factors) that ultimately influences your health, your weight, your risk of disease, and your carbon footprint. And, whatever your plate looks like, employing the three fundamental tenets of variety, balance, and moderation will go a long way towards building a healthy diet.

Variety, Balance, Moderation

Certainly you've heard that variety is the spice of life. So, too, is variety the spice of a salubrious diet: the greater the diversity in color and

SPRING

THE START OF SEASONAL PRODUCE
CELEBRATING SPRING DELIGHTS

Spring in Boston marks the opening of the seasonal markets that last until November. A time of transition, my meals feature ephemeral delicacies like asparagus, fava beans, and strawberries. Whether part of a garden party luncheon or a light supper, these dishes celebrate spring and welcome warmer days to come.

BEVERAGE
Infusions bursting with berries, flowers, and herbs are my go-to beverage, perfect for a sunny afternoon. Serve with a lemon wedge or sprig of mint for a delightful drink that's calorie- and sugar-free.

BEAN SALAD
A labor of love, I prepare fresh favas every spring. Dress with olive oil, lemon juice, salt, pepper, and whatever herbs strike your fancy. Watermelon radishes with their pink and green center are a gorgeous complement. (Parmesan shards optional.)

GREEN SALAD
Juicy berries, scallions, and toasted pecans lie atop a bed of spinach, glorious with an orange-balsamic vinaigrette. (Add farro or blue cheese for variety, or try other spring lettuces like mesclun or arugula.)

VEGETABLE
Simple as can be, just toss asparagus with olive oil, lemon zest, and crushed garlic; season with a bit of salt and ground black pepper; and toast in a hot oven until crisp-tender. Be on the lookout for purple asparagus!

DESSERT
Not for everyday eating, gelato is a special treat I make only when sumptuous local berries are at their best: red, sweet, and delicious. Simply amazing. Serve with a mint sprig garnish for a pop of color.

ICED HIBISCUS AND WILD BERRY HERBAL INFUSION

FAVA BEAN SALAD WITH WATERMELON RADISHES AND HERBS

SPINACH SALAD WITH STRAWBERRIES, SCALLIONS, AND TOASTED PECANS

LEMON-SCENTED ASPARAGUS WITH SPRING GARLIC

STRAWBERRY GELATO

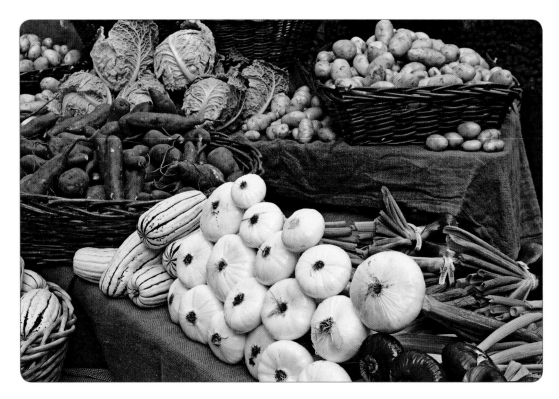

kind of foods we eat, the healthier our diet tends to be. No doubt this is why humans evolved as omnivores. Because each food contains different components, we increase the probability of avoiding nutritional deficiencies by consuming a wide array of foods. As some nutrients are toxic at high amounts, loading up on just a few foods can even be fatal. Therefore, treating a single food or nutrient as a magic pellet is not the road to health if other foods are neglected: forget the "superfood" du jour and focus on eating broadly.

Balance in diet, as in life, can be a tricky concept to put into practice, in part because there are different paths to a healthy diet. Sardinians consume a Mediterranean diet high in fat, primarily due to olive oil, with moderate wine intake; Okinawans enjoy a high carbohydrate diet filled with soy foods and green tea; and Seventh Day Adventists in Loma Linda, California, are vegetarians who eat a high fiber diet and don't drink alcohol. While all three groups eat primarily plant-based diets, the range of foods and beverages consumed vary greatly and are nestled firmly in their distinct geography, culture, traditions, and beliefs. As a result, the balance of the key energy-containing macronutrients fat, carbohydrate, and protein also differs. Nonetheless, these three diverse groups from three different parts of the globe share one important feature: the greatest longevity among the world's populations. Happily, there are numerous ways to achieve balance; one size does not fit all when it comes to diets that will get you to your hundredth birthday.

Moderation is the third pillar of the dietary triad, and it's arguably the most fun to implement when we're reveling in some of our favorite foods. Unlike vegetables and fruits, which should be eaten in abandon given most of us don't consume nearly enough, there are

◆ SUMMER ◆

Summer's Bounty
A SALAD BUFFET FOR A HOT DAY

From colorful squashes and lettuces to luscious berries and stone fruit,
I can make almost my entire supper from local produce
during the height of summer. Below is selection of favorites
I might serve as part of an evening buffet on a balmy day.
(Can you tell I eat a lot of salad?)

APERITIF
Mix puréed cucumber—
keep the skin for fiber
and color—with fresh
lime juice, basil simple
syrup, and sparkling
water for a flavorful,
pretty drink. For an
alcoholic version,
substitute gin.

Cucumber Basil Sparkler

✤

Warm Scallop Salad with Grilled Peaches and Baby Chard

STARTER
Grilled peaches are sublime
in summer (and make a
terrific dessert). Plate with
seared sea scallops and
baby chard and dress with
a peach vinaigrette for a
salad that is as lovely as it
is nutritious.

CORN SALAD
Top thinly sliced
squash with a
mixture of sun gold
cherry tomatoes,
corn, white onion,
and parsley dressed
with olive oil, white
balsamic vinegar, and
garlic. Summer on
a plate, made even
more divine with a
scattering of chèvre.

✤

Corn Salad with Sun Gold Cherry Tomatoes

✤

Herbed Quinoa Salad with Blueberries and Pignolis

GRAIN SALAD
Toss a selection of
lettuces and herbs
together with quinoa,
blueberries, and
toasted pine nuts for a
dinner salad that won't
leave you wanting.
Dress with a lemon-
herb vinaigrette, or
keep it simple with oil
and vinegar.

✤

Poached Rhubarb and Blackberries with Mascarpone

DESSERT
I put these together when I found both at the market one
spring day. Poached in port, orange peel, and spices and
topped with a dollop of mascarpone, this is a wonderful
dessert that can be served at room temperature.

other foods and dishes in which a moderate approach is best. Chocolate and alcohol come to mind, and you can easily envision dishes you adore that fall under the heading of "moderation." Your beloved, high-calorie dishes should not be totally eschewed, and complete denial can lead to an unhealthy relationship with food for some. Moderation is indeed part of a healthy diet and allows you to savor the divine pleasures of food and drink.

Plant-Based Diets

Building a diet that suits your palate and preferences upon a foundation of variety, balance, and moderation will go a long way toward creating healthy habits. Yet the one principle of nutrition and sustainable eating that will ultimately transform your health—and if billions of human beings do it, will in time restore the Earth—is following a plant-based diet. In Albert Einstein's words, "Nothing will benefit human health and increase chances for survival of life on Earth as much as the evolution to a vegetarian diet."

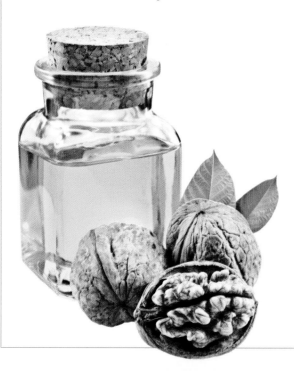

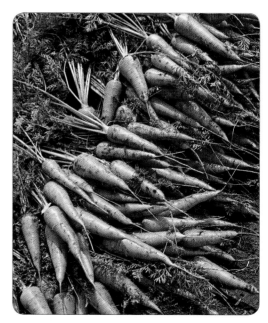

But with all this talk of variety, balance, and moderation combined with the recognition that the diet of early humans was omnivorous, must plants really take the lead in today's twenty-first century diets?

In fact, decades of research have shown the beneficial effect of diets high in plant foods such as vegetables, fruits, whole grains, beans, and legumes when it comes to human health, longevity, and disease prevention. While there are numerous forms a plant-based diet may take, paramount is the high intake of a variety of plant foods consumed in balance with each other and with physical activity to maintain a healthy body weight. Although science has shown it is not necessary to shun meat completely to obtain positive health benefits, filling our plates with plant foods of all kinds is vital.

A Healthy Planet

Science is also clear that plant-based diets are best for the health of our planet, primarily due to the high cost in fuel, feed, land, and water in producing animal foods. It's

AUTUMN

SHIFTING SEASONS
HARVESTING BOSTON'S BEST

As the days grow shorter and temperatures begin to drop,
late summer produce is still around at the markets,
but my attention turns to fall fare. These selections are early
autumn favorites that bridge the seasons, comprising here a
buffet for a board of directors' meeting for my theater company.

WINE

KALE SALAD WITH CARAMELIZED BRUSSELS SPROUTS AND TOASTED ALMONDS

SMOKED MUSSEL AND CORN CHOWDER

WARM HEIRLOOM TOMATO SALAD WITH MUSTARD GREENS AND GORGONZOLA

BUTTERNUT SQUASH SALAD WITH DRIED CRANBERRIES, TOASTED WALNUTS, AND CHIVE BLOSSOMS

GREEN SALAD
I fell in love with kale a few years back, greatly expanding my salad horizons. Chop the crucifer into thin strips and toss in a cider vinaigrette with caramelized Brussels sprouts. Top with sliced scallions and a sprinkle of dry roasted, unsalted almonds.

WINE
Alongside water at dinnertime, heart-healthy wine is a common libation for me. I keep bottles of red, white, and rosé on hand so people can select what they like.

CHOWDER
Traditional corn chowder is made with bacon and loaded in cream. My version substitutes smoked mussels for richness and includes diced zucchini and red peppers. Freshly shucked corn and stock made from the cobs makes all the difference.

TOMATO SALAD
A selection of brightly colored heirlooms needs little else but a drizzle of olive oil and vinegar, salt and pepper. Take things up a notch by roasting, plating over mustard greens tossed in a balsamic vinaigrette, and scattering with gorgonzola.

SQUASH SALAD
No autumn menu would be complete without winter squash. Cubes of roasted butternut pair beautifully with ruby red cranberries and toasted walnuts; pretty chive blossoms add elegance and flavor. Dress with maple-Dijon vinaigrette.

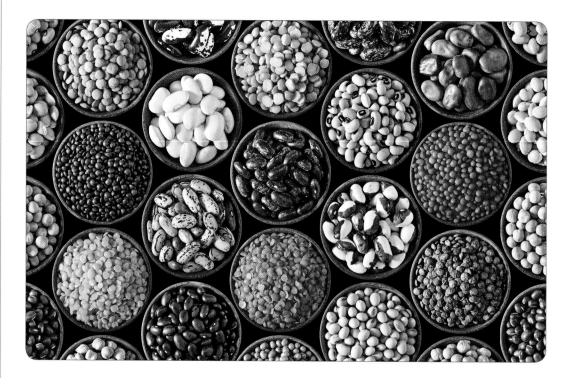

sorely inefficient to transform precious natural resources into meat and wreaks a greater burden on the environment. Further, there are numerous externalities associated with meat production that do not occur when growing plants, including the production of methane from ruminant animals, a greenhouse gas twenty-one times more powerful than carbon dioxide. For this reason, the impact of "food miles"—the environmental cost of how far a food travels to get to your plate—must be considered in the context of other more potent drivers of environmental damage. In general, food transportation affects climate change far less than food production: the "what" is usually more important than the "how far" when it comes to greening up your diet. While there are plenty of fantastic reasons to support your local farmers market

and select fresh foods in season, reducing your consumption of animal products will go much further in limiting the deleterious effects of your diet on the earth's soil, waterways, and atmosphere.

The time has arrived for you to embark on your journey into *National Geographic Foods for Health: Choose and Use the Very Best Foods for Your Family and Our Planet*. Drink in each chapter. Ponder how you might incorporate these teachings into your own diet to achieve variety, balance, and moderation. Recall that the whole food—and the whole diet—are greater than the sum of their individual parts. Give plants the starring role in your diet, remembering that moving toward a plant-based diet is better for your own health as well as the planet.

Be inspired. Get into the kitchen. Begin here. Start now.

From farm to fork, what you eat indeed matters.

WINTER

MIDWINTER GATHERING
TANTALIZE THE TASTE BUDS, WARM THE SOUL

Winter markets arrived in Boston a few years back, so I get fabulous food that supports Massachusetts farmers all year long. And did I mention there's a fishmonger who provides local oysters? I'm a lucky woman indeed. These are some of my favorite dishes I might serve as part of a multi-course dinner party to celebrate the holidays.

STARTER
Oysters are one of the most sustainable foods you can consume. I serve these tasty mollusks with a mignonette including sriracha (Asian chili sauce) and a touch of agave. Simple yet sublime.

OYSTERS ON THE HALF SHELL WITH SPICY-SWEET MIGNONETTE

BEET SALAD
My dad adores beets, which is how I learned to love them when I was a little girl. Roasted beets and orange segments on bed of arugula are terrific when dressed with an orange-balsamic vinaigrette; add toasted hazelnuts or pistachios for crunch.

ARUGULA SALAD WITH BEETS, ORANGES, AND TOASTED HAZELNUTS

SOUP
Roasting cauliflower maximizes flavor, and the addition of artichokes, leeks, garlic, and a touch of Romano cheese and cream make this soup dinner-party worthy. Add whole grain croutons for a satisfying dinner all on its own.

CAULIFLOWER-ARTICHOKE SOUP WITH LEEKS

SLOW-ROASTED SALMON WITH OLIVE OIL, HERBS, AND WARM LENTIL SALAD

ENTRÉE
Select whichever fish is in season and sustainably caught: most will work just fine when slow-roasted in olive oil and fresh herbs. (Include a splash of white wine and lemon juice, too, if you like.) Serve atop a warm salad of brown lentils, red peppers, parsley, and onions.

HOT TEA

BEVERAGE
A habit I learned from my mother, I often enjoy a cup of hot tea in the evening. Whether green or an herbal infusion like chamomile or peppermint, it's especially welcomed on a cold winter's night.

VEGETABLES

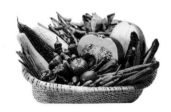

In 2007, during a campaign stop in Adel, Iowa, then–U.S. presidential candidate Barack Obama made a remark about the price of arugula. Some media pundits seized upon that comment as proof that the Illinois senator was elitist and out of touch with middle America, because who buys arugula in Iowa? Who even knows what it is? But you can indeed purchase arugula in Iowa, where it is commonly known as rocket. Many Iowans enjoy eating this leafy green, technically an herb, and they grow it in that state as well.

While not everyone may be aware of it, the United States is in the midst of a fresh-food revolution. If you need convincing, take a stroll through the vegetable aisle at your local supermarket. You will find a greater assortment of produce on display there than was available at any previous time in the nation's history. Supermarkets in every state in the country now stock an extensive variety of vegetables, both conventionally raised and organically grown.

Abundant and Available

You might see heirloom tomatoes, enoki mushrooms, bok choy, radicchio, purple potatoes, and yes, even arugula, at your grocery store. Seasonal produce, such as asparagus and tomatoes, that once made a cameo appearance in supermarkets only at certain times of the year are now imported from warmer climates, or grown hydroponically, and have become available year-round. In response to consumer demand for fresh local produce, the number of farmers markets in the United States has surged, growing almost 10 percent from 2011 to 2012. There's plenty of room to grow from there: Food from farmers markets accounts for less than half a percent of national consumption, though the figure is significantly higher when accounting for locally sourced produce sold through groceries.

Another sign of the shift in consumers' attitudes toward what they eat: Sales of vegetarian foods have doubled in the United States. Ten percent of Americans now say that they follow a "vegetarian-inclined" diet, and though strict veganism is still relatively uncommon, the practice of "Meatless Mondays" is a growing phenomenon. Supermarkets serve burgeoning immigrant communities by regularly stocking so-called ethnic foods, such as daikon radishes, yucca, lemongrass, plantains, and seaweed, and the average American palate has become more adventurous by virtue of being exposed to so many intriguing new ingredients.

Heirloom Legacy

Yet, in the midst of this bounty, Americans have never been so unhealthy. Today, U.S. citizens have shorter life spans and experience

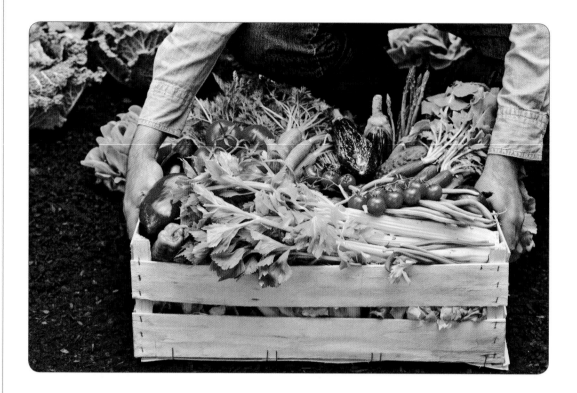

more illness than people in other comparably affluent countries. Two-thirds of American adults are obese or overweight, and childhood obesity has grown into a national epidemic. The reasons for this national health crisis are complex, but a sedentary lifestyle with large portions and eating habits that exceed caloric needs combined with the low cost and convenience of energy-dense foods that are high in sugar and fat are likely at the core of the problem.

Many people are convinced that part of the solution may be found in the vegetable aisle—not in one particular plant, but in the bountiful and healthful array of produce now available to most Americans. It seems as if every day a new study comes out that has media outlets touting one plant or another as a miracle food that can cure cancer, restore memory and sexual prowess, trim thighs, and sculpt and strengthen muscles. Pop-up ads

singing the praises of the latest vegetable du jour, from kale to kohlrabi, skitter across our computer desktops.

The truth is that food fads come and go just as quickly as those annoying Internet ads, and a single food has yet to be discovered that will help you live forever—and probably never will be. In fact, it can be dangerous to rely solely on any one food, no matter how healthy and nutrient-dense it may be.

Planetary Consciousness

As is true in most areas of life, variety, balance, and moderation are essential. Many vegetables have unique health properties, but eating an array of healthy foods in appropriate portions every day is the best way to ensure that your body gets all the nutrients it requires. Based on many decades of research, the consensus among nutritionists

*For the sake of our national health,
it's time we moved veggies to the center of the plate.*

is that a plant-based diet that incorporates a variety of nutrient-dense, minimally processed foods can promote health and physical well-being and substantially reduce the risk of obesity, heart disease, type 2 diabetes, stroke, and many cancers, as well as other chronic maladies ranging from arthritis to depression.

Adopting a plant-based diet may also be the single most important thing a person can do to combat global warming. The practices of commercial livestock production in the United States undermine the health of the planet every day by producing greenhouse gases, using vast amounts of water, and generating animal and chemical waste. Choosing "forks over knives" represents a commitment to a more sustainable way of life, and over time relatively simple choices such as what we eat can have a huge cumulative impact.

Earth's Abundance

Nonetheless, while vegetarianism isn't for everyone, the good news is that even the most devoted carnivores will benefit from adding more plant foods to their diet, particularly vegetables. Despite growing up with the repeated commandment to "Eat your vegetables" resounding in their ears, most Americans eat far fewer than the recommended amount of two and a half cups of vegetables per day. This is a low bar to reach. Current guidelines of the U.S. Department of Agriculture and Harvard School of Public

Health are for filling half your plate with veggies. And don't overlook dark-orange, red, yellow, and green plants.

In the following pages, you will find information about many vegetables from artichoke to zucchini, including a profile on seaweed and other sea vegetables, relatively new arrivals on the American culinary scene. Each entry features a current nutritional profile, detailed information about well-established health benefits and significant nutritional studies, and suggestions for food storage and preparation. You'll find information on the origins and history of each plant and learn about the vegetable family to which it belongs.

One of the most satisfying ironies of food history is that the parts of plants typically discarded or used only as food for slaves, peasants, and animals were eventually found to possess the most nutritional value. The following entries stress the benefits of consuming the whole vegetable, root to leaves, and offer tips on how to use all portions of the plant.

Finally, you will learn that not all convenience foods are unhealthy: Many vegetables come prepackaged or precut, frozen or canned, without significant loss of health benefits, enabling you to put a nutritious meal together quickly when life awaits. And vegetables, on the whole, are quite a bit more nutrient-dense than fruit.

So make room on your plate for vegetables. They will do wonders for your health.

ARTICHOKE

The giant bud of a plant that produces blue or pink thistle-like flowers, the artichoke was regarded as a delicacy in some cultures and as an aphrodisiac in others. In 1533, when Catherine de Medici left Italy to wed Henri II of France, she brought along a supply, since she couldn't bear to be without them. Today, nearly all artichokes grown commercially in the United States come from California, primarily from the foggy coastal climate of Monterey County. The Green Globe variety is the most prevalent; baby artichokes and purple varieties can sometimes be found at U.S. farmers markets.

Choose and Use

Look for tightly closed heads that squeak when you squeeze them. To prepare, wash well and trim an inch off the stem and the top and remove the tough leaves (bracts) around the base. Steam over boiling water, bud end down, until tender. To test, insert a sharp knife into the base of the artichoke—it should be soft and yield to the knife easily. Delicious both hot and cold, whole artichokes are eaten by removing one leaf at a time and scraping off the base with one's teeth before discarding the remainder. The hairy, inedible *choke* at the center must be removed before enjoying the fleshy base or *heart*—the prized part of the plant. Artichokes are often served with melted butter or mayonnaise for dipping; a healthier preparation is to dress lightly with olive oil and lemon juice. Halved, with the chokes removed, artichokes may be grilled or roasted after being steamed. Two naturally occurring chemicals present in artichokes, cynarin and chlorogenic acid, can make foods consumed after these delicacies taste sweet. But this reaction does not occur in all people and is temporary and harmless.

GIVES YOU
Dietary fiber
Folate
Vitamin C
Magnesium
Manganese
Potassium
Phosphorus
Copper
Phytonutrients
    flavonoids, phenolic
    acids, flavonolignans)

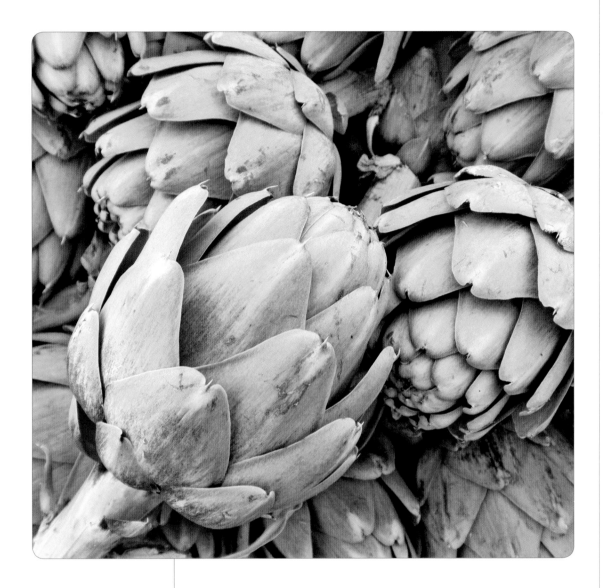

For Your Health
A large artichoke contains just 75 calories, and more antioxidants than any other cooked vegetable. This low-calorie food is high in dietary fiber and potassium and contains the phytonutrients cynarin and silymarin, both good for the liver.

For Our Planet
Almost all of the commercial U.S. artichokes are from California and require frequent irrigation, but you may find them at your local market in spring. The spiny exteriors allow for shipment without packaging, which reduces waste.

✦ TAKE AWAY

Artichokes make a tasty, low-calorie snack or side dish.

ARUGULA

Also known as rocket, rucola, and Italian cress, this edible herb grows wild in the Mediterranean. In ancient times arugula was grown for its leaves and seeds, used for flavoring oil, and was reputed to be an aphrodisiac. Arugula's distinctive peppery flavor is similar to watercress and dandelion greens. A member of the broccoli and cabbage family, arugula shares some of the cancer-fighting properties of other cruciferous vegetables.

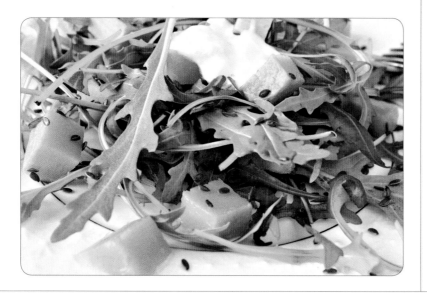

GIVES YOU

Vitamin K
Vitamin C
Folate
Calcium
Iron
Potassium
Magnesium
Phytonutrients
  (glucosinolates,
  flavonoids,
  carotenoids)

CONSIDER ✦ SALAD IN A BAG

Health-conscious grocery shoppers love bagged, prewashed salad mixes for their convenience. However, as with most convenience foods, all this packaging creates waste. Arugula and other salad greens often come in plastic containers that end up in the garbage or recycling bin. Due to the popularity of packaged greens, bunched arugula is sometimes not available. When you can find it, perhaps at a local farmers market or food coop, it's worth the trouble to wash your own. Just be sure to wash it well. You can then store it in the refrigerator in a reusable vegetable bag so that it's ready when you need it.

FOOD SCIENCE ✦ MESCLUN

Mesclun, a Provençal word meaning "mixture," is an assortment of young salad greens that began cropping up in U.S. supermarkets (loose and bagged) in the 1990s. Mesclun traditionally contains equal portions of arugula, chervil, endive, and lettuces, but now may include radicchio, mâche (or lamb's lettuce), frisée, baby spinach, and other tender greens. It's a great choice for adding diverse tastes, textures, and nutrients to your salads.

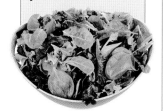

✦ **TAKE AWAY**

Add this peppery herb to your dishes for both flavor and essential vitamins.

Choose and Use

When not prebagged arugula is typically sold with roots attached. Choose bunches with fresh green leaves with no signs of wilting or yellowing. Once refrigerated, the leaves should be consumed within a day or two and must be rinsed well just before using to remove grit. Pesticides penetrate these delicate greens and cannot be washed away. The amount of residue is negligible for most healthy adults, but if slight amounts pose a particular concern for you, or out of concern for the environment, you might choose organic. Try combining with sliced red pears, blue cheese, toasted nuts, and a walnut vinaigrette for an elegant salad. (Dress with a light hand and don't toss until right before serving, since the tender leaves break down quickly.) Arugula can also be sautéed, like spinach. It also makes an excellent pesto and pairs wonderfully with eggs when added to frittatas and omelets.

For Your Health

Though tender, arugula's greens pack a nutritional punch. Unlike romaine and iceberg lettuce, which are less nutritious than darker-hued lettuces, raw arugula is an excellent source of the vitamin K, critical for bone health, as well as vitamins C and A. The leaves also contain glucosinolates, flavonoids, and carotenoids, which help boost the human immune system. Full of flavor, this fast-growing salad green has become widely available in U.S. markets.

For Our Planet

Because arugula does not attract many insects, much of the plant grown in the western U.S. is cultivated without pesticides, great news for maintaining soil quality and protecting farmworkers.

ASPARAGUS

Cultivated and enjoyed the world over for thousands of years, the elegant green spears of the asparagus have always signaled spring's arrival. A flowering perennial plant that produces edible shoots, asparagus is actually a member of the lily family. Commercially grown in the United States since the mid-1800s, asparagus is a labor-intensive crop, since each spear must be cut by hand. China is currently the world's largest producer of this vegetable.

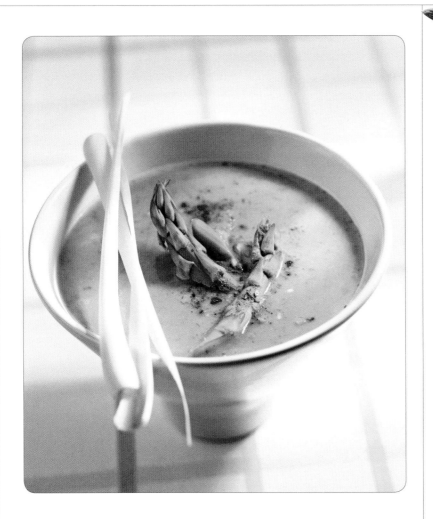

GIVES YOU

Vitamin K
Vitamin E
Folate
Vitamin C
Tryptophan
Riboflavin (vitamin B2)
Dietary fiber
Phytonutrients
    (carotenoids,
    flavonoids, saponins)

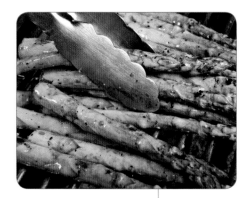

Choose and Use

This springtime favorite is now available year-round, though it costs less in season. Choose bunches of long, bright green spears with closed, compact tips. Spears are available in varying thicknesses, but thicker spears are generally more succulent. Green asparagus is most common in U.S. markets, though sometimes one finds purple too. White or light green asparagus, grown without sunlight, is more popular in Europe than the green variety. Immerse the base of a bunch in an inch or two of water and store upright in the refrigerator until use. Best consumed within two days of purchase, asparagus may be parboiled, steamed, stir-fried, roasted, pickled, or eaten raw. Thin spears require less cooking time; choose thicker spears for grilling and roasting. Try roasting asparagus with a little olive oil and then wrapping the spears in savory smoked salmon for a treat. A traditional French preparation, roasted asparagus also makes a wonderful bed for fried eggs.

For Your Health

Asparagus contains vitamin K, a fat-soluble vitamin that aids in blood clotting and bone health. Just four spears contain almost 40 percent of vitamin K needed for the day. Serving asparagus with a heart-healthy salad dressing made from polyunsaturated fats like vegetable and nut oils helps in vitamin absorption, as with any vegetable with fat-soluble nutrients. Low in calorie and high in fiber and protein, asparagus is also an excellent source of glutathione, one of the body's best cancer fighters. It is rich in beta-carotene. An excellent source of the antioxidants lutein and zeazanthin, asparagus is also high (for a plant) in choline. Some people notice their urine has a pungent odor after they eat asparagus—a harmless reaction to the body's metabolizing of sulfur.

For Our Planet

In North America, the growing season for asparagus extends from January to June, and it's a vegetable that for many marks the arrival of spring. According to the Environmental Working Group, asparagus is one of the "Clean 15" crops with the fewest pesticide residues if you can't access organic.

PREP TIP ✦ IT'S A SNAP

The bottom of asparagus stalks can be tough and fibrous. Trim them by hand rather than with a knife by bending each stalk until it snaps; it will naturally break at the point where it becomes tender. But don't throw out the ends! The asparagus stubs make a fine soup: simmer in water with some chopped onion, then puree with a few tablespoons of yogurt.

AVOCADO

Sometimes called the alligator pear because of its shape and pebbled skin, the avocado is botanically a fruit that masquerades as a vegetable due to its common culinary use. Avocado pits have been found in pre-Incan tombs, and evidence suggests avocado trees were cultivated in the Americas as early as 5000 BC. Available year-round, the creamy green flesh may be processed into avocado oil and used in cooking and cosmetics.

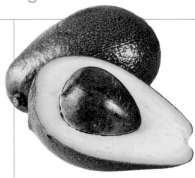

Choose and Use

Avocados sold in markets are usually hard, but they are climacteric fruits that will ripen in a day or two when left on a kitchen counter. Store at room temperature. A ripe avocado yields slightly to the touch; avoid those with soft or brown spots. Bisect the avocado lengthwise with a knife; when the blade hits the pit, rotate the knife around the avocado, then twist the two halves in opposite directions to separate. Sinking a blade carefully into the pit and twisting will dislodge it. Use a soupspoon to easily remove all the fruit cleanly from the skin. Lime or lemon juice rubbed on the cut surface prevents browning. Avocados are usually eaten raw.

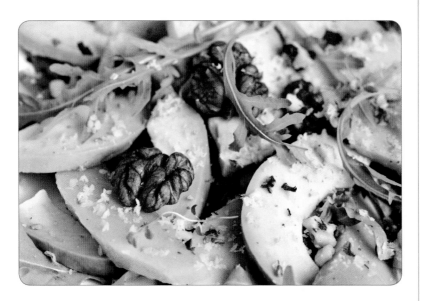

GIVES YOU

Dietary fiber
Vitamin K
Vitamin E
Riboflavin
Niacin (vitamin B3)
Folate
Vitamin C
Pantothenic acid
Potassium
Pyridoxine (vitamin B6)
Copper
Monounsaturated fats
Phytonutrients
   (carotenoids,
   phytosterols,
   polyhydroxylated
   fatty alcohols)

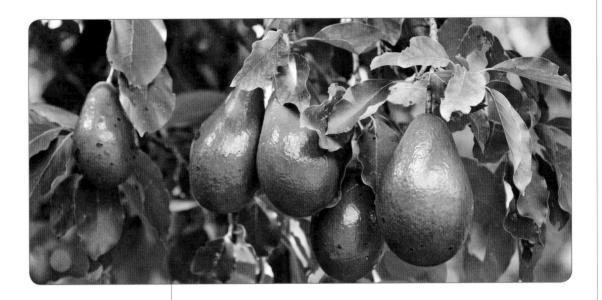

Avocado's heart-healthy fats add a rich texture to salads and meals.

Serve sliced into salads, or spread on bread. The buttery texture also pairs beautifully with citrus. Guacamole is a cinch to make too, including only mashed avocado, chopped onion, garlic, and lemon juice; it stays green longer when you leave the pit in the bowl. Cover the mixture with plastic wrap directly covering the puree to prevent oxidation.

For Your Health

Though high in calories (about 200 in a single avocado), avocados are rich in a protein that contains all the essential amino acids. Studies have shown that avocados contain an abundance of oleic acid, another heart-healthy fat, this time monounsaturated, which also contributes to the vegetable's satiating power. Avocados also have a small amount of heart- and brain-healthy polyunsaturated omega-3 fatty acids. Of the two types available in the U.S., the California avocado is richer in oil than the Florida variety.

For Our Planet

A place to consider the complexities of carbon emissions, while avocados grown in California may be closer (for some), they require extensive irrigation compared to those from Mexico.

BEET

A folk belief says that two people who eat from the same beet will fall in love. Typically a deep garnet-red—though ranging from golden to purple and even striped like a candy cane—beets have been long associated with physical passion: pictures of the root adorned the walls of a brothel in ancient Pompeii. Originally, the beet's root resembled a carrot, but preference through the centuries for a plumper juicier shape eventually resulted in the modern, swollen root one finds on market shelves today. Both roots and greens are good to eat.

Choose and Use

Beets are at their most tender from late June through early October, when they are picked fresh. The most flavorful are small to medium size, with the greens still attached. If selecting beets with the greens removed, check that some portion of the stem is still attached, the root is firm, and the skin smooth with no cracks. Separate the greens from the root and refrigerate both until ready to use. Rinse well under running water before preparing.

Highly versatile, beets add vivid color and sweetness to various recipes. Eastern Europeans make borscht, a traditional cold beet soup. The root may be grated and served raw or pickled in salads, or cooked by boiling or steaming. Roasting in particular concentrates the flavors. Cook beets whole, rub off the skins with your hands, and slice afterward on a cutting board

PAIRINGS ✦ GREAT WITH NUTS

Beets make a fine side salad, especially when teamed with chopped walnuts. Cut up roasted beets and toss with olive oil and a little balsamic vinegar, add crumbled cheese such as feta or goat cheese (chevre), then sprinkle with toasted nuts. Beets also pair well with arugula, anchovies, and sour cream.

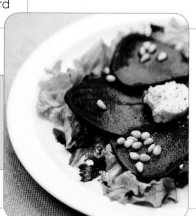

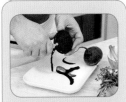

The raw beet's skin can be removed with a vegetable peeler or a paring knife, but an easier trick is to roast or boil the beet until tender, cool slightly, then rub off the skin with your hands or a clean kitchen towel you don't mind getting stained. The cooked skin should slip off easily.

GIVES YOU

ROOTS:
Folate
Manganese
Dietary fiber
Potassium
Tryptophan
Phytonutrients
 (betalains)

GIVES YOU

GREEN:
Vitamin K
Ascorbic acid
Potassium
Manganese
Riboflavin
Magnesium
Dietary fiber
Calcium
Iron
Copper
Phytonutrients
 (carotenoids,
 phenolic acids)

you don't mind staining; latex gloves will protect your hands. Root vegetables grown in contaminated soil will appropriate those contaminants (such as lead), a good reason to choose organic. Try sliced or grated beets with your favorite greens, toasted pecans or walnuts, and blue cheese for a colorful salad.

Too often discarded, beet greens are actually the most nutritious part of the vegetable. They may be cooked like any other dark leafy green such as Swiss chard or spinach; they are wonderful simply sautéed with olive oil and garlic.

For Your Health

Beets have the highest sugar content of any vegetable but are low in calories. Raw beets contain folate, a vitamin beneficial in cancer and heart disease prevention, but cooking diminishes this nutrient. Nutritional studies indicate that table beets are rich in antioxidants that promote cardiovascular health. They are also a good source of fiber. Consuming these roots may turn urine and stools red, a harmless (though alarming) condition. Beet greens contain almost nine times the recommended daily value of vitamin K, a bone nutrient and heart protector.

For Our Planet

Beets with attached greens are often sold bundled in markets with no additional packaging, reducing the carbon cost of processing. Consuming both the greens and roots also reduces unnecessary methane-producing food waste.

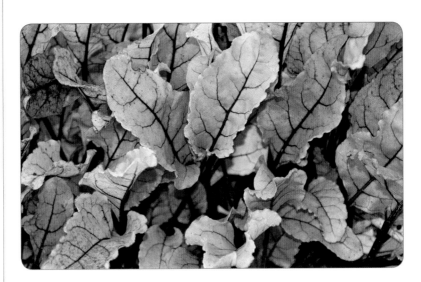

BOK CHOY

Also called Chinese white cabbage, *pak choi*, and white mustard cabbage, bok choy has been grown in China for more than 6,000 years and is still associated primarily with Asian cuisine. Bok choy means "white vegetable" in Cantonese, a reference to the snowy white stalks of the plant.

Choose and Use

Now available in the United States, Canada, and the Philippines, bok choy has been slower to catch on elsewhere in the world. Two varieties commonly found in U.S. markets are Shanghai bok choy with its white stalks and tender dark green leaves, and light green baby bok choy. In Hong Kong, one may find 20 different varieties of this vegetable.

Choose bunches with firm white stalks and crisp green leaves. Refrigerated, bok choy will keep for three to four days in the refrigerator. This mild-tasting leafy green may be steamed, braised, stir-fried, or added to soups. The stems take longer to cook than the leaves. The Korean pickled cabbage known as kimchi is sometimes made with bok choy. Used raw, it adds a pleasant crunch to salads.

GIVES YOU

Vitamin C
Vitamin K
Folate
Calcium
Iron
Phytonutrients
  (carotenoids,
  glucosinolates)

PREP TIP ✦ USE IT LIKE CABBAGE

Bok choy may be used as you would cabbage: think steamed or shredded finely for a coleslaw-like presentation. This vegetable also benefits from grilling. First, trim the base of each bunch and remove and clean the stalks. Lightly oil and season both sides with salt and cracked black pepper and grill until leaves are crisp at the edges.

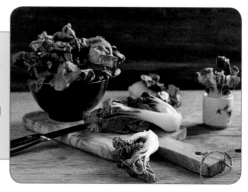

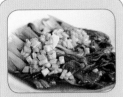

Like other Asian greens, bok choy is wonderful when prepared simply, with garlic and olive oil. For bigger flavors, try peanut oil and a pinch of crushed red pepper. Combining bok choy with other vegetables, like carrots and red peppers, makes a colorful and delicious side dish or bed for a piece of fish. Or toss with pasta for a quick, nutritious dinner.

✦ **TAKE AWAY**

For centuries this Chinese cabbage has added flavor, nutrients, and a satisfying crunch to meals.

For Your Health

Bok choy is an excellent source of carotenoids and vitamins C and K, as well as folate and calcium. It is low in oxalate, which binds calcium and impedes absorption, so the calcium in bok choy can be more readily absorbed than that in other leafy greens. This relative of the cabbage also contains carotenoids like beta-carotene, which may help prevent heart disease and stroke as well as some cancers. As with other cruciferous vegetables, chopping bok choy before cooking increases the bioavailability of cancer-preventive compounds.

For Our Planet

Imported bok choy seems to have fewer pesticides than domestic, but today many small farmers have begun growing and selling this Asian treat at local markets.

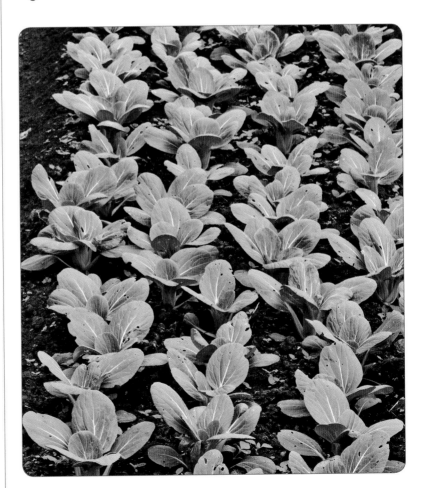

BROCCOLI

Beloved by ancient Romans who consumed it several times in the course of a single banquet, broccoli was sometimes referred to as "the five green fingers of Jupiter." Native to Italy, this leafy green vegetable was first commercially cultivated in the United States by Italian immigrants in the 1920s. When overcooked, broccoli can be sulfurous and mushy, traits that have led to the plant's periodic bouts with unpopularity. Today, many celebrate broccoli, and its star rides high again in the vegetable firmament.

Choose and Use

Fresh broccoli can be found in markets year-round, though peak season is October through April. Choose bunches with sturdy stems and compact, bluish green heads; pass on those with cracked bases and yellowing florets. Sometimes purple and white varieties become available, as well as the astonishing lime-green Romanesco broccoli, a living fractal, with its cluster of spiraling heads. Frozen broccoli is just as nutritious as fresh. The stems are edible and nutritious and are particularly tender in "baby" broccoli varieties. This vegetable can be steamed, sautéed, stir-fried, or roasted. Slice the stem into pieces and prepare along with the separated florets. Cooked broccoli may also be pureed into a soup; roasting with olive oil and garlic first brings in the most flavors. A member of the mustard family, broccoli is most healthful when cooked as little as possible, until crisp-tender and retaining its bright green color, and served simply—without calorie-laden sauces.

For Your Health

It is difficult to overstate the benefits of broccoli. This cruciferous vegetable is rich in beta-carotene as well as lutein and

GIVES YOU

Vitamin C
Vitamin K
Folate
Manganese
Dietary fiber
Tryptophan
Potassium
Pyridoxine
Riboflavin
Thiamine
Phosphorus
Calcium
Phytonutrients
   (carotenoids,
   flavonoids [higher in
   raw], glucosinolates,
   phenolic acids, lignans)

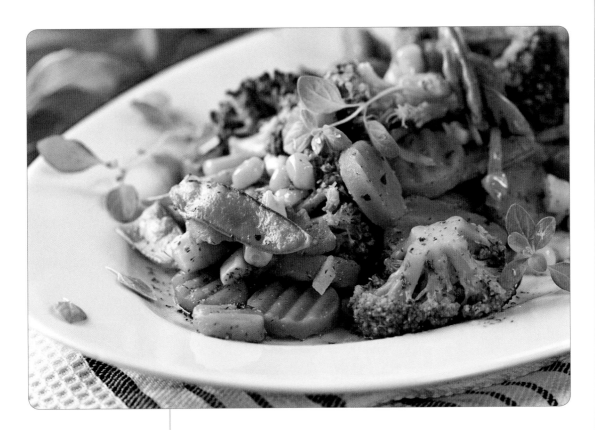

zeaxanthin, meaning it helps prevent age-related macular degeneration, and it promotes heart health. People who eat an abundance of broccoli appear to have a reduced incidence of bladder and prostate cancer. Although most people prefer it cooked, raw broccoli also makes a great salad addition.

For Our Planet

A sturdy vegetable, broccoli is often found with relatively little packaging—which reduces the resources used to process broccoli and cuts down packaging waste.

PREP TIP ✦ DON'T FORGET THE GREENS!

The neatly trimmed heads of broccoli displayed in most produce aisles bear only a partial resemblance to the living plant itself: the large mass of flower heads grows surrounded by leaves that can be prepared just like broccoli rabe or collard greens, with delicious and healthy results. If you find the discarded greens at your local farmers market, ask if you can take some home for your supper table.

BROCCOLI RABE

Related to both the cabbage and the turnip family, broccoli rabe (pronounced *rahb*), also called rape, or rapini, is used in the cuisines of southern Europe, Portugal, the Netherlands, and China. Many Americans are unfamiliar with this leafy green, though it is a favorite vegetable in Italian immigrant communities throughout the United States. The plant has six- to nine-inch stalks, ruffled green leaves, scattered clusters of broccoli-like buds, and a distinctively bitter taste that complements starchy foods such as pasta and rice.

Choose and Use

Broccoli rabe makes its appearance in the market from late summer through the fall and winter, though it may be elusive in some regions. Look for bunches of slender stems, crisp green leaves, and compact florets; avoid wilted or yellowed broccoli rabe, though a few yellow flowers should not trouble you. Store in the refrigerator in a reusable plastic container for no more than five days, and wash well before cooking. The stems of this vegetable tend to be tough, so trim off a couple inches before use. One method for reducing the bitter flavor of this green is to quickly blanch it in boiling water, followed by an ice-water dip; then it can be sautéed, stir-fried, or braised. Serve broccoli rabe on its own as a side dish, combine with potatoes or pasta, or add to broth. The chopped leaves may be added to salads.

✦ TAKE AWAY

Broccoli rabe adds a flavorful variation to rice or pasta.

PREP TIP ✦ BRAISE LONG AND SLOW

For many, broccoli rabe can be a tough vegetable to love, but braising slowly tames its bitterness. Heat some sliced onions in a small amount of olive oil, then add the chopped broccoli rabe and a couple tablespoons of raisins. Add some water, cover, and let simmer for an hour or more. Finish with a handful of chopped almonds right before serving. For those less sensitive to bitter flavors—taste buds differ among humans—a simple sauté in olive oil and garlic is a quicker, easier preparation.

FOOD SCIENCE ✦ THE BRASSICA GENUS

Brassica is a genus of plants in the mustard family and one of the most popular food crops worldwide. Collectively known as cruciferous vegetables (Latin for cross-bearing, because of the shape of their flowers), this family includes cabbage, cauliflower, broccoli, kale, Brussels sprouts, bok choy, turnips, and other nutritional green leaf vegetables—generally considered to be healthy foods with cancer-fighting properties. Cruciferous vegetables are rich in sulfuraphanes, which help protect arteries from disease by boosting the body's own natural defense mechanisms. Plants in this beneficial family contain isothiocyanates and phytochemicals known as organosulfur compounds, which are powerful anticarcinogens.

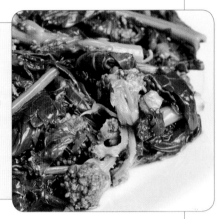

GIVES YOU

Vitamin K
Vitamin C
Folate
Vitamin E
Thiamine (vitamin B1)
Niacin
Riboflavin
Pyridoxine
Manganese
Iron
Calcium
Phosphorus
Potassium
Tryptophan
Phytonutrients
   (carotenoids,
   glucosinolates)

For Your Health

Broccoli rabe is a rich source of glucosinolates, which the body converts to cancer-fighting compounds. Studies credit nutrient-dense broccoli rabe with many other benefits as well, such as strengthening bones, lowering the risk of heart disease, and detoxifying the liver.

For Our Planet

The entire plant of broccoli rabe can be enjoyed, which means less ends up in landfills.

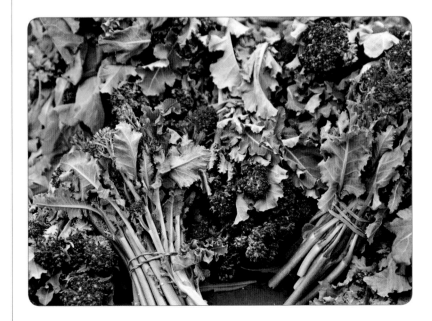

BRUSSELS SPROUTS

Another member of the cancer-fighting family of cruciferous (*Brassica*) vegetables, which include cauliflower and broccoli, Brussels sprouts grow along a towering stalk, crowned with a cabbage rose. Ancient Romans called them *bullata gemmifera* (diamond-making bubbles) because they were reputed to increase mental clarity. The modern Brussels sprout was first extensively cultivated in Belgium and named after that country's capital city. Alas, many English and American cooks boiled this highly nutritious vegetable into a sulfurous lump, earning it a reputation as culinary Kryptonite. Today, the practice of oven roasting them is gaining in popularity and the much-maligned Brussels sprout seems to be enjoying a renaissance.

Choose and Use

Brussels sprouts are usually trimmed and sold in net bags or baskets, though they can increasingly be found on their impressive stalks at farmers markets. Look for small, bright green sprouts with tightly packed leaves. Use soon after purchasing since they begin losing their sweetness as soon as they are picked. Frozen sprouts are a good option as they retain most of their flavor and nutrients. This fall/winter crop often appears on Thanksgiving menus paired with chestnuts.

To prepare, rinse, pull off any loose outer leaves, and trim a bit off each base. An X cut into the base of each will hasten cooking. Leave sprouts whole, or halve them, or just use the individual leaves. They may be roasted, boiled, steamed, pan fried, or chopped finely and used raw in a slaw. Overcooking greatly reduces their nutritional value and creates bitter flavors. Roasting Brussels sprouts coaxes out a nutty sweetness from

GIVES YOU

Vitamin K
Vitamin C
Manganese
Folate
Dietary fiber
Potassium
Pyridoxine
Tryptophan
Thiamine
Iron
Phosphorus
Phytonutrients
   (flavonoids,
   glucosinolates,
   carotenoids, lignans)

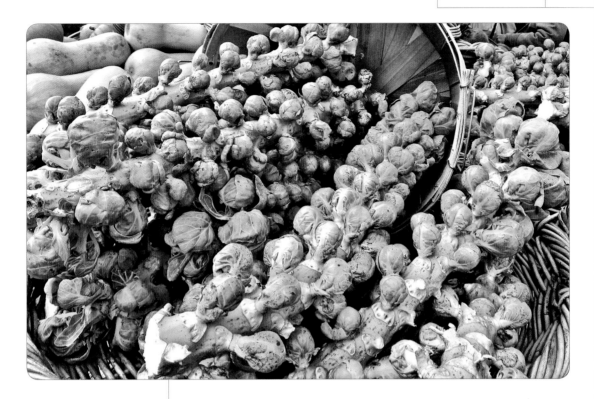

the caramelized sugars in the plant. Finish under the broiler to lightly char the outer leaves. Brussels sprouts pair beautifully with nuts, mustard, garlic, caraway seeds, and lemon.

For Your Health
Brussels sprouts offer the same benefits as other members of the *Brassica* genus and contain more antioxidants than broccoli ounce for ounce. The carotenoids lutein and zeaxanthin, present in Brussels sprouts, promote eye health.

For Our Planet
Most U.S. production is in California, but many small farms also grow Brussels sprouts, a great opportunity to support your local farmer come autumn.

✦ TAKE AWAY

You can roast, boil, steam, or fry Brussels sprouts, but be careful not to overcook them.

PREP TIP ✦ **ROAST UNTIL NUTTY AND SWEET**

Roasting coaxes out a wonderful nutty sweetness that even a lifelong sprout hater may find impossible to resist. Finish under the broiler if desired to lightly char the outer leaves.

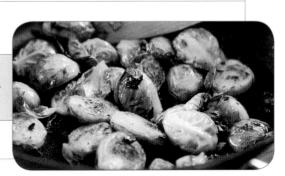

CABBAGE

Nutritionally rich, cabbage has been used throughout history as both a medicine and a food. In preparation for a night of overindulgence, ancient Romans ingested it to ward off hangovers, and 17th-century explorers brought it along on ocean voyages to prevent scurvy, since the vegetable is a good source of ascorbic acid, or vitamin C. Cabbage has also served as a subsistence food in many cultures. As a result, the privileged classes have tended to look down their noses at it, and the unpleasant smell of overcooked cabbage has contributed to its disfavor. Still, the humble cabbage with its pleasant crunch deserves a place at every health-conscious table.

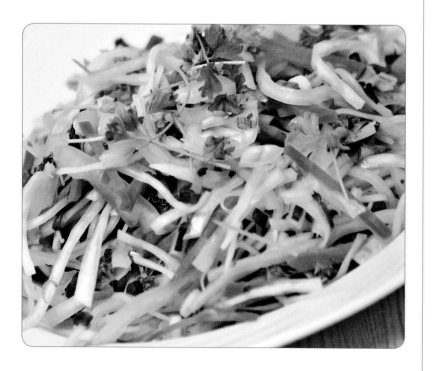

GIVES YOU

Vitamin K
Vitamin C
Folate
Dietary fiber
Manganese
Pyridoxine
Potassium
Phytonutrients
  (carotenoids,
  glucosinolates,
  phytosterols,
  flavonoids/phenolic
  acids [in red
  cabbage], lignans)

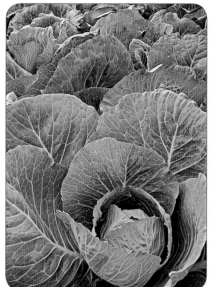

Choose and Use

When selecting a head of cabbage, choose one that is firm, glossy, and feels heavy for its size. Cabbage keeps in the refrigerator for about a week but tastes best when eaten right away. To prepare, first discard any wilted outer leaves and rinse. Cabbage may be boiled, steamed, braised, or stir-fried, as well as stuffed and baked; the quickest cooking methods will preserve the most nutrients. Do not cook cabbage in an aluminum pot—a chemical reaction will discolor the vegetable. Finely chopped or grated, raw cabbage adds a spicy crunch to salads and slaws. The nutritious core, which people often discard, may be grated into a slaw.

For Your Health

Along with broccoli and Brussels sprouts, cabbage is a cruciferous vegetable with proven cancer-fighting properties. The three main types are green, red/purple, and Savoy, all of which are low in calories and high in fiber (red has more fiber than green, and Savoy has the most). Since the different colors contain different cancer-fighting glucosinolates, it's wise to eat a mix. Chopping cabbage and then allowing it to aerate for five minutes on the cutting board enables an enzyme in the vegetable to convert these glucosinolates into isothiocyanates, which enhance the body's natural detoxification systems. Steam cabbage to increase its cholesterol-lowering powers.

For Our Planet

Conventionally grown cabbages retain fewer pesticide residues than many other fruits and vegetables. Cabbages also transport well from farm to purchase, so they are usually sold unwrapped, which reduces unnecessary packaging waste.

✦ **TAKE AWAY**

Use many types of cabbage to make your meals more colorful and nutritious.

PREP TIP ✦ **HOLD THE MAYO**

Classic coleslaw recipes tend to drown shredded cabbage in a sea of mayonnaise, which adds a lot of extra calories and dilutes the crunch and flavor cabbage provides. Try substituting a smaller amount of nonfat Greek yogurt for the mayo for a change. Sliced cabbage can also be served simply with vinegar and, if left to sit, will quickly pickle for an interesting side dish.

CARROT

A carrot's greens might tip you off that this root is a member of the parsley family, related to Queen Anne's lace. The earliest carrots were actually skinny and purple or yellow, and probably originated in Afghanistan. We have Dutch horticulturalists to thank for the large bright orange carrots so common in markets today, which they fed to cows to ensure that butter made from their milk had a rich yellow hue, imparted from the orange-hued carotenoids found in carrots.

Choose and Use

Harvested beginning midsummer through fall, carrots are available year-round. They are often sold trimmed and packed in plastic bags, or in bunches with the greens attached. Choose bunches with firm carrots and fresh-looking greens, and avoid those with cracks or hairlike rootlets. Green tops rob the root of nutrients, so remove before refrigerating. (They can be stored in the freezer for use in a homemade vegetable stock.) Carrots keep for weeks but do lose some flavor as they sit. Also avoid storing them near apples, pears, and potatoes, which emit ethylene gas that can give carrots a bitter taste. As long as carrots are washed thoroughly their skins can be eaten.

GIVES YOU

Vitamin A
Dietary fiber
Vitamin C
Potassium
Phytonutrients
   (carotenoids,
   polyacetylenes,
   phenolic acids,
   lignans)

FOOD SCIENCE ✦ PURPLE CARROTS

A purple carrot might look like a science fair project gone awry, but it harks back to the original carrot, which was not orange but purple. Today, carrots are bred in a rainbow of colors, including purple, maroon, red, orange, yellow, and white. Different colors signal the presence of different phytonutrients. The anthocyanins in purple carrots act as powerful antioxidants. This pigment may also reduce the risk of heart disease by slowing blood clotting. Alas, they lose much of their color during cooking but make a gorgeous addition to salads when served raw.

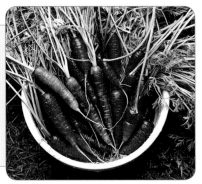

CONSIDER
✦
THAT'S NO BABY

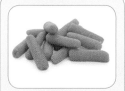

The bagged carrots that now dominate the market are not "baby" carrots at all, but mature carrots milled down to a uniform small size, then soaked in water containing chlorine. The waste products from this process are used to make shredded carrots and the peel for cattle feed. Simply prepared carrot sticks you cut yourself are more flavorful and avoid unnecessary packaging and energy use.

This versatile tuber may be prepared any number of ways: boiled, steamed, sautéed, stir-fried, or grated raw over salads. As with other vegetables, roasting deepens their flavor and converts some of their starches into sugars. Spices such as caraway, dill, cumin, cinnamon, and coriander all enhance this vegetable. The carrot's natural sweetness makes it a favorite in cakes and muffins too.

For Your Health
A ten-year-long study conducted in the Netherlands on the impact of different-colored fruits and vegetables on cardiovascular disease determined that those with darker shades of orange and yellow offered the most protection, with carrots ranking highest in this category. Eating these roots as part of a plant-based diet also guards against cancer and diabetes. Beta-carotene, which the body converts into vitamin A, improves night vision and protects skin from sun damage. Alpha-carotene, also present in carrots, has been shown to significantly reduce one's risk of death from cardiovascular disease, cancer, and other diseases. Carotenoid value may increase when carrots are boiled rather than steamed. Dressing carrots with olive oil or butter aids in absorption of the fat-soluble nutrients in these vegetables.

For Our Planet
Carrots can be enjoyed root to leaf, so reduce your personal food waste by keeping the skins on—make sure to wash well—and use the bright-tasting greens in a pesto or stock.

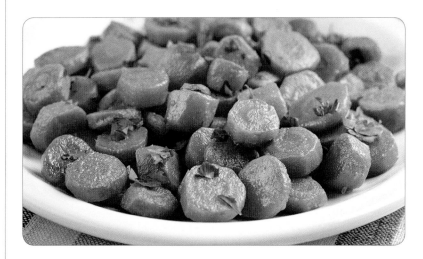

CAULIFLOWER

This member of the *Brassica* genus is well named, since it truly is a flower, or rather thousands of tiny flower buds packed into larger buds that make up the head's snowy bouquet. The outer leaves of the cabbage-like plant are tied closed over the young heads of white cauliflower to block sunlight and "blanch" them as they grow, making cauliflower one of the most labor-intensive crops. This delicately flavored winter vegetable, which pairs wonderfully with spices, is a staple of Indian cooking as well as classic French cuisine, but it leaves many American cooks cold. Eye-catching new varieties in orange and vivid purple pigments may help raise the profile of this nutritious, delicious, low-calorie vegetable.

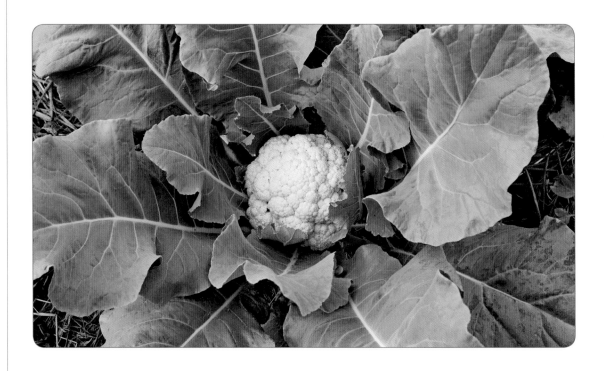

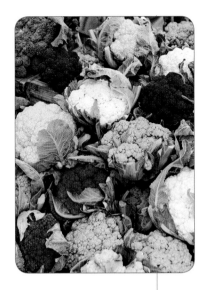

Choose and Use

Choose cauliflower with compact florets, no discoloration, and fresh green leaves (which are edible). Wrapped in plastic, it will keep for up to two weeks in the crisper. Rinse and pat dry, then cut out the large core on the underside of the head, or curd. Avoid cooking cauliflower in aluminum or iron pots, which will discolor it. Cauliflower may be divided into florets and steamed, boiled, sautéed, or eaten raw. The whole head may also be steamed (stem end up), or baked. Different colors vary slightly in taste, but all cauliflowers taste delicious with sharply flavored ingredients such as mustard and spices. Roasting at a high heat makes it crispy and sweet, and mashing it with a little garlic and olive oil is a lower-calorie and more healthful alternative to potatoes.

For Your Health

Low in calories and high in fiber, this cruciferous vegetable may reduce the risk of bladder, breast, colon, prostate, and ovarian cancer, thanks to sulforaphanes, the compounds responsible for many of its health benefits. Cauliflower also contains a compound called glucoraphanin, which protects the stomach and intestines. Different colors of cauliflower provide different nutrients in varying amounts—for instance, orange cauliflower contains 25 times more beta-carotene than the white variety.

For Our Planet

Cauliflower is a great choice to conserve your food dollars and reduce your food waste by eating the whole vegetable: core, flowers, and leaves. If possible, choose organic to invest in sustainable farming.

GIVES YOU

Vitamin C
Vitamin K
Folate
Choline
Pyridoxine
Potassium
Dietary fiber
Manganese
Phytonutrients
(glucosinolates, phytosterols, carotenoids, phenolic acids, lignans)

PREP TIP ✦ ROAST IT, MASH IT

If you've never tried it before, roasted cauliflower is a revelation. Preparing it this way also seems to reduce the bloating and flatulence that some people experience after eating this vegetable. Cauliflower cooked until soft and mashed with yogurt and some extra-virgin olive oil also makes an excellent, low-calorie substitute for mashed potatoes.

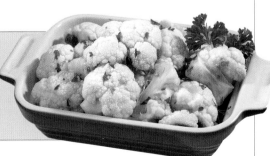

CORN

Maize, known in the United States and Canada as corn, has been so essential to human survival in North American cultures that native peoples regarded the plant as a deity. Originally a wild grain, corn was domesticated thousands of years ago in Mexico. Today, it's the number one field crop in the United States and the source of more than 800 processed foods, including breakfast cereals, flour, grits, syrup, and oil. Ethanol fuel, ink, medicine, and plastic containers are also made from corn. Sweet corn, the type categorized and consumed as a vegetable, is a sugar-rich variety of grain harvested when immature. Dried corn, including popcorn and corn flour, is considered a grain.

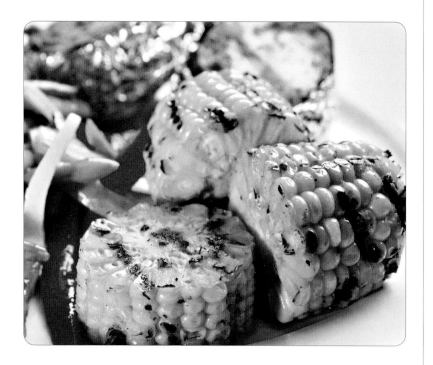

GIVES YOU

Dietary fiber
Folate
Vitamin C
Niacin
Pantothenic acid
Phytonutrients
    (flavonoids [in purple
    corn], carotenoids,
    phenolic acids)

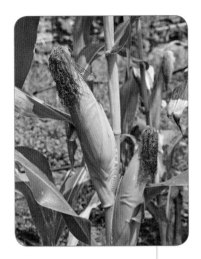

Choose and Use

Eat fresh corn as soon off the stalk as possible, when it's the sweetest: Corn that sits in the refrigerator will still be good to eat but will become less tasty as some of its simple sugars are converted to starch. Choose ears with bright green, snugly fitting husks, and gold-brown silk. Peel back the very top of the husk and look for plump, evenly spaced kernels. This vegetable comes in a variety of colors, with yellow and white the most common; "butter and sugar" corn, with its combination of yellow and white kernels, is a summer favorite. Corn tastes best when cooked until just tender, either by immersing the husked cobs in unsalted water and bringing just to a boil for a few minutes, steaming, or by cutting off the cob and sautéing. You can also soak the ears and then grill corn in its husk, a tasty summertime treat. Place corn in its husk directly on the middle rack of the oven and bake at 350 degrees for approximately half an hour for an infallible side dish. Eventually, the kernels will caramelize, resulting in a delicacy for corn aficionados.

For Your Health

A good source of dietary fiber, corn can help boost weight loss by making one feel full. It also contains lutein and zeaxanthin, antioxidant phytonutrients that keep the eyes healthy as they age.

For Our Planet

The United States produces more corn, by far, than anywhere else in the world. Forty percent of this crop is used to produce ethanol, a corn-based biofuel. Overall, U.S. corn production has become more sustainable. According to the Field to Market alliance for sustainable agriculture, corn production saw a 30 percent decrease per bushel in greenhouse gas emissions between 1987 and 2007.

✦ TAKE AWAY

Choose the freshest ears available, and boil, steam, or grill them.

CONSIDER ✦ CORN IN THE FOOD CHAIN: ANIMAL FEED

Only a small percentage of the U.S. corn crop is destined for human consumption. Most of the corn grown in North America is dent, or field corn destined for livestock feed because it's cheap and plentiful. Ruminants such as cattle have trouble digesting corn; this leads to a host of physical problems that then need to be controlled with antibiotics, another problem with conventionally raised cattle.

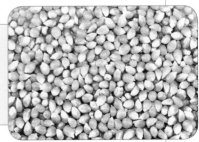

EGGPLANT

Eggplants belong to the nightshade family, as do potatoes and tomatoes, and initially people in many world cultures believed them to be poisonous. The Italian word *melanzana* derives from an older name: *mela insana,* or "insane apple," but the eggplant is actually a large berry—botanically a fruit that is categorized and consumed as a vegetable. The original American eggplant was small and white, hence the name; in the U.K. and in France they are called aubergines. Eggplant today lends its silky texture and bulk to Mediterranean, Chinese, Indian, and Middle Eastern cuisines.

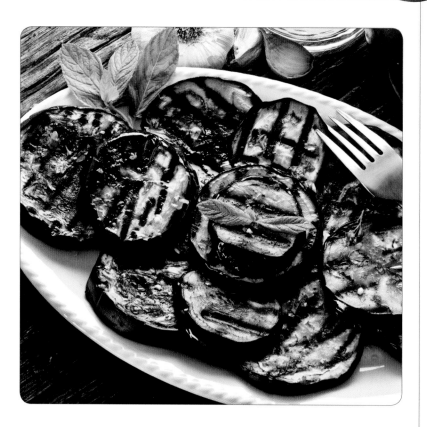

GIVES YOU

Dietary fiber
Thiamine
Pyridoxine
Phytonutrients
   (phenolic acids,
   flavonoids, nasunin)

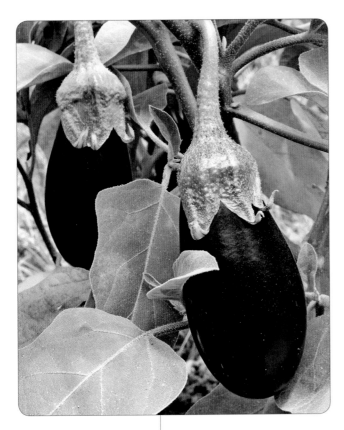

Choose and Use

The best-tasting eggplants tend to be smaller, since larger ones may be seedy and bitter. The large, deep purple variety is most commonly seen in U.S. markets, but one also finds smaller white eggplants, striped varieties, and the slender, purple kind known as Japanese eggplants. A green cap and firm, unblemished skin signal freshness. This summer vegetable should be stored in the refrigerator crisper drawer. Slice or cube the vegetable (leave the edible skin on for an extra nutritional boost). Large eggplants may also be baked whole and then mashed, or sliced and grilled. Smaller types have more tender skins and may be stir-fried, sautéed, or roasted.

For Your Health

Eggplants get their rich purple color from anthocyanins, antioxidants that may lower the risks of cancer and heart disease. A powerful antioxidant, nasunin is found only in the skin of eggplants and is responsible for its purple color. Eggplant's high fiber and meaty texture create a feeling of fullness with very few calories.

For Our Planet

Keep the skin for maximum nutrition and to avoid food waste.

✦ TAKE AWAY

Try roasted or baked eggplant instead of meat—its thick texture will leave you satisfied.

PAIRINGS ✦ A SIMPLE RATATOUILLE

Eggplant tastes delicious teamed with other summer vegetables, such as tomatoes and zucchini. A simple version of ratatouille can be made by cutting eggplant into chunks and braising it with tomatoes and garlic. Finish with some chopped fresh basil. More adventurous cooks might enjoy using eggplant in a traditional Indian dish such as curried eggplant.

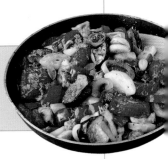

FENNEL

Over millennia, a host of medicinal and magical benefits have been attributed to this hardy perennial herb. Revered by the ancient Greeks and Romans as an appetite suppressant, fennel was also reputed to increase strength, improve vision, stimulate lactation in nursing mothers, and ward off evil spirits. According to Greek mythology, when Prometheus stole fire from the gods, he hid it in a fennel stalk. The type of bulbous fennel found in most markets is called Florence fennel, which lends its licorice flavor to absinthe. Fennel seeds, a popular herb, are actually the dried fruits of another variety of the fennel plant.

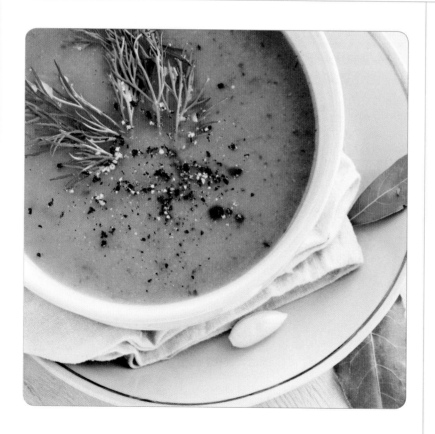

GIVES YOU

Vitamin C
(especially the fronds)
Dietary fiber
Potassium
Manganese
Folate
Calcium
Phytonutrients
  (anethole, flavonoids)

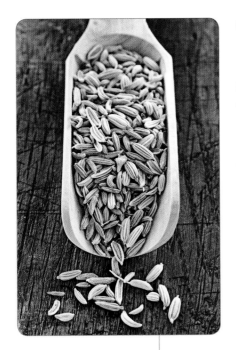

Choose and Use

Look for fennel with stalks intact and clean, crisp bulbs. Refrigerate, tightly wrapped, until ready to use. All parts of the plant are edible and can be eaten raw or cooked in a variety of ways, including braising, baking, and sautéing. The feathery fronds may be snipped like dill and used as a garnish or as part of a delightful herb salad. Closely related to carrots, parsley, dill, and coriander, fennel marries well with all of these ingredients. Its anise-like character diminishes when cooked; sometimes chefs add a little anisette to boost the licorice flavor. Fish, especially salmon, taste wonderful with this vegetable.

For Your Health

Far more nutritious than celery, fennel provides the same low-calorie crunch. The folate in fennel aids in brain function and limits the risk of heart disease and stroke. When consumed by pregnant women, fennel can also reduce brain and spine defects in newborns. The high amount of ascorbic acid supports the immune system, and its flavonoids contribute antioxidants. Anethole, the primary component of fennel's volatile oil, has been shown to have anti-inflammatory and anticancer properties. In India, fennel seeds are traditionally offered after meals to freshen breath and aid in digestion.

For Our Planet

Reduce your food waste by enjoying the entire fennel plant: bulbs, roots, stems, seeds, and fronds. Fennel's distinct aroma seems to discourage insect pests, which means fewer pesticides are used to grow it. Most fennel sold in markets is in bulk, which reduces packaging waste.

✦ TAKE AWAY

Use all parts of the fennel plant to boost flavor and add essential nutrients.

PAIRINGS ✦ COLESLAW WITH AN ADULT FLAIR

Shaved very thin with a mandoline or a sharp kitchen knife, fennel makes a wonderful substitute for cabbage in a twist on traditional coleslaw, especially when dressed with lemon juice and a sprinkling of fennel seeds. The addition of the fronds to an herb salad is also a refreshing change.

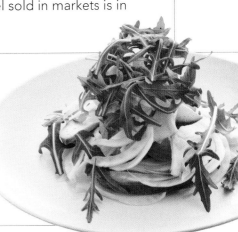

GARLIC

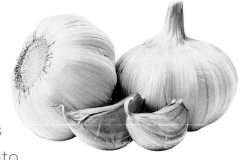

One of the oldest cultivated plants on earth, garlic belongs to the lily family, along with chives, leeks, and onions. Heads of garlic have been discovered tucked into the tombs of Egyptian pharaohs, and the slaves who built these tombs ate garlic to increase their physical strength and endurance. In the Middle Ages, people believed that ingesting garlic could render one immune to the bubonic plague. Proponents of herbal medicine prescribe garlic to prevent colds, the flu, and other infectious diseases, and around the world people enjoy the aromatic range of flavor that it brings to food.

Choose and Use
Purchase bulbs, or heads, of garlic with firm, plump cloves and dry skins. Avoid garlic with small green sprouts or mold, both signs of age. Stored in an open container in a cool, dark place, a head of garlic will keep about eight weeks. The individual cloves are usually peeled before use, and they may be eaten raw or cooked, depending on the flavor desired. Pressing garlic produces a sharper flavor than chopping or slicing it. When cooking

GIVES YOU
Manganese
Vitamin B6
Vitamin C
Selenium
Calcium
Tryptophan
Phytonutrients
   (organosulfur
   compounds, lignans)

(PREP TIP ✦ ROAST THE WHOLE HEAD)

Roasting garlic radically changes its character, transforming it into a sweet and caramelized paste that can be used in a broad range of dishes, from flavoring mashed potatoes or smashed cauliflower to spreading on a sandwich. Fill an ovenproof casserole with a half-inch of water, then place several heads of garlic upright inside and cover. Roast for 30 minutes, or until soft, in a 375-degree oven. Or drizzle with extra-virgin olive oil and put in a dish or wrap in foil before roasting. Water will leach off some nutrients, and the oil preparation will add more calories; it's a matter of taste and trade-offs.

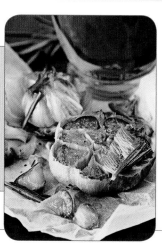

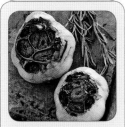

Crushed or sliced garlic is a super way to add robust flavor to a wide variety of foods and dishes. But have you ever seen it take on a bluish-green hue in a hot oven, or when it's pickled? This is because of an enzymatic reaction due to the sulfur components in garlic (and other aromatics), which breaks down in high heat or acidic environments. Don't worry, though: the colorful garlic may take you by surprise, but it's perfectly safe to eat.

garlic at high heat, take care not to let it burn or it will turn bitter. Garlic can enhance all sorts of savory dishes. Raw garlic may cause indigestion in some people.

For Your Health

One hears many grandiose claims about the health benefits of garlic. While some have been bolstered by science, other studies have proved inconclusive. The widely held folk belief that garlic helps ward off the common cold has yet to be fully substantiated. Sulfur-containing compounds in garlic, specifically hydrogen sulfide, are the source of many of its health-promoting effects. Colorectal and ovarian cancer rates drop in populations that regularly ingest a lot of garlic. There also appears to be a correlation between allium foods and reduced gastric cancer risk. And not the least of garlic's benefits is its ability to elevate the taste of bland food. Chopping or crushing garlic helps release a chemical called allicin; wait at least 15 minutes before using to increase its healthful properties.

For Our Planet

Heads of garlic are typically transported and sold without additional packaging waste. But chemicals are heavily applied to fumigate the soil in which garlic is grown, so buying organic if possible is a more sustainable option to protect the Earth.

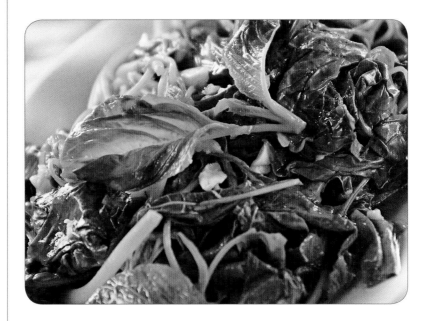

GREEN BEAN

Though consumed throughout the Americas, green beans were not raised commercially in the United States until 1836. These legumes became so popular that growers once marketed them as "The Ninth Wonder of the World," and they still rank high on Americans' list of favorite vegetables. Also called string beans or snap beans, green beans are related to other so-called common beans, including kidney, navy, pinto, and black beans. Harvesting earlier results in the fresh green character of this vegetable, which pairs well with lemon, vinegar, dill, parsley, garlic, and almonds. Other varieties include pale yellow wax beans and purple beans.

Choose and Use

Green beans are available year-round, with peak season between May and October. Look for bright green beans that snap, not bend. The freshest beans have slightly fuzzy skins; avoid bumpy looking ones where the beans are visible under the pod. Unwashed green beans stored in a plastic bag will keep for about five days in the crisper. As with any vegetable, rinse well before using. The entire bean pod is edible and may be consumed raw or cooked by steaming, boiling, braising, and stir-frying. Pickled green beans taste great too. In many Middle Eastern recipes, green beans are slow-cooked until meltingly soft, but they retain more of their phytonutrients, vitamins, and minerals when steamed quickly just until tender-crisp. An ice bath after cooking preserves their bright green color and prevents overcooking. Green beans are also sold frozen and canned; make sure to choose brands with no added sodium or sugar.

For Your Health

Green beans contain a wide variety of carotenoids (such as lutein and beta-carotene) and flavonoids (such as quercetin),

GIVES YOU

Vitamin C
Vitamin K
Manganese
Dietary fiber
Folate
Molybdenum
Magnesium
Iron
Phytonutrients
(carotenoids,
flavonoids, lignans)

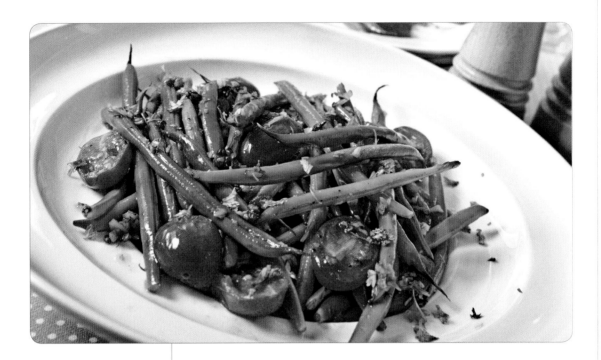

which have antioxidant properties that have been shown to support cardiovascular health. They also afford a good source of the mineral silicon, which can help build strong bones and support the growth of connective tissue in the body.

For Our Planet

Sixty percent of all conventionally produced green beans are grown in the United states, in Illinois, Michigan, New York, Oregon, and Wisconsin. Food miles is just one part of the carbon emissions equation, though: efficiently transported green beans from afar can sometimes have a smaller footprint.

PREP TIP ✦ THINK CELERY SUB

If you're craving a green, crunchy snack, skip the celery and try some raw green beans. They taste great and offer far more nutritional benefits than celery, and you don't have to cut them into sticks. For a real treat, see if you can find purple pole beans at your local market, which are similar in flavor to green beans. Toss with a little olive oil, vinegar, and garlic and lightly season with salt and pepper for a colorful, snappy salad.

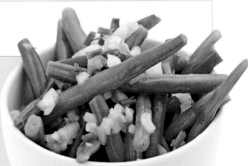

HEARTY GREENS: COLLARD, MUSTARD, CHARD

Easily cultivated, fast growing, and highly nutritious, cooking greens provided sustenance for the many enslaved persons, sharecroppers, and migrants who labored on U.S. plantations. Inexpensive and available year-round, mixed greens are most popular in the American South, where they are typically cooked with butter, lard, or oil and flavored with fatback, also called salt pork, or a ham hock. Often lumped together as a "mess" of greens, each has a distinct flavor, with chard being the mildest and mustard the most peppery. While they can be consumed raw, making for a robust if somewhat bitter salad green, slow cooking (braising) or sautéing is more common. The practice of cooking down the leafy greens and drinking the juices, or "pot likker," stems from African heritage. All cruciferous vegetables, these greens are nutritional powerhouses.

Choose and Use

Greens wilt easily, so select the freshest-looking bunches with the greenest leaves. Unwashed greens may keep longer than a week if wrapped in dampish paper towels and stored in the crisper. Rinse thoroughly before cooking to flush out the dirt trapped between the ribs of the collard and chard, in particular. Both stems and leaves are edible, and the quickest preparation is to chop and cook the entire plant together; the slower-cooking stems will yield a satisfying crunch. Swiss chard has white stalks and glossy green leaves; ruby chard has red ribs and stalks and a stronger flavor. Sometimes varieties are bunched together and labeled "rainbow chard." The oxalic acid in chard will discolor an aluminum pot. Collards may be prepared in the same manner as spinach or cabbage. Raw mustard greens add a peppery bite to salads, but may also be steamed, braised, or sautéed.

GIVES YOU

Vitamin K
Vitamin C
Folate
Manganese
Calcium
Potassium
Copper
Iron
Phytonutrients
   (glucosinolates, phenolic
   acids, flavonoids,
   carotenoids)

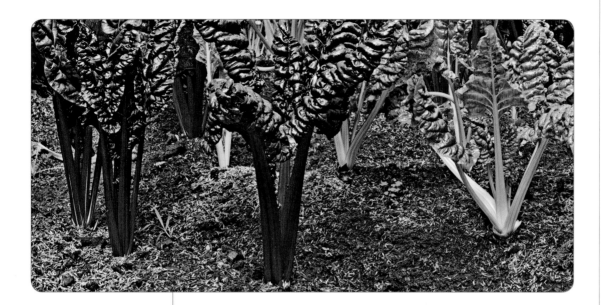

✦ TAKE AWAY

Hearty greens provide a range of flavors and promote heart, bone, and digestive tract health.

For Your Health

Greens are rich in vital minerals, such as iron, copper, and manganese, and bone-building vitamin K and calcium, which help ward off osteoporosis. Mustard greens, which stave off breast cancer and heart disease and keep bones healthy when consumed as part of a plant-based diet, may be especially beneficial for menopausal women. Chard also helps prevent cancers, especially those of the digestive tract. Collard greens outrank all other common cruciferous vegetables in their ability to lower cholesterol.

For Our Planet

Especially prone to damage, conventionally grown leafy greens often require lots of chemicals—especially troublesome for farmers growing them for your dinner table. Selecting organic is an investment in sustainable growing practices and also protects farmworkers.

PAIRINGS ✦ **A HEALTHIER MIX**

Southern greens are traditionally cooked with fatty meats, which reduces their healthfulness. A more nutritious preparation for both you and the planet is to sauté them—either mixed together or singly—in a little olive oil with freshly chopped garlic and a bit of salt and pepper. A splash of lemon juice or vinegar adds a bright finish.

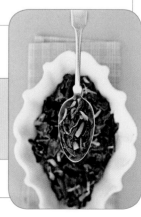

KALE

Modern kale, which resembles collard greens with frilly leaves, comes in many varieties and colors, including red and purple. It still bears a striking resemblance to fossils of wild grasses that grew on Earth billions of years ago. A member of the mighty *Brassica* genus, kale thrives in a cold climate. This hardy winter vegetable is usually harvested after the first frost, which intensifies its flavor, making it sweeter and more tender. Kale was the most widely eaten green vegetable in Europe until the end of the Middle Ages, when it was eclipsed by its cousin the cabbage.

Choose and Use

Choose relatively small bunches with sprightly leaves and no wilting or discolorations. The unwashed greens will keep for several days in a cold refrigerator. Wash well and cut out the tough midrib of each leaf before use—these can be simmered in water to make a broth, or sliced thinly and served with the greens. To preserve its rich stores of vitamins K, A, and ascorbic acid, it's best to cook kale quickly in minimal water or, better yet, sauté it with olive oil and a bit of garlic. Steaming kale concentrates its cholesterol-lowering powers. Brighten the flavor of kale with a splash of lemon juice or vinegar.

✦ TAKE AWAY

Add kale to salads and dishes for its cancer-fighting antioxidants.

PREP TIP ✦ **GREAT ON THE GRILL**

For a more tender salad, dress the kale and let it sit overnight (less time will suffice), which helps tenderize the leaves. First remove the large rib, which can be tough unless sliced thinly, and cut the leaves very thin, then toss with a vinaigrette. Sprinkling with lemon juice before letting it sit enhances kale's phytonutrient concentration.

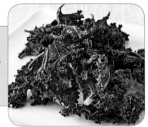

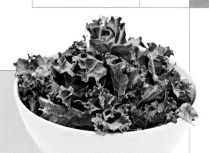

PAIRINGS ✦ A HEALTHIER SALAD GREEN

A hearty green, kale's colors include red, green, and purple. Texture also varies, including a flatter leaf or one with crinkles. Whichever you choose, kale makes a beautiful salad when paired with toasted nuts and cheese. Topped with a piece of grilled fish or tofu, it makes a fine dinner on its own.

GIVES YOU

Vitamin K
Vitamin C
Manganese
Dietary fiber
Copper
Tryptophan
Calcium
Pyridoxine
Potassium
Iron
Folate
Phytonutrients
  (carotenoids,
  flavonoids,
  glucosinolates,
  lignans)

For Your Health

Of late, kale has been hailed as a superfood, and the label seems largely justified. A 2010 study published in the *American Journal of Clinical Nutrition* showed that eating a diet rich in the antioxidant vitamin K reduces one's risk of developing or dying from cancer. Studies have also shown that ingesting kale can slow cognitive decline, prevent rheumatoid arthritis and heart disease, and slow age-related macular degeneration. The carotenoids, flavonoids, and vitamin K in kale are fat-soluble nutrients and must be eaten as part of a meal including fat to increase absorption. Try consuming as part of a winter salad with a heart-healthy vegetable oil such as olive or canola.

For Our Planet

Like other greens, conventionally grown kale often requires a lot of pesticides to obtain a thriving crop. If you are able to find and afford organic, buy it to protect the earth as well as those who grew it for you: the farmers.

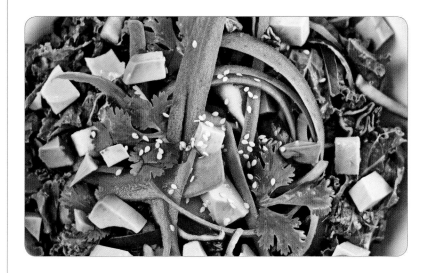

LEEK, ONION, GREEN ONION

For centuries, members of the pungent tribe known as the allium family have lent their versatile character to all manner of savory dishes, and countless recipes begin with the simple act of chopping an onion. Our ancestors worshipped onions long before they ventured to eat them, however. Egyptian tomb paintings depict onions more than any other plant. The word *onion* derives from the Latin *unus*, meaning "one," and ancient Romans regarded the plant's multilayered sphere as a symbol of the universe.

Today these noble bulbs are inexpensive and readily available, and they work all manner of magic in the cuisines of the world. "Dry" onions range in size and sharpness, from large yellow, white, and red onions to sweet varieties such as the Vidalia, to diminutive pearl onions. Green onions are slender onions without bulbs, a favorite ingredient in Asian dishes. The mildest-tasting member of this fraternity and the soul of vichyssoise, the leek has been cherished by gourmets for thousands of years, though it has yet to make much headway in American kitchens.

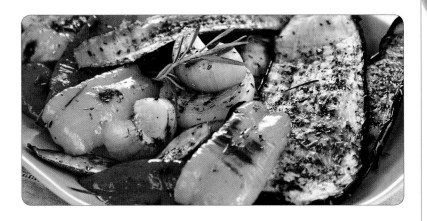

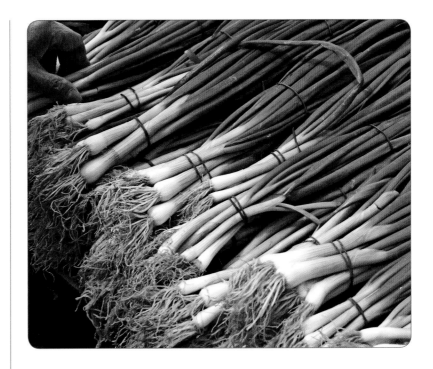

GIVES YOU

LEEK:
Vitamin K
Manganese
Vitamin C
Folate
Pyridoxine
Iron
Dietary fiber
Phytonutrients
  (carotenoids,
  flavonoids,
  organosulfur
  compounds)

ONION:
Vitamin C
Dietary fiber
Pyridoxine
Folate
Tryptophan
Phytonutrients
  (phytosterols,
  flavonoids,
  organosulfur
  compounds)

GREEN ONION:
Vitamin K
Vitamin C
Dietary Fiber
Folate
Calcium
Iron
Phytonutrients
  (flavonoids,
  carotenoids,
  organosulfur
  compounds)

Choose and Use

When choosing dry onions, look for firm bulbs with glossy papery skins. Avoid any that have sprouted or have soft or moldy spots or an odor. Onions should not be refrigerated. Kept in a cool, dry place with good air circulation, they should last approximately two months. Cutting onions causes tearing (a result of certain sulfuric compounds). If this bothers you, try wearing glasses or goggles made for this purpose. The sharper the knife, the fewer the tears. The onion adds flavor to almost anything you cook, and its culinary uses are practically infinite. This versatile vegetable may be fried, braised, boiled, sautéed, roasted, baked, or eaten raw. When cooked slowly, the high sugar content in onions

PREP TIP ✦ LEEKS: CUT, RINSE, REPEAT

Grown in sandy soil, the leek tends to trap dirt in its bulb and must be cleaned carefully before use. To ensure that no residual grit finds its way into the cooking pot, chop the white stalk (and the green leaves, if you plan to use them) and immerse the pieces in several changes of water to rinse away the grit, then toss in a colander to drain. A salad spinner is a useful tool for this task.

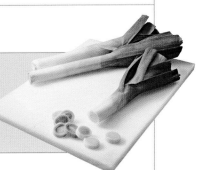

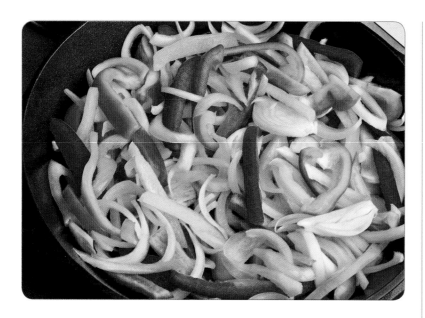

caramelizes, resulting in a wonderfully mellow flavor. The very sweetest varieties, such as Vidalia and Walla Walla onions, may even be eaten out of hand, like an apple.

Green onions are usually sold in bunches; the stalks should look fresh and crisp. Wrapped in plastic, they last up to two weeks in the refrigerator. Rinse before using, and trim off the rootlets. Sliced raw green onion may be sprinkled over foods or soups or added to salads, or stir-fried with other vegetables.

Leeks no larger than two inches in diameter with a slightly limber stem are the most tender. Choose those with brightly colored leaves and an unblemished white bulb. Bagged in plastic, leeks will last in the crisper for about five days. If using whole leek, trim off the root end, slit lengthwise, and rinse well under running water, to flush out the grit between the plant's many layers. People often discard the green leaves and use only the bulb, but the leaves are edible too—though they take longer to tenderize. Leeks have a more delicate flavor than dry onions. They may be braised, steamed, and grilled, or chopped and added to soups or salads.

For Your Health

Ingesting onions can boost immunity, lower blood pressure, help prevent stroke, and decrease one's risk of developing colorectal, ovarian, pancreatic, and prostate cancer. An onion's

FOOD SCIENCE ✦ ALLIUM

A genus of the lily family, alliums include garlic, chives, shallots, and scallions, which look almost identical to green onions but are a distinct variety. Many plants in this group were cultivated as herbal medicines long before they were used to flavor food. Research shows that eating alliums adds anticancer, anti-inflammatory, and antioxidant compounds to one's diet. With all of their shapes, sizes, colors, and flavors, mix them up in your diet to gain the maximum health benefits.

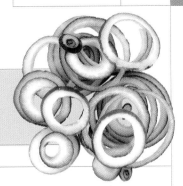

PREP TIP ✦ **USE RED ONIONS WHEN USING ONIONS RAW**

Raw onions can have a sharp taste that some people find unpleasant. In recipes calling for raw onion, opt for the red ones, which are sweeter and have a more balanced flavor than yellow or white onions. They are especially wonderful on salad, where they add flavor as well as color.

cancer-fighting power is directly related to its pungency: The strongest-tasting onions, such as the New York Bold, prove most effective at reducing one's cancer risk. Onions are rich in cancer-fighting antioxidants called flavonoids. Because many of these flavonoids are concentrated in the onion's outer layers, overpeeling can result in a significant loss of these phytonutrients. Take care to remove only the onion's papery outer skin. Onions can also help improve bone density. One study showed that eating an onion a day helped postmenopausal women reduce their risk of hip fracture.

For Our Planet

Some commercial onion producers, notably Gills Onions in California, have pioneered sustainability practices to reduce plant waste in onion production. This grower converts 100 percent of its daily onion waste (unusable tops, tails, and skins) into emissions-free electricity and uses drip irrigation systems to conserve water.

✦ **TAKE AWAY**

Onions add a range of flavors and essential nutrients to many dishes.

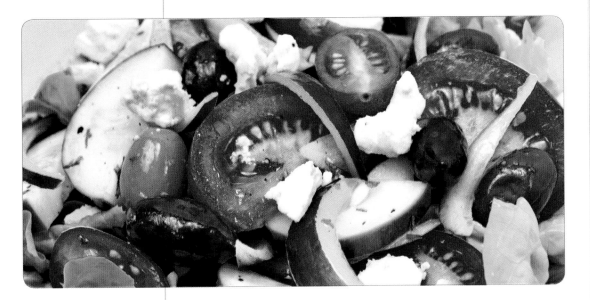

MUSHROOM

Neither animal nor plant but something in between, the mysterious mushroom is classified as a fungus. Mushrooms come in a fantastic array of sizes, shapes, and colors. People in every age and culture have eaten them as food, but they have also served as medicines or as hallucinogens in religious ceremonies. Most of the mushrooms eaten in the United States are cultivated inside darkened buildings where temperature and humidity are controlled. Wild mushrooms, which may be cultivated or foraged, offer a more exotic range of flavors than the typical white supermarket mushroom, with a higher price tag.

Choose and Use

Medium-sized white button mushrooms and brown criminis (baby portobellos) are the most common varieties stocked in supermarkets. Select firm mushrooms with tightly closed caps and no gills showing, and store in the refrigerator for as much as a week. To clean, brush off caps with a damp paper towel. Mushrooms can be eaten raw in salads, or sautéed and added to pasta, omelets, soups, and other dishes to impart a wonderful earthiness to a recipe. The larger portobello mushroom grills beautifully and provides an excellent substitute for meat in a vegetarian diet. Try one as part of a vegetarian "burger." More exotic varieties, such as the shiitake, oyster, and chanterelle, can be found in many markets, along with canned mushrooms and dried wild mushrooms.

GIVES YOU

Selenium
Riboflavin
Copper
Niacin
Pantothenic acid
Potassium
Phosphorus
Vitamin D
Ergothioneine
Phytonutrients
    (beta glucans)

FOOD SCIENCE ✦ WASHING MUSHROOMS

Despite kitchen folklore, it is a myth that mushrooms absorb excess liquid and become soggy when cleaned in water. While they should not be submerged, rinsing mushrooms gently but thoroughly under water, like other vegetables and fruit, will ensure your fungi are free of dirt and ready to be used in your favorite recipe.

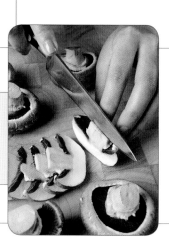

PREP TIP
✦
MUSHROOM DIVERSITY

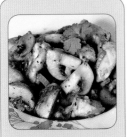

Fresh and dried mushrooms are found in a wide array of shapes and sizes, textures and flavors. Some mushrooms, like shiitake, have tough stems that should be trimmed and composted. Dried mushrooms are a shelf-stable food that will last for months in your pantry. Once the mushrooms are rehydrated in a hot water bath, the soaking liquid can be used in your favorite soup or stew.

✦ TAKE AWAY

Raw or cooked, mushrooms can enhance the flavor and texture of your dishes.

For Your Health

Studies show that mushrooms may play a role in both cancer prevention and treatment. The B vitamins and antioxidants in mushrooms support cardiovascular health, and they also represent one of the few food sources of bone-building vitamin D. Mushrooms also contain glutamic acid, a nonessential amino acid that the body makes on its own but that helps brain function and muscle recovery. This low-calorie but filling food can aid in weight loss by satisfyingly replacing meat in regular meals. Cultivated mushrooms provide the same benefits as more expensive wild varieties.

For Our Planet

Mushrooms are a crop that grows rapidly and yields high returns. Many organizations regard mushroom cultivation as playing an important role in moving the planet toward sustainability.

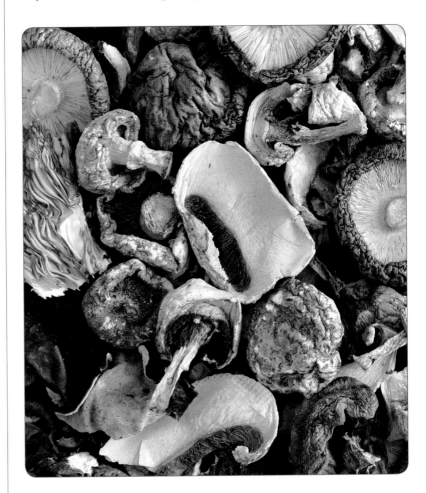

PEPPERS: RED, ORANGE, YELLOW, GREEN

Native to the Americas, and related to the eggplant, potato, and other edible members of the nightshade family, these colorful vegetables are also called sweet peppers to distinguish them from their fiery cousins, the chilis. Each color signals a different stage of maturity: green bell peppers turn yellow, orange, and then red as they ripen and grow sweeter. Peppers can also be found in white and purple varieties.

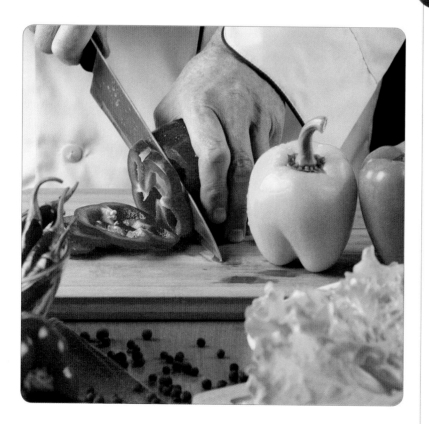

GIVES YOU

Vitamin C
Pyridoxine
Folate
Dietary fiber
Vitamin E
Potassium
Phytonutrients
  (flavonoids,
  carotenoids, phenolic
  acids, phytosterols,
  lignans)

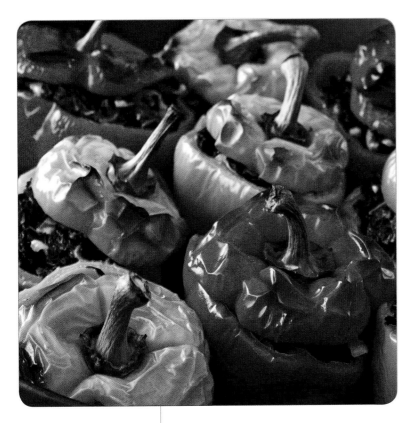

Choose and Use

Look for firm peppers that feel heavy for their size and have shiny skin and bright green stems. Leave the stem intact and store in a crisper for a week or longer, then rinse well before use. Sliced raw peppers add a pleasant crunch to salads. With the top sliced off and seeds and ribs removed, peppers may be stuffed and baked. Add them to stir-frys or grill them. To roast peppers, spear one with a fork and rotate slowly over a gas flame until the skin blackens and blisters. Let the roasted pepper sweat in a sealed paper bag until cool, then peel off the skin (don't wash off the juices), and remove the stem and seeds. Olive oil, onions, and tomatoes all pair well with peppers.

For Your Health

Although red peppers are lower in the carotenoids beta-carotene and alpha-carotene than green peppers, they have more vitamins and nutrients, including the antioxidant lutein, a potential agent for cancer prevention. Red peppers contain more than three times the vitamin C of oranges. Pairing them with iron-rich foods helps increase absorption of this mineral. Peppers of all colors are very high in antioxidants.

For Our Planet

All colors of commercially grown bell peppers have been classified by the Environmental Working Group as one of the "Dirty Dozen" vegetables that retain high levels of pesticide residues. If you're able, selecting organic is a good choice.

✦ TAKE AWAY

Prepare peppers in a variety of ways to benefit from their antioxidants and sweet, tangy taste.

RADICCHIO

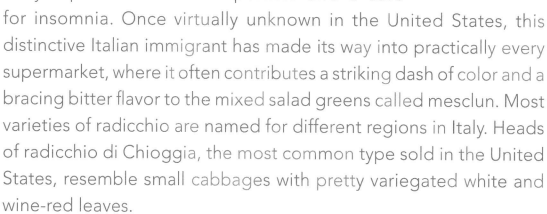

Radicchio (pronounced *ra-DEE-kyoh*) is a type of red-leafed chicory related to both endive and escarole. It was listed in an ancient Roman encyclopedia as a blood purifier and a cure for insomnia. Once virtually unknown in the United States, this distinctive Italian immigrant has made its way into practically every supermarket, where it often contributes a striking dash of color and a bracing bitter flavor to the mixed salad greens called mesclun. Most varieties of radicchio are named for different regions in Italy. Heads of radicchio di Chioggia, the most common type sold in the United States, resemble small cabbages with pretty variegated white and wine-red leaves.

Choose and Use

Choose heads with crisp-looking outer leaves with no discolorations. This cool-season plant may be purchased year-round and will keep for many weeks in the vegetable crisper. Green salads can benefit from the color and pleasantly bitter taste of radicchio leaves. It tastes good baked with rice or mixed into risotto, or braised on its own as a side dish. Radicchio pairs well with balsamic vinegar or dressings with a touch of sweetness. The leaves may be brushed lightly with olive oil and grilled or roasted, which mellows their flavor.

GIVES YOU

Vitamin K
Copper
Folate
Vitamin C
Vitamin E
Potassium
Phytonutrients
   (flavonoids,
   carotenoids)

PAIRINGS ✦ RADICCHIO SALAD

The pretty purple and white leaves of radicchio are lovely to look at but the bitter flavor can be too much for some. Combining it with sweeter salad greens like spinach alongside avocado, pears, or toasted nuts keeps the pleasing color and provides balance.

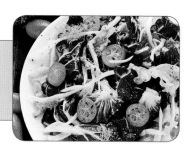

For Your Health

Radicchio is an excellent source of vitamin K, important for bone health and which may play a role in the treatment of Alzheimer's disease. This leafy vegetable contains the antioxidants zeaxanthin and lutein, which help protect the eyes against age-related macular degeneration. Radicchio gets its bitter flavor from lactucopicrin, which has a sedative and pain-killing effect in the body.

For Our Planet

If you enjoy gardening, radicchio is easy to raise and requires less water than many other crops. And, if you're really adventurous, enjoy the whole plant: its roots can be used to brew chicory coffee.

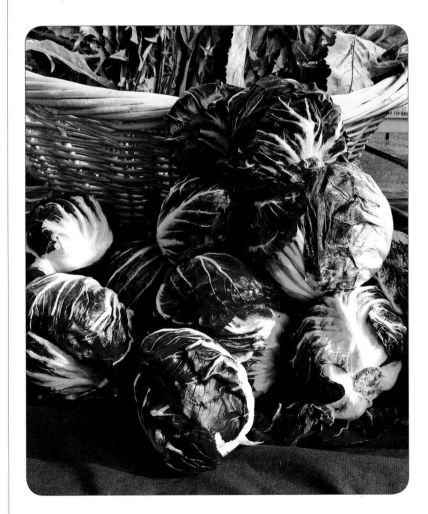

PREP TIP
✦
GRILLED RADICCHIO

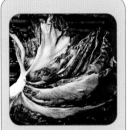

Everyone loves to barbecue during summertime but few are familiar with grilling lettuce. Grilled radicchio is beautiful and the high heat cuts down its bitter flavors. Cut the heads in half length-wise, drizzle with olive oil, and season with salt and pepper then toss onto the grill at high heat. Enjoy as a side dish on its own, or toss with whole wheat pasta, garlic, and parmesan for a quick supper.

✦ TAKE AWAY

Radicchio adds a tasty bitterness to salads and is a traditional ingredient in risotto.

RADISH

First cultivated in China, the radish is the edible root of a mustard-like plant, which accounts for its peppery flavor. A close relative of the cabbage, turnip, and cauliflower, this crucifer is often relegated to the status of a decorative garnish on American plates—a regretful waste of a beneficial and flavorful vegetable. Varieties include the red globe, and the black radish, widely used in eastern Europe. The large white daikon radish has multiple uses in Asian cuisine.

Choose and Use

Red globe radishes, the pretty red ones sold in bunches at the market, have a mild peppery flavor. Bright color and crisp green leaves indicate freshness. Avoid the largest ones, which may be pithy, and any with cracks. Remove the green tops, which leach off nutrients, and store in the refrigerator. Most radishes grow more pungent as they mature, so use them within a few days of purchase, although they last in the fridge for weeks if stored in a plastic bag. Many people discard radish tops, but they are nutritious and tasty, either eaten raw in salads, sautéed along with the radishes, or used as you would other greens. Wash roots and tops well before using, to rinse away any residue and grit. Raw

GIVES YOU
Vitamin C
Potassium
Pyridoxine
Phytonutrients
    (glucosinolates,
    phenolic acids,
    flavonoids)

PREP TIP ✦ WATERMELON RADISH

An heirloom variety of the daikon radish that originated in China, the watermelon radish masks its wonders inside an unassuming white exterior. Slicing one open reveals a striking magenta core, which tastes mild and sweet and resembles the beloved summer fruit. Watermelon radishes lose their brilliant color when cooked, so you may prefer to showcase them raw in salads or pickle them.

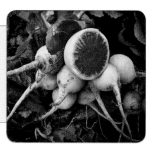

✦ TAKE AWAY
Add radish greens or the red bulbs to your salads, or eat the spicy roots as snacks.

radishes make a low-calorie snack or an unexpected addition to salsa. Cooked (by braising, stir-frying, or steaming), they lose their bite and taste more like turnips. Chopped daikon added to soups and sauces softens during cooking and adds texture.

For Your Health

Radishes offer many of the same cancer-fighting benefits as other vegetables in the *Brassica* genus. They are also a good source of vitamin C, an antioxidant that boosts the immune system. Don't peel radishes, since many of the antioxidants are thickly concentrated in the peel.

For Our Planet

Radishes are grown in most U.S. states, with California and Florida being the largest producers. Enjoy green tops in addition to the root to reduce your food waste. These plants are easy to cultivate and grow quickly, so anyone with a vegetable plot can raise their own.

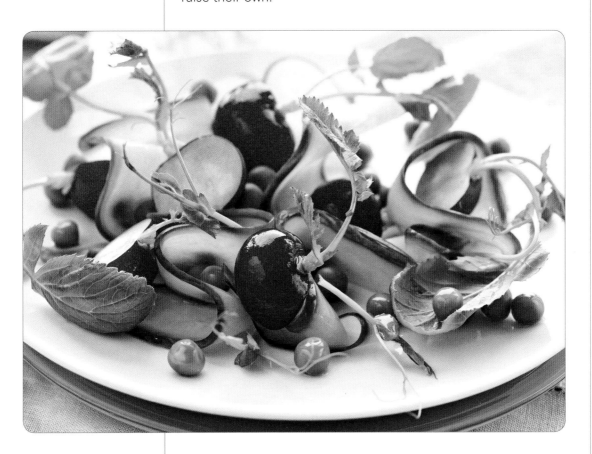

SEAWEED

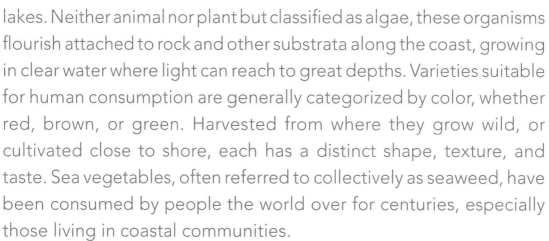

Thousands of varieties of seaweed grow in the Earth's oceans as well as in freshwater lakes. Neither animal nor plant but classified as algae, these organisms flourish attached to rock and other substrata along the coast, growing in clear water where light can reach to great depths. Varieties suitable for human consumption are generally categorized by color, whether red, brown, or green. Harvested from where they grow wild, or cultivated close to shore, each has a distinct shape, texture, and taste. Sea vegetables, often referred to collectively as seaweed, have been consumed by people the world over for centuries, especially those living in coastal communities.

Today, seaweed makes up 25 percent of the Japanese diet. It can also be found in the cuisines of Scotland, Ireland, and Wales, as well as in China, Korea, Vietnam, and Malaysia, where people welcome the range of flavors and abundant nutrients sea vegetables bring to the table. Nonetheless, most Americans are still largely unfamiliar with seaweed, though they have been unknowingly ingesting it all their lives. Additives made from seaweed are used as stabilizers, emulsifiers, and thickening agents in processed foods such as ice

FOOD SCIENCE ✦ CARRAGEENAN

While most people don't know exactly what carrageenan is, they might recognize the term from an ingredient list. Carrageenan is extracted from some red seaweeds and its various forms are used as thickeners, gels, and stabilizers in a wide variety of foods. Incredibly versatile, its properties vary according to type, important to know if you're using it in home cooking. Agar-agar is one form of carrageenan known for its exceptional gelling properties.

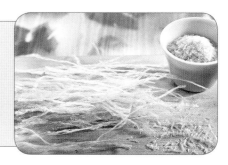

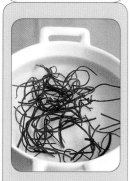

Rehydrating dried seaweed is a cinch: separate the dried pieces, being careful not to prick your hands; place in a large pan; and cover with water. Seaweed will swell as it absorbs water, rehydrating completely in about 30–40 minutes; add more water as needed. Plain water works perfectly, but you could use a no-sodium seafood or vegetable stock for more flavor.

cream, pudding, and pie fillings, like the familiar carrageenan found on so many ingredient labels.

The most popular sea vegetables include nori, used to make edible wrappers for sushi rolls; kombu and wakame, simmered to flavor broth, such as for miso soup; and hijiki, which resembles black, wiry pasta. Kelp, the North American equivalent of kombu, is often roasted and processed into flakes. Dulse, harvested from the frigid waters off the north Atlantic and the northern Pacific coast, is soft and chewy and is sometimes sold as a snack food. The Western palate has become more cosmopolitan, and adventurous cooks will doubtless find ways to add this versatile, healthy, and highly sustainable food to their diets.

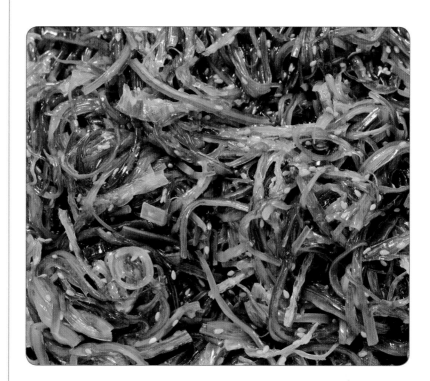

GIVES YOU

Vitamin K
Folate
Magnesium
Calcium
Iron
Iodine
Phytonutrients
(fucoidans, flavonoids)

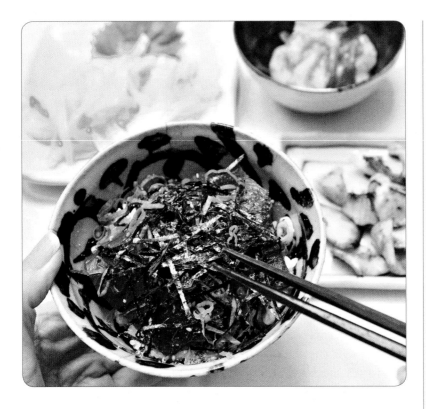

Choose and Use

Sold in many health food and specialty stores, sea vegetables also may be ordered online. As with any food sourced from the sea, water quality is a concern—it's wise to purchase from suppliers who guarantee the purity of their seaweed. In the future, different varieties will likely become more widely available in supermarkets. Look for this food in various forms, such as in sheets (nori), whole pieces (dulse), or in flakes (kelp). Stored at room temperature in tightly sealed packages, it should keep for at least six months. A versatile and convenient food, seaweed needs no cooking, but many varieties require soaking for five to ten minutes, depending on the desired consistency. To prepare, follow the directions on the package.

For anyone unfamiliar with this food, incorporating it into the diet can pose a challenge. Using seaweed as a seasoning is a great place to start. Sea vegetables come in flaked and powdered forms that can be added to other foods, to impart a fifth taste, umami, a savory flavor that is neither sweet, salty, sour, nor bitter. Flaked kelp may be used as a seasoning at the dinner

---

PAIRINGS
✦
SEAWEED SALAD

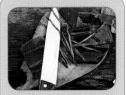

The familiar seaweed salad served in sushi restaurants is easy to prepare at home. The healthiest option is to rehydrate dried seaweed. (You can buy seaweed that's ready to go, but watch out for added sodium.) Chop the seaweed into strips and toss with a simple dressing of rice vinegar, sesame oil, soy sauce, grated ginger, and garlic. Thinly sliced cucumber and a sprinkle of toasted white sesame seeds add color and crunch.

PREP TIP ✦ **SIMMER INTO SOUPS**

Given how healthy and sustainable seaweed is, it's time to start simmering it into some of your favorite stews and soups. The most traditional dish is miso soup, but it can be added to any Asian-style recipe for flavor and body.

table. (Certain seaweeds have a high sodium content.) Try sampling a few varieties to learn which ones you like best. Experiment with adding chopped sea vegetables to salads, rice, pasta, stir-frys, and soups. Dulse makes a tasty bacon substitute, since it turns crispy when fried.

For Your Health

One of the healthiest foods on earth, sea vegetables contain the same range of minerals that the human body requires, in quantities far exceeding those in land vegetables. Seaweed can also protect against radiation. Kelp has a beneficial isotope that prevents the thyroid from absorbing radioactive iodine-131, a byproduct of nuclear energy production. The sodium alginate in this sea vegetable also helps the body excrete radiation and heavy metals. Unique phytonutrients found in seaweed have anti-inflammatory, antiviral, and anti-cancer properties, and reduce the risk of blood clots in addition to lowering blood LDL ("bad") cholesterol. Seaweed is also a natural source of iodine, necessary for the proper functioning of the thyroid gland, which regulates the body's metabolism.

✦ **TAKE AWAY**

Experiment with seaweed, which has higher amounts of essential nutrients than any land vegetable.

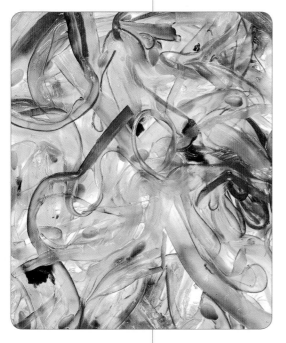

For Our Planet

Sea vegetables represent the ultimate sustainable food. A World Bank study showed that the production process of seaweed farms could actually have a *negative* carbon footprint, since they could potentially absorb 20 percent more carbon dioxide than they emit. In the future, seaweed may be one of the key foods sustaining the world's growing population.

SPINACH

Spinach grew wild in ancient Persia (modern Iran) before the Moors introduced it to Spain. Related to Swiss chard and beets, this dark leafy green became known across Europe as the "Spanish vegetable." Today, people everywhere associate spinach with super strength, thanks to its well-known evangelist, the cartoon character Popeye.

Choose and Use

Spinach is often sold in bunches. Look for crisp, fresh-smelling leaves, with no wilting or yellowing. Wrapped in plastic, this leafy green may keep well for a week in the vegetable crisper. Stems are edible but can be trimmed if tough. Immerse in several changes of water to remove sand. Rinse well even when the package says, "triple washed." These greens may be cooked by steaming or sautéing, and eaten on their own or combined with many other ingredients. Spinach cooks quickly and reduces considerably in volume, so allow one-fourth to one-half pound of raw spinach per person. Raw spinach also makes a fine salad, especially wonderful when served with sliced avocado, citrus, and toasted nuts. Frozen spinach is handy to have around for addition to stews and sauces; make sure to select a no-sodium variety if using canned spinach.

✦ **TAKE AWAY**

Spinach, high in protein and other nutrients, is delicious raw or cooked.

CONSIDER ✦ A SWEETER SPINACH

Like other salad and cooking greens, spinach can be purchased as large, often curly leaves or as its smaller, sweeter, and more tender counterpart known as "baby spinach." Adding spinach to a salad, whether for lunch or dinner, will give you a boost of vitamins and nutrients that paler salad greens won't provide. If you're not used to the stronger flavor, combine it with other lettuces while your palate adjusts.

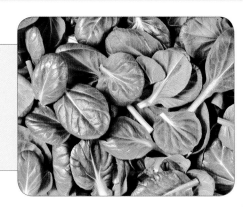

PREP TIP ✦ NUTRITION BOOST

Spinach from the frozen food aisle is just as nutritious as fresh, as it's picked and processed at the height of ripeness. It's great to keep on hand to help your children eat more vegetables. Adding spinach to soups, stews, and tomato sauce will add nutrition and flavor—and your kids probably won't even notice.

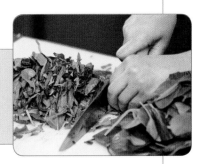

GIVES YOU

Vitamin K
Manganese
Folate
Magnesium
Iron
Vitamin C
Riboflavin
Calcium
Potassium
Pyridoxine
Tryptophan
Vitamin E
Dietary fiber
Protein
Phytonutrients
(carotenoids,
flavonoids, phenolic
acids, phytosterols)

For Your Health

Popeye was right: Spinach is good for you. Rich in vitamin K, for bone health, spinach also protects against various forms of cancer and promotes cardiovascular and eye health. It is also a good source of vegetable protein. Spinach loses some nutrients when cooked, but heating makes the protein in spinach easier to break down, and one can eat considerably more cooked spinach than raw at a sitting due to its high water content.

For Our Planet

Particular prone to pests, pesticide residues in convention-ally grown spinach have earned it a spot on the Environmental Working Group's 2013 "Dirty Dozen" list. Buying organic is a good idea, but if you can't it's still better to be like Popeye and eat your spinach—however grown.

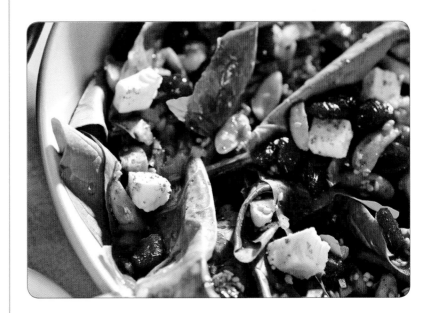

SUMMER SQUASH: ZUCCHINI, PATTYPAN, YELLOW

We know that early farmers in Mexico and Central America cultivated summer squash more than 10,000 years ago, because the preserved seeds of these vegetables have been found in ancient caves. Native Americans referred to them as one of the "three sisters," along with corn (maize) and beans. Related to the hard-shelled winter squash, as well as to melons, cucumbers, and other cucurbits, summer squashes are actually a type of gourd with a thin, edible skin and high water content. The most common varieties are the zucchini (known as courgette in the United Kingdom and France), the bright yellow crookneck, and the pattypan or scallop squash, which comes in a variety of colors. Formerly called Italian squash, the versatile zucchini is a relative latecomer to American kitchens, but it is a featured ingredient in many of the world's cuisines.

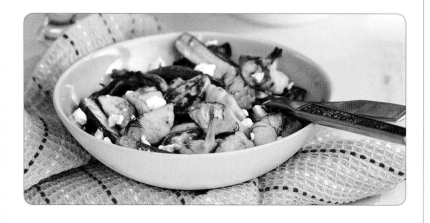

GIVES YOU

Vitamin C
Molybdenum
Pyridoxine
Riboflavin
Potassium
Folate
Dietary fiber
Phytonutrients
　　(carotenoids, lignans)

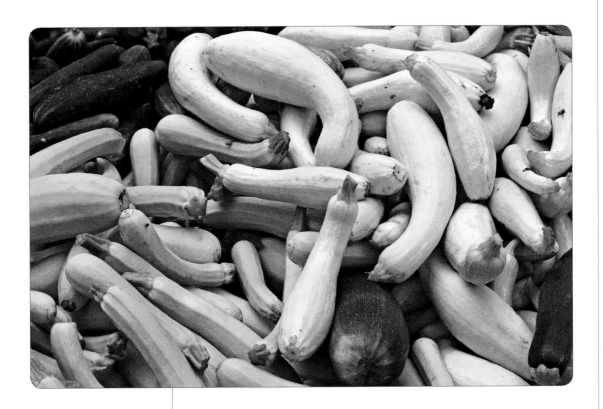

✦ TAKE AWAY

Delicate in flavor, summer squash pairs well with herbs and other summer vegetables.

Choose and Use

Available all year, these vegetables are especially plentiful during the summer months. Choose brightly colored small- to medium-sized squashes, which have more flavor. Their cut ends should look fresh, and their skin should be smooth and unbruised. Wash them well, but don't peel them before cooking. Unlike their tough winter sisters, summer squashes are highly perishable and won't usually last longer than a week in the refrigerator. Mildly flavored, and slightly sweet, they pair well with many other foods and may be eaten raw or cooked.

PREP TIP ✦ ZUCCHINI'S VERSATILITY

The most popular of summer squashes, zucchini also bears brilliant orange flowers. They make a delightful side dish when stuffed simply with goat cheese and herbs or with a combination of grains, nuts, cheese, and diced zucchini. Or use them as a garnish for a special dish. No matter what, zucchini makes a great summer dish.

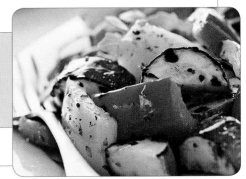

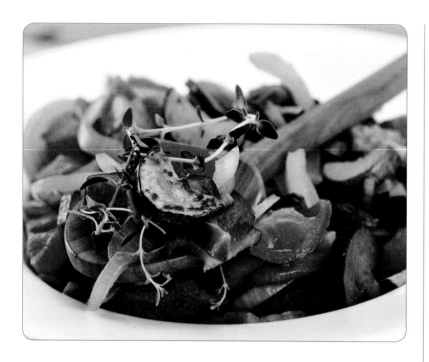

Squash can be sliced and steamed, sautéed, fried, roasted, broiled, or grilled. The most common variety of zucchini has dark green skin, but a bright yellow variety is sometimes available. All summer squash cooks quickly, and the line between crisp-tender and mushy is a fine one, so stay vigilant. All parts, including the flowers, are edible, and stuffed squash blossoms are considered a special seasonal treat. Summer squash retain much of their antioxidant values after steaming, which is not the case when they are boiled or microwaved. Squash tastes lovely garnished with herbs such as parsley, dill, and basil, and paired with other summer vegetables such as tomatoes.

For Your Health
The bright green and yellow skins of different varieties of summer squash are an advertisement for the many nutritional benefits found in their colorful phytonutrients. Recent studies have highlighted the antioxidant benefits from lutein of summer squash, which protects the eyes against age-related macular degeneration and the development of cataracts. To obtain full antioxidant benefits, one needs to ingest the skins and seeds of

---

PAIRINGS
◆
SUMMER STIR-FRY

The height of summer is the perfect time to feature the local bounty—and nothing's more plentiful than squash. Select a combination that pleases you to create a colorful array, and grab a red pepper, onion, and garlic to add texture and flavor. For a quick stir-fry, just sauté with garlic and olive oil. More adventurous cooks might try a combination of soy, ginger, and sesame oil and garnish with toasted almonds for Chinese flair.

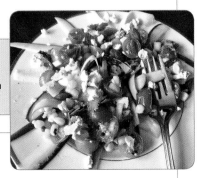

the squash. Of the many varieties of summer squash, zucchini are especially low in calories and contain no saturated fats; adding them to your diet can help support weight loss as part of a high fiber, plant-based diet.

For Our Planet

Summer squashes are usually sold in bulk, which limits packaging waste. Many are commercially grown in the United States, but quantities are also imported from Mexico. If you opt to grow your own, remember that zucchini is a notorious overproducer—better find a good recipe for zucchini bread and some neighbors for sharing the harvest.

✦ **TAKE AWAY**

Add summer squash to your dishes to incorporate valuable antioxidants.

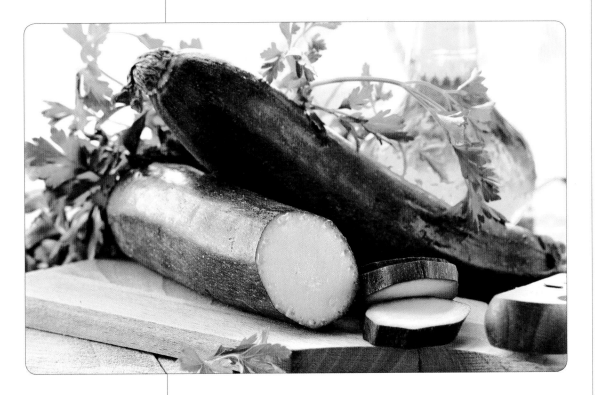

SWEET POTATO

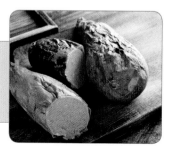

The sweet potato travels under various aliases. Not a potato at all but a large edible root belonging to the morning glory family, it is sometimes called a yam, though it bears no botanical relation to the true yam, a tuber native to Africa. Two varieties of this New World plant are common in U.S. supermarkets: one with reddish brown skin and orange flesh (the so-called yam) and one with tan skin and pale yellow flesh. Red and purple varieties are often harder to find but worth the effort. Growers subject both kinds to a curing process: once unearthed, the tubers are held in a heated, high-humidity environment for four to six days to increase their sweetness and retard spoilage.

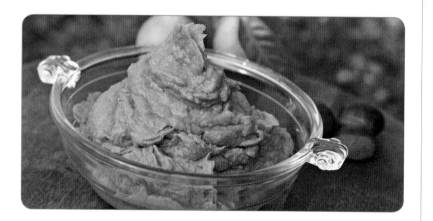

✦ TAKE AWAY

More nutritious than white potatoes, sweet potatoes cook quickly and are delicious chopped or mashed.

PREP TIP ✦ **THE OTHER BAKED POTATO**

Sweet potatoes aren't just for Thanksgiving all dressed up fancy. They can be prepared the same way as a baked potato—piercing and cooking in a hot oven—for a more nutritious alternative to white. Eat the skins, too: they're loaded in fiber and nutrients.

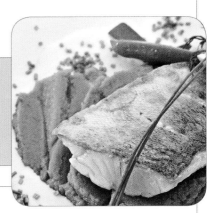

PAIRINGS ✦ A BED OF SMASHED POTATOES

Like white potatoes, sweet potatoes are terrific mashed or, if you leave some in larger chunks, smashed. You can keep the skins on, too. Add a bit of olive oil, cumin, and garlic, and you've got a satisfying, tasty side dish. Smashed potatoes also make a colorful bed for a piece of fish or chicken. For an elegant (and indulgent) alternative, add a bit of truffle oil and goat cheese.

GIVES YOU

Vitamin C
Manganese
Pyridoxine
Tryptophan
Potassium
Dietary fiber
Pantothenic acid
Copper
Thiamine
Riboflavin
Niacin
Phytonutrients
(carotenoids,
flavonoids [in purple])

Choose and Use

Available year-round, these tubers taste best in fall and early winter. Sweet potatoes are more perishable than they appear and should be used within a week of purchase, if possible. Until then, store them in a cool, dry place. Older potatoes can be used in soup or mashed for a more nutritious alternative to white potatoes. Choose medium-sized ones with smooth skins that taper at the ends. The flesh of the red variety is sweeter and more moist than that of the starchier yellow type. Both can be roasted whole and eaten hot from the oven or enjoyed cold the next day. Cut in pieces and boiled or steamed, they cook quickly. Puréed sweet potatoes make a rich-tasting side dish. The skins are perfectly edible and fiber-rich. People often blanket their "yams" with marshmallows in typical Thanksgiving attire, but these naturally sweet roots don't really require additional sugar.

For Your Health

Like other yellow-orange vegetables, sweet potatoes are an excellent source of beta-carotene, which the body converts to vitamin A. Consuming them as part of a preparation or meal that includes fat aids in absorption of this nutrient, which is fat soluble. Though sweet, these tubers are not high in calories—just higher than most vegetables. Look for purple-fleshed varieties, which are rich in anthocyanins with anti-inflammatory and antioxidant properties.

For Our Planet

North Carolina produces about 40 percent of the U.S. sweet potato crop, followed by California. A planet-friendly vegetable, sweet potatoes can be conventionally grown without a lot of pesticides and require little nitrogen (a common fertilizer) or irrigation.

TOMATO

Like its cousin the eggplant, the tomato is an anomaly—botanically speaking it is a fruit, but it is consumed as a vegetable. Europeans were slow to welcome this edible member of the nightshade family into their diet, fearing it was toxic. Eventually, it became a cornerstone of Italian cuisine. Today the average American ingests 22 pounds of tomatoes a year, mostly processed into ketchup and tomato sauce. For decades, commercially grown tomatoes have been selectively bred for firmness and uniformity, resulting in a practically tasteless product. Efforts to restore the tomato's flavor have led to the increasing availability of heirloom varieties.

Choose and Use

Available all year in many different shapes, sizes, and colors, the tomato is a summer fruit that tastes best in season. Ripe tomatoes should be used soon after purchase. Store at room temperature, since refrigeration causes enzymatic reactions that compromise its sweetness and kill flavor. The versatile tomato may be eaten raw or cooked in countless ways, including broiling, stewing, or sautéing. Roasting intensifies its flavor. Tomatoes can be stuffed and baked, or made into hot and cold soups or condiments such as ketchup and salsa. Sun-dried tomatoes taste great in salads or egg dishes.

GIVES YOU

Vitamin C
Vitamin K
Potassium
Molybdenum
Dietary fiber
Glutamic acid
Phytonutrients
(flavonoids, phenolic acids, carotenoids, phytosterols)

PREP TIP ✦ **KEEP CANS ON HAND**

Nothing beats a sweet, summer-fresh tomato when in season. But there are a whole host of canned tomato products that contain even more lycopene (the tomato's main antioxidant) than fresh. Always keeping an array of canned tomatoes in your pantry, including crushed, diced, sauce, whole, and paste, is a good way to help you get a meal together in a flash.

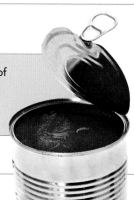

Fresh tomatoes taste delicious and bring acidity and texture to a dish. However, research has shown that cooking tomatoes, including canned products, boosts their nutritional value, specifically the carotenoid lycopene; the bioavailability of this fat-soluble phytonutrient further improves in the presence of oil. But you can feel great about substituting healthful canned tomatoes for fresh in a recipe, so keep these products handy in your pantry shelves. Canned tomatoes are also a low-cost way to enjoy these summer plants out of season.

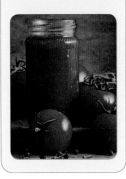

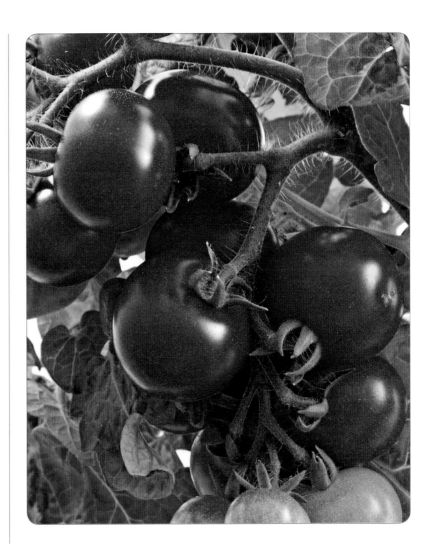

For Your Health

In addition to many other phytonutrients, the low-calorie tomato is rich in lycopene, a carotenoid associated with prostate cancer risk reduction and cardiovascular health. A recent study indicated that the lycopene in orange tomatoes may be more readily absorbed than that in red tomatoes. Eating tomatoes may also help prevent pancreatic and colorectal cancer.

For Our Planet

Buying sweet tomatoes at the height of summer treats your taste buds and supports local farmers. Or try your hand at growing your own tomatoes, easily raised in your garden or on your windowsill.

TURNIP

A hardworking yeoman of the vegetable kingdom and part of the cruciferous family, the humble turnip has many virtues. Easily grown, even in nutrient-poor soil, turnips provide a nourishing food during the cold winter months. They filled our ancestors' bellies when other food was scarce, and served as fodder for their farm animals. Sometimes this pale root with the purple shoulders even provided a source of illumination, since (according to an Irish myth) the very first jack-o-lantern was a turnip.

Choose and Use

Choose turnips that are smooth and firm. Smaller equals sweeter—all the better if fresh green leaves are still attached. Turnip roots keep for a few weeks in the refrigerator, but the greens lose their nutrients rapidly and should be eaten right away. The root is hard, and should be peeled unless the turnip is very small, and you'll need a heavy knife to chop it into pieces. Then it may be braised, roasted, boiled, or steamed. The earthy flavor of the turnip blends well with other root vegetables in stews, or puréed into a creamy soup. Roasting brings out its sweetness, but if cooked using other methods it may benefit from a little added sugar, such as honey. Eaten raw, a baby turnip tastes peppery, like a radish.

PAIRINGS ✦ ROASTED TURNIP "FRIES"

Mild in flavor, turnips are particularly good when roasted. Cut into wedges or strips, toss with oil, season lightly with salt and pepper, and roast at high heat until tender. For more flavor, add cumin or chili powder or a selection of fresh herbs.

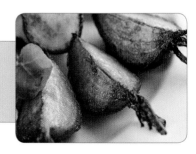

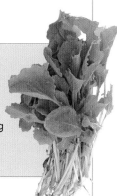

PREP TIP ✦ TURNIP GREENS

Those accustomed to discarding their turnip tops on the compost heap should be advised that the majority of a turnip's nutrients are concentrated in its nutritious greens. Cooked, the greens provide more than six times the recommended daily value of bone-building vitamin K, as well as high levels of vitamins A and C, folate, manganese, and fiber. The presence of calcium gives the greens their bitter flavor. Turnip greens contain even more cancer-preventing glucosinolates than cabbage, kale, and broccoli. A quick sauté with a little vegetable oil and garlic is all that's needed to enjoy turnip greens, or add them to your next soup or stew.

✦ TAKE AWAY

Turnips are full of antioxidants; include green tops for added nutritional benefits.

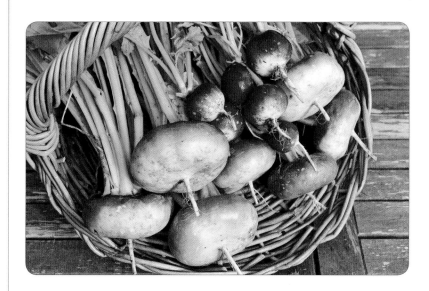

GIVES YOU

Vitamin C
Dietary fiber
Potassium
Manganese
Copper
Potassium in greens
Calcium
Pyridoxine
Folate
Phytonutrients
(glucosinolates/
organosulfides,
flavonoids,
carotenoids in
greens)

For Your Health

Adding these crucifers to your diet can lower your risk of developing cancer of the breast, bladder, lung, and prostate. Turnip tops contain flavonoids, antioxidants that neutralize free radicals in the body and help protect against these cancers. They also provide a rich source of Vitamin C (diminished somewhat by cooking), which boosts cardiovascular health. Even more benefits may be gained by eating the turnip greens.

For Our Planet

Eating turnips roots to leaves is another fantastic way to save your food dollars and reduce your personal food waste. This way, edible food doesn't end up in landfills—where it creates methane, a potent greenhouse gas.

WINTER SQUASH: BUTTERNUT, ACORN, SPAGHETTI, PUMPKIN

This uniquely American plant is actually a type of gourd, a fleshy fruit protected by a tough rind. Thousands of years of cultivation culminated in the sweet, dense squash we enjoy today. However, the first squash grew wild in Central America, where it was loved only for its seeds, since its flesh was thin and bitter. Traveling north with migrating peoples, squash became a staple of Native American agriculture, and European colonists soon recognized the value of a crop that could last through the winter in a cellar without spoiling.

Harvested when fully mature, winter squashes have harder shells, larger seeds, and more nutrients than summer squash. They vary widely in appearance and flavor: the large, pear-shaped butternut, the compact green acorn, the familiar Halloween pumpkin, and more

FOOD SCIENCE ✦ ROASTED SEEDS (IT'S NOT JUST FOR PUMPKINS)

When it comes to squash seeds, most people think only of pumpkins. Yet a variety of squash seeds can be roasted and enjoyed any time of year. Butternut squash has a smaller, rounder seed that creates a wonderful topping to soups and salads. Whether dry roasted or prepared with a kick of flavor from cumin and a drizzle of maple syrup, enjoy the seeds for extra crunch and nutrition while also reducing your food waste.

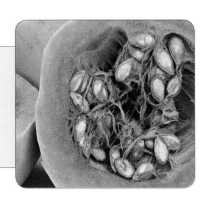

GIVES YOU

Vitamin C
Dietary fiber
Manganese
Pyridoxine
Potassium
Vitamin K
Vitamin E
Phytonutrients
  (carotenoids)

decorative varieties such as the striped delicata, the turban, and the homely Hubbard, all herald the arrival of autumn, massed in decorative heaps at the market. The spaghetti squash, a relative newcomer whose interior separates into pasta-like strands when cooked, was first grown in Manchuria, China, in the 1890s.

Choose and Use

Choose squashes with dull rinds that are firm, heavy for their size, with no soft spots. Store them in a cool, dark place. Winter squash are far more durable than summer squash and will keep from a week to six months, depending on the variety and storage conditions. Wash under cold water before cutting.

The thick rinds of winter squash demand a heavy knife, and the various shapes of squash can make cutting and peeling a challenge. First slice off the stem and then cut the squash in half (you may have to lean your weight on the back of the knife to accomplish this). Scrape out the seeds, boil them till soft, and

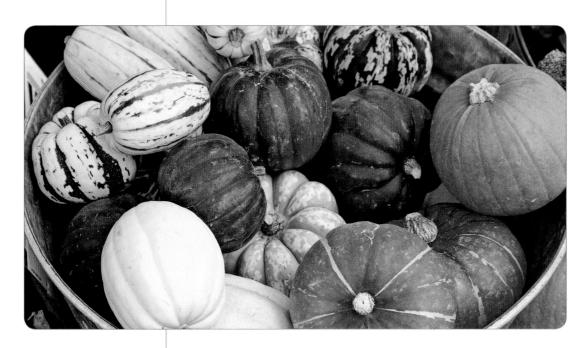

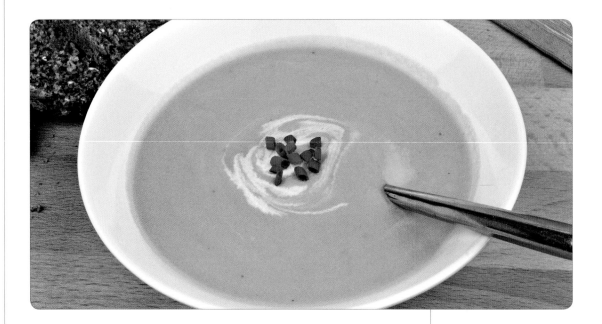

then roast with a little oil and salt for a crunchy and nutritious snack or topping for soups. The rest of the squash may then be cut into manageable pieces, or left in halves for roasting. Since winter squash arrive in their own easy-to-cook containers, this is a classic preparation. Simply coat with vegetable oil, season with salt and pepper, and roast approximately one hour, depending on size. For a lower-calorie option, place each cut side in a shallow pan of water and bake in a 400-degree oven. Spaghetti squash (known as vegetable spaghetti in the U.K.) is the exception: roast this whole, then separate the strands with a fork. Its mild flavor combines well with pasta sauces for a healthful noodle alternative. You may leave the skin on some squash before steaming; other types must be peeled. The sunny flesh of the butternut makes a lovely soup on a gray winter day, or try a mix of squashes for variety. Unlike their warm weather counterparts, winter squashes have distinct flavors, so if one variety doesn't appeal, try another.

Don't despair if this prep work seems daunting: squash is also available precut and frozen, perfect for roasting, steaming, or simmering. Add canned pumpkin to sweet breads, muffins, and pies; a high fiber, lower calorie option is to mix some puréed pumpkin with plain Greek-style yogurt and a sprinkle of cinnamon for a protein-rich autumn snack. Winter squash can stand

✦ **TAKE AWAY**

Each winter squash has a distinct flavor— experiment to find the ones you like best.

PREP TIP ✦ **GOTTA ROAST**

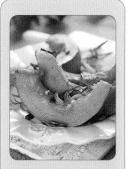

When it comes to bringing out the best in winter squash, nothing beats roasting. Wash and dry the squash then carefully cut it in half and remove the seeds. Season with oil and a bit of salt and pepper and bake for 20–40 minutes. (Time varies by size.) When the squash can be pierced easily with a knife, it's done. Scooping out the flesh and mashing makes a quick side or throw into a pot with sautéed onions, garlic, and vegetable stock, simmer, and purée for soup. Spaghetti squash strings when dragged with a fork, creating a pasta-like shape.

up to an assertive array of seasonings, including nutmeg, cardamom, ginger, rosemary, and thyme.

For Your Health

Winter squash, like many orange-fleshed vegetables, is a great source of health-supportive carotenoids, including alpha-carotene and beta-carotene. The soluble fiber in the flesh can help lower cholesterol. The seeds from any of the squashes can be toasted and consumed; pumpkin seeds are particularly rich in magnesium and heart- and brain-healthy omega-3 fatty acids; together, the two work together to stabilize blood sugar and blood pressure.

For Our Planet

Nothing says the arrival of autumn more than a colorful selection of winter squash. Particularly tasty when in season, a trip to the farmers market may be worthwhile, and eating the seeds reduces your food waste. And, armed with its own protective shell, winter squash can be shipped and stored without the need for excess packaging, great news from a petrochemical perspective.

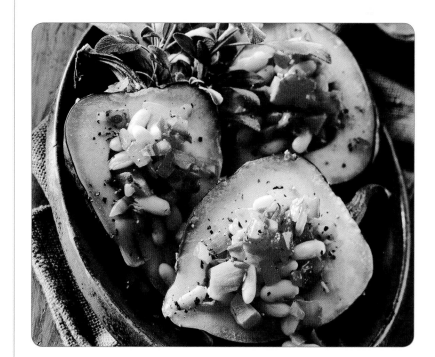

FRUITS

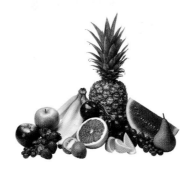

The peach and plum with their pits as hard as a nutshell, the kiwi with its ring of black specks in green flesh, the apple with shiny dark teardrops enclosed in a fibrous core—all fruits represent the ingenious strategy of a plant to disperse its seeds and perpetuate its kind. Birds and mammals eat the fruit and later sow the undigested seeds (complete with natural fertilizer) at some distant location by defecating on the ground.

Plants gain nothing when animals feed upon their roots, leaves, or stems—the parts we call vegetables. But the life cycle of many plants absolutely depends on this pas de deux between fruit and beast. Thus fruit has evolved over many millions of years to attract and please would-be seed dispersers. At just the right season for sowing, the fruit ripens, flashing brilliant color to contrast with surrounding foliage, and sending out a plume of fragrance.

For tens of millions of years, human ancestors have responded to this promise of a sweet, nutritious, and highly seasonal meal. Our closest living relatives, the great apes, prefer fruit. And the diets of many Paleolithic hunter-gatherers certainly included fruits.

Humans' preference for sweetness and accessible calories may be responsible for latter-day misadventures in the baked-goods aisle of the local supermarket. One researcher even suggests that alcoholism may have evolved from an ability to recognize and locate ripening fruit by the odorous ethanol it emits. But seeking out the fruit itself gave people of the Stone Age a survival advantage—and the same holds true today.

Relatively mobile hunter-gatherers suffered less malnutrition than the farming peoples who succeeded them, largely, scientists believe, because hunter-gatherers ate a variety of plant foods, while early agriculturalists relied on just a few foods.

Enjoy More Fruits

Today, the nutritional variety offered by whole, seasonal fruits remains every bit as important to good health. Scientists have observed, time and again, that people who routinely eat plenty of fruits and vegetables as part of a plant-based diet are less likely to develop heart disease, type 2 diabetes, and certain cancers—diseases that are largely preventable through diet.

In many contemporary societies, grocery stores offer nutritional variety. Gone are the days when residents of New York or London might lose their teeth from scurvy for lack of a vitamin C–rich fruit in wintertime. Indeed, modern consumers have access, year-round, to an unprecedented array of fruit, from tropical bananas to North Woods blueberries, including off-season produce grown locally in hothouses or warehouses. However, only a third of American adults consume the minimum two servings of fruit per day recommended by the U.S. Department of Agriculture.

The antidote, according to many nutritionists, is for each of us to adopt dietary changes that mesh with our lives, choosing fruits that are appealing, reasonably convenient, and affordable. You like canned peaches? Add some to warm breakfast cereal or toss them in a salad. Dried apricots? Munch them on your evening commute. If the high calories of dried fruit are an issue, pack an apple. Fresh strawberries are a pleasure, but frozen are lovely too, especially when fresh berries are out of season and shipped unripe from distant ports. Organic fruit give you sticker shock?

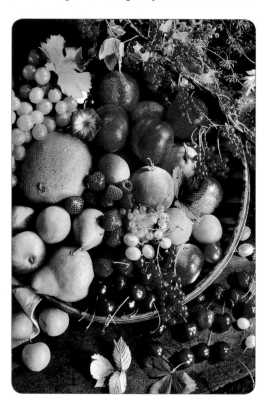

Buy it occasionally or when shopping for products that are particularly burdensome on the environment. Don't let anything limit your enjoyment of fruits and vegetables, which, even when conventionally grown and/or processed, are among the healthiest and most environmentally sound foods you can eat.

Eat a Variety of Fruits

Ironically, while Americans on average consume too little fruit, fads regularly surface that encourage people to binge on "super fruits" or identify the one element in, say, cranberries or pomegranates that imparts optimal health, which they then swallow in high-dose supplements. Again, variety is the key, and that includes all of the vitamins, minerals, fiber, and phytonutrients that, working together in the body, make a whole fruit good to eat. Consuming more of one particular component is not necessarily better, as science has shown.

It's fascinating to learn that colorful pigments in some fruits may help prevent vision loss, heart disease, and cancer, or that vitamin C helps arrest cell damage that results naturally when the body reacts with oxygen, a contributor to aging. But much of this evidence is produced in the laboratory, and individual plant components, when tested in human trials using supplements, have often proved disappointing. In short, although diets rich in fruits, vegetables, and beta-carotene can reduce the risk of heart disease and cancer, studies have shown that long-term use of beta-carotene supplements increases lung cancer risk for smokers.

Fruit isn't medicine, but something far more valuable. If we live by Hippocrates's words "Let food be thy medicine," food is

"Let food be thy medicine."
—Hippocrates

also something elemental. The way we produce, market, and consume fruit today affects human health in the broadest sense, by impacting our bodies, our natural environment, and our cultures, both globally and locally.

Local and Seasonal

Today's high crop yields and worldwide distribution bring to our tables a luxuriant supply of fruits that Americans a century ago might never have glimpsed, let alone eaten regularly. But this comes with a cost. Turning over vast tracts of land to a single crop—monoculture—often damages local ecosystems and increases susceptibility to pests, which increases the use of pesticides. Certain crops and intensive land use in general require more fertilizer. Manufacturing these chemicals produces the emissions that are warming our planet. Shipping all that fruit around the world by sea, air, and land—even trucking it from orchard to roadside stand—churns out even more greenhouse gases. Given economies of scale and different growing and transportation methods, it's not always the case that a local food has a smaller carbon footprint than does a food shipped from afar. And to keep prices down in a competitive international market, growers must hold down labor costs; farm workers are among the most impoverished in the world. Finally, uneaten fruit ends up in landfills, contributing to the release of methane, a greenhouse gas twenty-one times more potent than carbon dioxide.

All this tends to recommend an updated version of an old-fashioned way of life. Yet, it's not practical to eat only locally grown fruits. (Some 19th-century Bostonians did without fruit through the winter and got through on salt cod and beans—hardly desirable.) But it makes sense to be aware of which fruits grow locally and when they're in season. Pass up the flavorless midwinter cantaloupe from Central America for a New York apple or a California navel orange when in season; they'll taste far better. Supplement liberally with frozen and canned fruits (with no added sodium or sugar), often harvested and processed at peak nutritional value. Sure, processing increases the carbon footprint, but plant foods generally are far more eco-friendly than animal products. It's a balancing act. What's most appetizing, nutritious, affordable, and responsibly produced doesn't always come together in one satisfying bite. Then again, sometimes it does—when you find a basket of berries at the farmers market or roadside stand, fragrant and ripened on a stem not far away. Enjoy their sublime taste in good health.

APPLE

Today's cultivated apple—crisp, fleshy, and sweet—comes to us as a gift from the ancient human past. The apple tree with its gnarled limbs and blush-colored blossoms may be one of the first trees ever cultivated. The progenitor of today's commercial apples still grows in the forests of Kazakhstan in Central Asia. Centuries ago, traders carried its seeds along the Silk Road to Western Europe, the tree hybridizing with local wild varieties along the way. European colonists, in turn, brought their beloved apple varieties to the New World. Nurseryman Johnny Appleseed distributed seeds across the American Midwest.

Choose and Use

Though local apples bought soon after the autumn harvest may be especially tasty, apples store and ship well, holding their texture and nutritional value over months. Varieties with a hint of tartness, such as Jonathans, are often favored for baking, while a crunchy, sweet apple such as the newer Honeycrisp or Gala makes good eating. There are so many varieties available today outside of the supermarket, ask the farmers at your local green market for suggestions of new ones to try.

GIVES YOU

Vitamin C
Dietary fiber
Phytonutrients
(flavonoids,
phenolic acids)

CONSIDER ✦ APPLE SNACKS: CUT UP, PEEL ON

Cut and peeled apple wedges can be purchased at the store, but you'll reduce your packaging waste and get more flavor and nutrition by doing it yourself. Select a variety of colors and leave the peel on for a simple snack that kids love, best in autumn when apples are in season. For a protein and energy boost, serve with a nut butter like peanut, almond, or cashew.

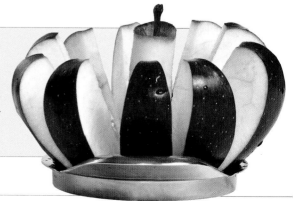

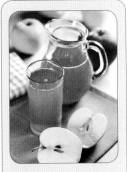

There's a downside to peeling: Antioxidants and fiber are concentrated in an apple's skin. Applesauce (homemade is best) retains much of the apple's nutritional value, and there's no reason to remove the skins, which add texture, nutrients, and color. Apple juice, on the other hand, is largely stripped of healthy phytochemicals and fiber found in the whole fruit.

✦ TAKE AWAY

Bite into a refreshing apple rich in flavor and antioxidants.

For Your Health

Apples are a major source of flavonoids and phenolic acids in the American diet. Together with vitamin C (an apple provides ten percent of the recommended daily allowance), these plant compounds make the apple a potent anti-oxidant package, helping the body resist cell damage that can result from natural metabolic processes involving oxygen and lead to cancer.

Will an apple a day really keep the doctor away? Population studies have indeed linked regular apple consumption to reduced risk of lung cancer, heart disease, asthma, and type 2 diabetes.

Apples are also especially high in pectin, a water-soluble fiber that turns to gel in the small intestine and takes up cholesterol and sugars, slowing their absorption into the bloodstream.

For Our Planet

Intensive pesticide use is the norm among conventional growers of the fruit, which is particularly vulnerable to bugs and disease. Washing and peeling helps but does not eliminate pesticide residues. In 2012, the nonprofit Environmental Working Group listed apples as the single most-contaminated produce item. That's one reason organic apples are among the top-selling organic products, accounting for about 6 percent of U.S. apple-growing acreage.

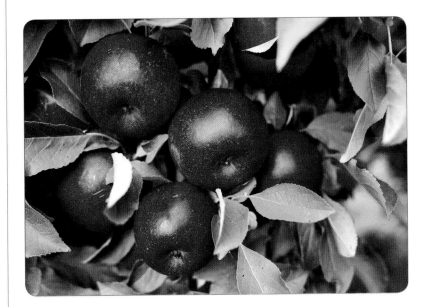

APRICOT

The apricot tree with its trim, tender-fleshed fruit is a close relative of the plum. It got its name, *Prunus armeniaca*, from the assumption among Europeans that it originated in Armenia. It has been cultivated there for at least two thousand years, but scientists believe it originated further east, perhaps in western China. The tradition of drying apricots goes back thousands of years in the area of the Fertile Crescent. Turkey and Iran are the world's biggest apricot growers today. Turkey is the largest exporter of dried apricots; the U.S. is its biggest customer. A tarter, less fleshy variety has entered the marketplace in recent years.

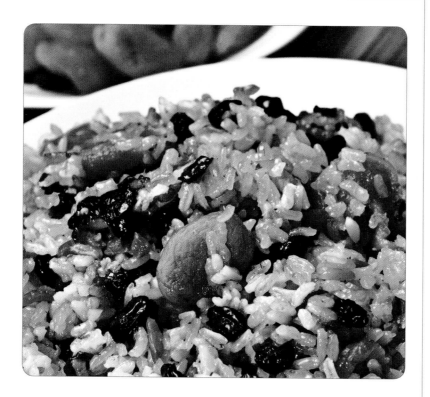

GIVES YOU

Phytonutrients
  (carotenoids)
Vitamin C
Vitamin E
Iron
Dietary fiber
Potassium

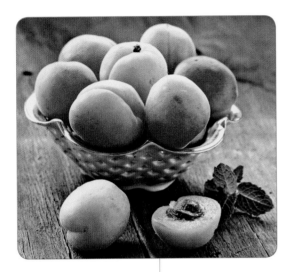

Choose and Use

Look to sweet scent, tender flesh, and sharp orange color in finding a good, ripe apricot during its May to July or August season. It will be excellent eaten raw as a dessert, or with nuts, cheeses, and whole-grain crackers. Dried apricots are often found in Middle Eastern stews featuring lamb or chicken or a whole grain pilaf such as rice or oats. Drying removes much of an apricot's vitamin C, but ounce for ounce, the dried fruit contains more iron, carotenoids, protein, and fiber than its fresh equivalent.

For Your Health

Ounce for ounce, a fresh apricot packs more ascorbic acid than a peach and provides roughly five times the carotenoids (including beta-carotene and lycopene), those orange, yellow, pink, and red pigments that, like ascorbic acid (vitamin C), act against cell damage from oxidation. This compact fruit also delivers twice the peach's fiber and potassium, one important in reducing cholesterol levels, the other a vital part of a diet to maintain healthy blood pressure.

For Our Planet

California is the source of most U.S. apricots, with roughly 40 percent of the crop going to processors for drying, freezing, canning, and juicing. The bulk of imports are Turkish dried apricots, with some fresh winter fruit coming from South America. California production on mostly small farms is in decline due to labor costs, less consumer demand for canned product, urban growth, and competition from cheaper imports.

✦ TAKE AWAY

Serve apricots as a stand-alone desert or as a tasty component in a wide range of dishes to experience this fruit's health benefits.

PAIRINGS ✦ **DRIED OR FRESH, PERFECT WITH CHEESE**

Sweet apricots are wonderful with cheese for a simple, French-inspired dessert. Choose dried in winter, which are loaded with even more vitamin A, and save the juicy, fresh version for when apricots are in season, at their best.

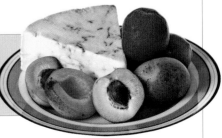

BANANA

The banana is native to Southeast Asia. The earliest evidence of banana cultivation dates to at least 6,500 years ago in the Western Highlands of Papua New Guinea. Portuguese sailors carried the first bananas to the Americas in the 16th century. After the U.S. Civil War came the rise of multinational banana companies growing the fruit in so-called banana republics of Central America. Cheap, conveniently packaged, and exotically sweet, the banana became America's most popular fruit by the 1920s.

Choose and Use

American groceries offer a single variety of banana—the robust, yellow-skinned Cavendish. Though less flavorful than some heirloom varieties, the Cavendish has come to dominate because of transport and storage concerns. Because bananas ripen naturally after picking, that's the factor to consider when choosing a bunch. Why does sealing them in a bag accelerate ripening? It traps in ethylene gas, a natural plant hormone produced by bananas that promotes ripening. Add hard peaches or pears to the bag, and the ethylene will ripen them too.

For Your Health

Scientists have found that a diet rich in potassium and low in sodium helps control blood pressure, a key risk factor for cardio-vascular disease. It's the ratio of these two minerals that matters, and, given that most Americans get way too much salt, a medium-sized banana offers an ideal balance: very little sodium, with 12 percent of an average adult's daily potassium needs. Bananas are generally higher in sugar than many fruits, but those that are not fully ripe are a source of resistant starch and release their energy into the bloodstream slowly, preventing blood-sugar spikes and crashes. Unlike most fruits, bananas are also a good source of

GIVES YOU

Potassium
Pyridoxine (vitamin B6)
Vitamin C
Dietary fiber
Magnesium

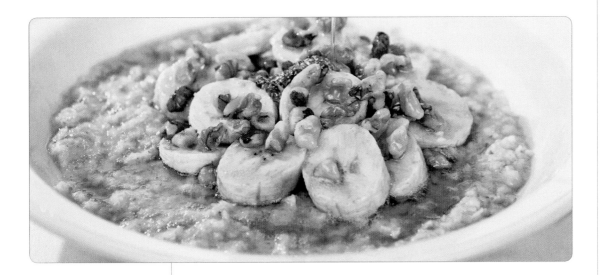

pyridoxine, a vital player in the breakdown of stored glucose and the synthesis of important chemical messengers in the brain.

For Our Planet

For decades the banana business was notorious for exploiting workers and replacing great swaths of Central American rainforest with chemical-intensive plantations—leading to erosion, flooding, and soil and water pollution. There have been improvements since the 1990s, with more than 15 percent of all bananas in international trade now certified by the nonprofit Rainforest Alliance as meeting environmental and social standards. Look for the green frog seal.

Banana monoculture is another problem. Growers' planting of a single variety of banana leaves plantations vulnerable to disease. Indeed a fungal wilt called Panama disease struck plantations in Southeast Asia during the 1990s, and there's great concern that it will sweep through Latin America and Africa as well, devastating international supply.

✦ TAKE AWAY

Add bananas to your diet for a sweet source of potassium and other vital minerals.

CONSIDER ✦ BABY BANANAS: PERFECT FOR KIDS

Baby bananas were once available only in places like Thailand. Often red but sometimes yellow, baby bananas are slowly making their way to America. About half the size of a regular banana, they're the perfect portion for kids.

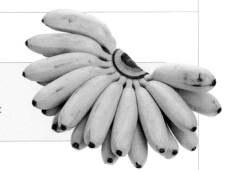

BLACKBERRY

Blackberries—a kind of bramble—grow wild in much of the Northern Hemisphere. Human foragers have likely plucked these purple berries from their thorny canes for millennia. Indeed it seems that no serious efforts at cultivating the berries were made until the 19th century.

Choose and Use

Blackberries should be plump and very nearly black; lighter red or blue berries are unripe. Though they are sturdier and less perishable than some other berries, to avoid spoilage they should not be washed until just before eating. Like dark foliage in a summer garden, blackberries add visual interest and intense flavor to a mixed-berry salad. Toss the berries with a light sprinkling of sugar and let them marinate, then add a small dollop of whipped cream and a sprig of mint for an elegant, healthful dessert.

For Your Health

These ink-dark, tart and seedy berries are an embarrassment of riches nutritionally. Endowed with multiple compounds thought to lower risk of cardiovascular disease, they boast the essential vitamins C, E, and folate as well as the purple pigments (anthocyanins) that are a type of flavonoid. One promising clinical trial testing the effects of berries themselves (as opposed to

GIVES YOU

Vitamin C
Vitamin K
Manganese
Dietary fiber
Vitamin E
Folate
Phytonutrients
  (flavonoids,
  phenolic acids)

PREP TIP ✦ THINK BEYOND SWEET

Like other berries, blackberries are often found in sweets but bring flair and elegance to a host of savory presentations. A handful of blackberries are terrific paired with citrus and fennel in an elegant dinner salad, or they can be combined with grains and herbs for a spa-like lunch. At the height of the season, try pickling blackberries in a simple brine to enjoy in colder months.

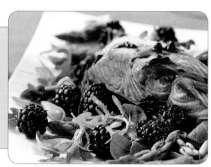

✦ TAKE AWAY

Enjoy this pleasantly tart berry full of essential vitamins.

supplements) found that, in 72 middle-aged subjects, eating a mixture of berries twice daily for two months lowered blood pressure, increased "good" HDL cholesterol, and slowed blood-platelet function (which can mean fewer blood clots).

For Our Planet

Oregon is the biggest blackberry-growing state in the U.S., with California second. Since blackberries grow well in many areas, local specimens may be available in the summer season. Off-season, the berries typically come from Mexico. Picking berries is hard, careful work performed mainly by migrant and seasonal workers, who may endure poor working conditions (including high pesticide exposure) and earn subpoverty wages.

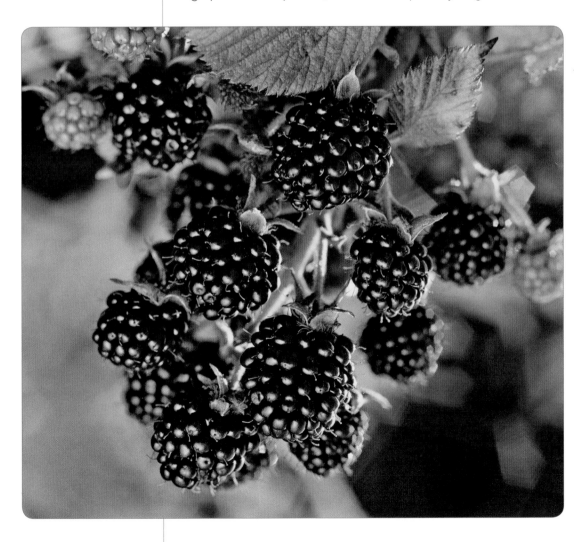

BLUEBERRY

This tender round berry of dusky hue is a native of North America. Indigenous peoples of the continent gathered it for food and medicinal uses.

It wasn't domesticated until the twentieth century, when a U.S. Department of Agriculture researcher, Frederick Colville, began the research that would lead to the "highbush" blueberry and its successful commercial cropping in 1908. The U.S. remains the fruit's biggest producer, with Maine the dominant grower of lowbush or "wild" blueberries and Michigan leading in the plump highbush type.

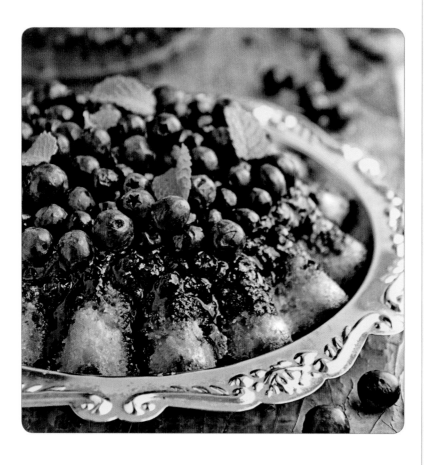

GIVES YOU

Vitamin C
Vitamin K
Manganese
Dietary fiber
Phytonutrients
(flavonoids,
resveratrol)

The indigo-colored juice from blueberries was once used as a textile dye. It's that same color that's responsible for many of the health properties of blueberries, perhaps why it's known as one of today's "superfoods." Loading up on a single food doesn't generally work when it comes to good nutrition, though: enjoy your blueberries along with other vegetables and fruits for the best health.

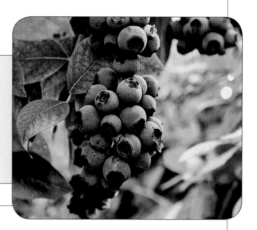

Choose and Use

Berries are ripe when wholly blue, not reddish; wrinkled skins suggest they're past their peak. Fresh, in-season berries taste best, but frozen are nearly as healthy, and even baked blueberries retain most of their nutritional value. Fresh berries keep in the fridge for up to two weeks; wash just before serving.

For Your Health

A cup of mild-flavored blueberries provides a quarter of the vitamin C you need in a day, and about the same proportion of the recommended intake of vitamin K and manganese, both of which are important for bone integrity. In addition, these berries boast a diverse mix of antioxidant phytonutrients linked with reduced risk factors for cardiovascular disease. They get their indigo color from a high concentration of anthocyanins, a type of flavonoid that, in laboratory experiments, has slowed the proliferation of cancer cells. Population research has also hinted that people who eat the most strawberries and blueberries experience slower cognitive decline as they age compared with those who consume few berries.

For Our Planet

The blueberry is native to North America. Many small farms grow and sell the berries locally or even invite customers to pick their own. Blueberries found in the supermarket will have been grown in the U.S. or in Canada during the summer months and in Chile or other South American countries from November through March. Interestingly, testing in 2013 by the nonprofit Environmental Working Group found that domestic blueberries had more pesticide residues than imports.

CONSIDER
✦
THE SAVORY SIDE OF BLUEBERRIES

The sweet, mild flavor of this beloved round berry make it a popular ingredient in baked goods like pies, muffins, and scones, but it's also a terrific addition to savory dishes, hot and cold. A salad including greens, nuts, herbs, and grains topped with fresh blueberries makes a nutrient-filled and satisfying supper on hot summer nights. Blueberries sautéed in oil with minced shallot and finished with balsamic vinegar will break down to create a zesty sauce for fish, chicken, or even tofu.

CANTALOUPE

This melon is so high in water that its pale orange flesh goes down like a refreshing drink on a summer's day. To produce the sumptuous fruit, vines need hot, sunny days, warm nights, and a long frost-free growing season. Such was the climate of ancient Persia, the cantaloupe's place of first cultivation some 5,000 years ago, and of Cantalupo, the Italian town where the fruit, planted in papal gardens in the 16th century, is said to have gotten its name.

Choose and Use

The sign of a good, ripe cantaloupe is its sweet fragrance. Look for a fruit that feels heavy for its size and is free of mushy spots. Go for U.S.-grown cantaloupes, available from late spring to early fall when in season, as these are generally tastier than the ones shipped from Mexico and Central America in winter. Because they grow in contact with the soil and have porous, netted rinds, cantaloupes are susceptible to hosting colonies of bacteria that can make you sick. Wash the outside thoroughly in hot water, and wipe it dry before cutting to avoid introducing bacteria inside the cantaloupe. Refrigerate cut melon to dis-courage bacterial growth.

GIVES YOU

Vitamin C
Vitamin A (carotenoids)
Potassium

PREP TIP ✦ KEEP WHOLE UNTIL USING

Tender cantaloupe is a summertime favorite and it's especially sweet when purchased in season. Once ripened on the countertop, however, it's best to store the melon in the refrigerator whole until ready to be used. Like other fruits and vegetables, pre-cutting fruit days before use will decrease its shelf life. And try snacking on frozen cubes, too, on a hot summer's day.

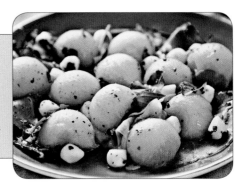

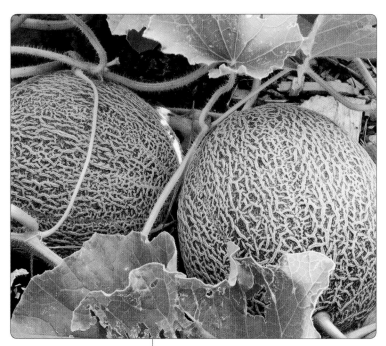

For Your Health

Due to its extremely high water content, cantaloupe is filling yet has vanishingly few calories. Plus, it's highly nutritious. It's full of vitamin C; a medium-sized wedge provides more than 40 percent of the recommended daily intake. And it's loaded with natural plant pigments called carotenoids, in particular, beta-carotene and alpha-carotene. These carotenoids have pro–vitamin A activity, meaning that the body can convert them to vitamin A; a wedge of melon helps provide nearly half the recommended daily supply of this essential vitamin. Though studies on the benefits of taking supplements have failed to show any benefit (indeed beta-carotene supplements boosted lung-cancer risk for smokers), population research shows that people who consume diets high in beta-carotene and other carotenoids are less likely to develop cardiovascular disease and certain cancers. It is also worth noting that, although honeydew melon shares many of the cantaloupe's nutritional benefits, its orange counterpart is much higher in beta-carotene.

For Our Planet

California is the biggest U.S. producer of cantaloupes, followed by Arizona and Texas. According to the Environmental Working Group's survey, cantaloupe flesh is low in pesticide residues, perhaps due to its thick rind. Varieties with lengthwise ridges and relatively little netting don't ship well but are delicious when available from local sources. Melon harvest is labor-intensive handwork often performed by low-paid seasonal and migrant workers.

✦ TAKE AWAY
Indulge multiple senses with this aromatic melon that is abundant in taste and nutrients yet low in calories.

CHERRY

The cherry as a cultivated food probably originated some 2,500 years ago in the area of present-day Greece or Turkey. With the rise of the Roman Empire and flourishing trade routes, the vivid, firm-fleshed fruit spread into the Mediterranean Basin and east through Asia. Early English and French settlers brought cherries to North America. Today, the U.S. is the world's second-largest producer of cherries, after Turkey.

Choose and Use

Sweet cherries like the plump red Bing are usually enjoyed fresh, while tart cherries such as the Montmorency are widely frozen and give intense flavor to traditional pies and jams. Both sweet and tart are available in dried forms. These are highly nutritious and a delight to the eyes and palate when sprinkled onto salads, savory rice dishes, and desserts. A small handful is also a healthy snack.

For Your Health

Sour cherries not only have a little more ascorbic acid than sweet cherries (a serving provides a quarter of the day's recommended consumption), they also are richer in carotenoids contained in red-yellow-orange pigments that can be converted to vitamin A in the body.

Both cherry types are rich in flavonoids like quercetin and the purple-tinting anthocyanins, thought to have anti-inflammatory

GIVES YOU

Vitamin C
Dietary fiber
Potassium
Phytonutrients
(flavonoids, phenolic acids, carotenoids)

PAIRINGS ✦ TRAIL MIX AND BEYOND

Dried fruit is a common addition to a trail mix. With its dark red hue, dried cherries add sweetness and color alongside a selection of mixed nuts and other fruits like raisins. Dried cherries are also wonderful in baked goods, and fresh or dried cherries pair especially well with dark chocolate when you want a little something sweet.

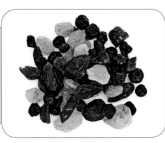

PREP TIP
✦
REHYDRATING DRIED CHERRIES

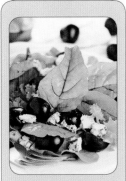

Dried cherries can be sweet or tart, depending on the variety. While often enjoyed out of hand as a snack, dried cherries also quickly rehydrate into a tender fruit if given a hot water bath. Or add them to porridge or pilaf and they'll rehydrate in the dish itself, adding sweetness and depth to the meal.

✦ TAKE AWAY

Satisfy an array of taste buds with cherries that range in flavor from sweet to tart.

properties. Small randomized, placebo-controlled human trials have found that regular consumption of tart cherry juice decreased blood markers for inflammation and lessened muscle pain after long-distance running. Another study suggests that consuming the fruit may reduce attacks of gout, a painful condition involving joint inflammation.

For Our Planet

These densely flavored summer fruits are a chance to go local, since few are imported off-season, and, when they are, they are quite expensive. Some orchards host pick-your-own events. The West Coast grows the great bulk of the sweet cherries available in the U.S., and Michigan produces the preponderance of tart cherries.

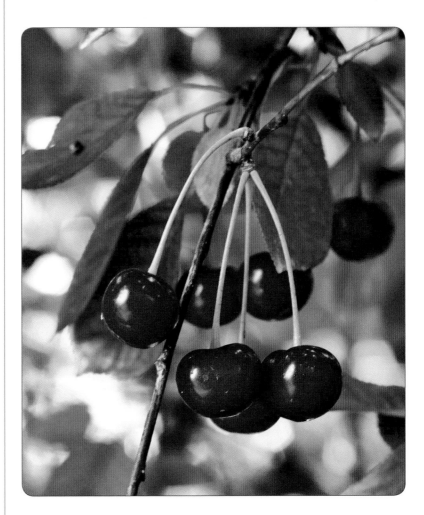

CRANBERRY

The Pilgrims likely did not savor cranberry sauce with their fowl during the first Thanksgiving dinner; for one thing, they had no sugar. But 19th-century founders of the holiday may be forgiven for not including cranberry, an authentic American fruit whose native range extends from North Carolina to Newfoundland. The tricky process of learning to cultivate the cranberry—it grows only in bogs layered with sand and organic matter—had been accomplished not long before Thanksgiving became a national holiday in 1863. It happened in 1816, when Revolutionary War veteran Captain Henry Hall first grew cranberries on Cape Cod.

Choose and Use

Fresh cranberries appear on shelves during their short autumn season, but the robust fruit holds up well to freezing. A versatile food suited to sweet and savory dishes alike, cranberries add a burst of color and flavor to relishes, chutneys, and compotes. They're great in pies and quick breads, and added fresh (or dried, although these are usually sugar-sweetened) to porridge.

For Your Health

Between traditional antioxidant nutrients, vitamin C, and manganese and a rich array of phytonutrients (some associated with

GIVES YOU

Vitamin C
Dietary fiber
Manganese
Vitamin E
Phytonutrients
(flavonoids, phenolic acids, resveratrol)

PREP TIP ✦ MAKE YOUR OWN SAUCE

Thanksgiving wouldn't be complete without tangy cranberry sauce. Store-bought brands of this sweet-tart sauce can be loaded in sugar or salt, though, and it's simple to make at home by boiling fresh cranberries with water, simmering, and sweetening with sugar, honey, or agave nectar. Adding orange zest or toasted walnuts is a nice variation.

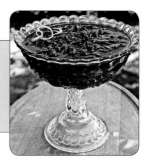

FOOD SCIENCE
✦
GOING WHOLE

More than bucolic, cranberries grown in bogs may also be healthier: there are more anthocyanins in cranberries at the water's surface due to their increased exposure to sunlight. A cranberry is more than the sum of its individual nutrients, though, and recent studies have found that consuming either juice or extract does not provide the same benefits as consuming the whole fruit.

the berry's brilliant color), cranberries have one of the highest antioxidant values of any fruit. Theoretically, at least, this could translate into protection against the "diseases of aging" associated with damage from free radicals, the volatile molecules produced as cells react with oxygen, and from the inflammation that results. Small human trials have hinted that consuming cranberry juice daily may affect risk factors for cardiovascular disease—reducing "bad" LDL cholesterol (oxidized) or increasing "good" HDL cholesterol, for example.

Cranberry juice has long been promoted as a remedy for urinary tract infections (UTIs). In the laboratory, the juice appears to prevent bacteria from sticking to the walls of the urinary tract. One 2012 systematic review of the evidence found that cranberry's effect on UTIs may not be as efficacious as originally thought, but more research is needed.

For Our Planet

Wisconsin produces more than half of the nation's cranberries, followed by Massachusetts. According to a survey by the University of Wisconsin, 98 percent of the state's cranberry producers are family owned. Most participate in recycling programs and test their soil and plants for nutrient needs to avoid overfertilizing, which would have a negative impact on the marine life found in the bogs.

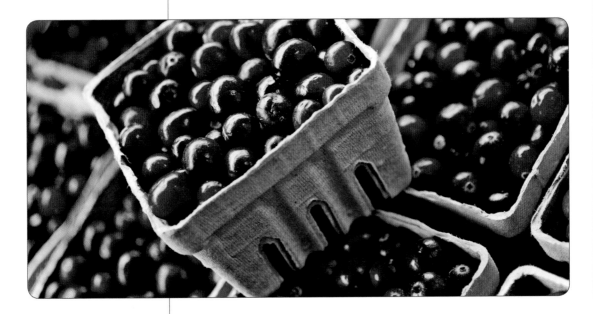

GRAPE

The fruit of the vine, first domesticated in the South Caucasus some 8,000 years ago, spread westward through the Middle East. From their earliest beginnings as a cultivated food, grapes have been fermented to make wine, a mainstay of the religious and daily lives of Ancient Israelites, Egyptians, Greeks, and Romans. "White" grapes evolved from red grapes by means of genetic mutations that switched off the grapes' ability to make anthocyanins, natural purplish pigments. Most but not all white wines are made with these light-colored grapes; the key difference lies in the fact that the white wines do not include the grape skin.

Choose and Use

Fresh grapes make a delightful finger food, especially if you partake of the many varieties available these days, from the popular Flame Seedless to the delicately flavored golden Muscat. Pair them with a hard cheese and whole grain crackers. Or take advantage of their high sugar content: Freeze them for a summertime dessert as tempting as an ice pop.

For Your Health

Americans dramatically upped their consumption of red wine in the early 1990s after researchers suggested the libation might explain why French people suffer relatively little cardiovascular disease despite their (relatively) high-fat diet. While red wine

GIVES YOU

Vitamin C
Vitamin K
Phytonutrients
  (flavonoids,
  resveratrol)
Dietary fiber

PREP TIP ✦ CHOKING HAZARD

Kids love the sweet taste of grapes, whether red or green, and they come in the perfect bite size package, easy for eating. But avoid giving them to toddlers whole: they are a choking hazard.

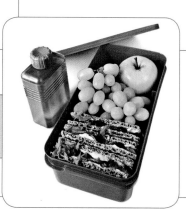

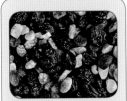

Fresh grapes are more than 80 percent water. Take away the water, and you've got a raisin. Although drying removes a significant amount of vitamin C, otherwise the raisin simply concentrates the grape's constituents—its antioxidants, sugars, calories, etc.—in a smaller, chewier package. Like other dried fruits, raisins are very slow to spoil and convenient to carry. Raisins and protein-rich nuts make the classic "trail mix," a lightweight, sweet and salty, high-energy snack. A little goes a long way.

✦ TAKE AWAY

Incorporate these nutritional fruits into another dish or eat them alone as a wholesome, juicy snack.

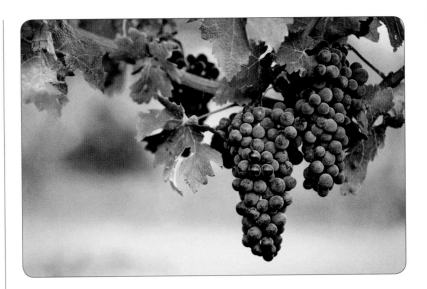

may be beneficial, animal studies have shown that the levels needed to evoke a protective effect are incredibly high, much greater than would normally be consumed as part of a diet including moderate alcohol consumption; the French Paradox probably has as much to do with such unglamorous factors as portion size and increased physical activity.

Still, in the laboratory, the flavonoids and resveratrol present in the skins of red grapes (and in red wine) have been found to combat inflammation, blood clotting, and oxidation of "bad" low-density lipoprotein (LDL) cholesterol—all factors in the buildup of fatty deposits in blood vessels. Research suggests purple grape juice confers similar benefits, helpful knowledge for those who don't consume alcohol. Grapes are also a great source of ascorbic acid, with a single cup providing a quarter of the recommended daily intake.

For Our Planet

Most fresh grapes you find in U.S. supermarkets hail from California, except in the off-season (January through April), when they're often shipped from Chile. Farmers markets are the best source for seasonal local grapes. Subject to rot, grapes are often liberally treated with fungicides and come in at number three on the Environmental Working Group's 2013 list of contaminated fruits and vegetables. Organic is a good way to go, if you can afford it. Always wash grapes before serving.

GRAPEFRUIT

Somewhere in the Caribbean islands, before the mid-18th century, the large, acid-green pomelo crossed with the Jamaican sweet orange. The result was grapefruit. In his 1750 *Natural History of Barbados*, the Rev. Griffith Hughes described it as "the forbidden fruit," and quite delicious.

In keeping with its status as a relative newcomer, the grapefruit is essentially an American fruit. In the 19th century, settlers planted grapefruit in Florida and, later, Texas, where it thrived as a commercial crop. The U.S. remains the largest producer and consumer of grapefruit worldwide.

Choose and Use

Look for a fruit that's heavy—bursting with juice—but not squishy, which may indicate it's overripe. Most grapefruits come from Florida or Texas, and their peak season is winter, roughly January through April. Peel and eat the bittersweet fruit like an orange for maximum fiber, slice it onto salads, or cut it in half along its equator and broil it with a little brown sugar and spices for a low-calorie dessert.

For Your Health

Sit down to a half a grapefruit in the morning, and you'll be spooning up 65 percent of the vitamin C you need for the day, but a mere 2 percent of the calories. (It makes a terrific dessert too.) Though vitamin C is much overrated as a cure for the common cold (high doses may slightly reduce symptoms), it is an antioxidant that's vital to tissue repair. The body neither makes nor stores it—excess amounts are flushed out in the urine—so it's important to get enough in your diet. Pink and red grapefruits provide much more of the pigments called carotenoids than do white grapefruit. Carotenoids are antioxidants and produce vitamin A in the body, required for normal vision, skin,

GIVES YOU

Vitamin C
Phytonutrients
   (carotenoids)
Dietary fiber
Potassium

Forbidden fruit seems an odd handle for such an apparently wholesome food, but grapefruit must indeed be considered off-limits by people taking any of more than 40 common medications. Natural compounds in the fruit, called furanocoumarins, interfere with liver and intestinal enzymes that break down drugs. This can lead to excessive blood levels of the medicine—drug toxicity—or block the drug from working. Drugs susceptible to this interaction include cholesterol-lowering, antianxiety, and some heart medications. Check with your doctor if you're not certain.

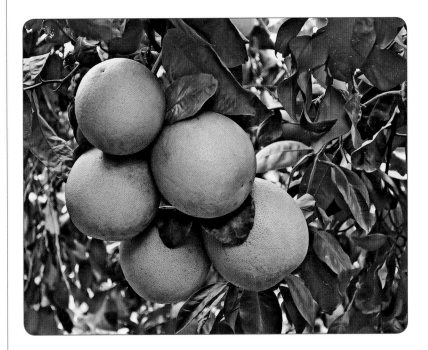

bones, and immune function. The flavonoid paringin found in white grapefruit has been linked to lower lung-cancer risk.

For Our Planet

Some of Florida's citrus groves are along the ecologically delicate Indian River Lagoon, which flanks 156 miles of Atlantic Coastline. Chemical-laden runoff can lead to smothering algae blooms, but government agencies, environmentalists, and growers are working to protect and restore the lagoon. The Environmental Working Group ranks grapefruit as one of the least pesticide-tainted fruits or veggies available, possibly due to its thick rind.

✦ TAKE AWAY

Quench your thirst and appetite with this nourishing fruit high in dietary fiber and restorative antioxidants.

KIWI

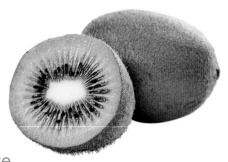

The kiwifruit is native to China's Yangtze valley. Chinese traditional medicine categorizes the "yang-tao" or "strawberry peach" as a "cooling" food that can balance digestion. But it remained exclusively wild-growing until about 300 years ago. New Zealand, which handily dominates production today, began cultivating the fruit in the twentieth century, naming it kiwi, or kiwifruit as a marketing effort in the 1960s. Before, it had been known as the Chinese gooseberry.

Choose and Use
Fresh fruit from California arrives October through May, with imports from New Zealand and Chile available April to November. Purchase kiwis that are firm but not hard; they will ripen (and sweeten) if left at room temperature for a few days. The Hayward variety that dominates U.S. groceries has a thin skin that can be eaten along with the succulent flesh for added nutrients and fiber.

GIVES YOU
Vitamin C
Vitamin K
Vitamin E
Potassium
Dietary fiber
Folate
Phytonutrients
   (flavonoids,
   carotenoids)

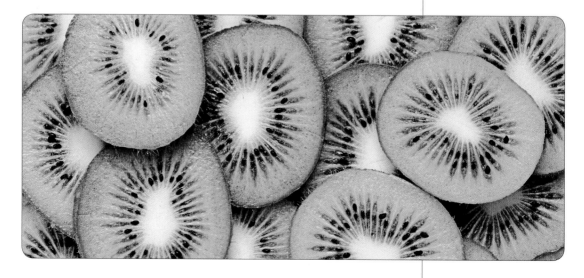

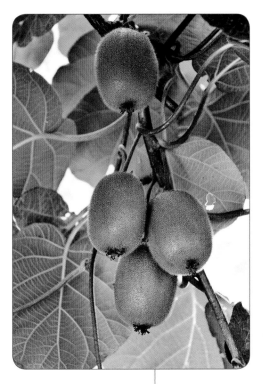

For Your Health

This strange little fruit of translucent green flesh dotted with tiny black seeds boasts a significantly higher density of vitamin C than an orange—along with significant amounts of potassium and vitamin E. All are considered important to healthy blood vessels. Kiwi also contains two carotenoids, lutein and zeaxanthin, linked to improvement of age-related macular degeneration, an eye disease affecting many older people.

In the lab, a kiwi extract proved better than an (vitamin C) solution at protecting DNA from oxidative damage, suggesting there are components beyond its ascorbic acid that make the kiwi a power fruit important in the prevention of cancer. (Of course, extracts tend to concentrate nutrients and provide much larger amounts than would ordinarily be consumed in a serving of the actual fruit.) Another study found that eating two or three kiwis per day for a month lowered plasma triglycerides (an undesirable fat found in the blood) and inhibited the clumping of blood platelets, both factors in cardiovascular diseases like atherosclerosis.

For Our Planet

Zespri, the world's largest marketer of kiwis from New Zealand and other countries, reports that shipping accounts for 35 percent of its total emissions. The company is taking steps to reduce greenhouse-gas emissions by maximizing use of space on vessels, using very large vessels, and shipping at slow, fuel-efficient speeds.

✦ **TAKE AWAY**

Throw an exotic twist into your daily diet with the kiwi's distinct texture and flavor.

PREP TIP ✦ EAT THE FUZZ

With their fuzzy exterior and speckled green interior, kiwis are a fun fruit for children. No need to peel the edible skin, either: teaching kids to eat the fuzz early on will help them learn to enjoy it and avoids unnecessary food waste.

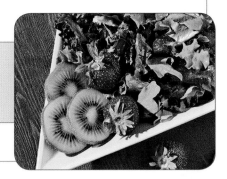

LEMON AND LIME

Lemons and limes are so closely linked in food culture that they seem almost like varieties of a single fruit. Both are small citrus fruits not often eaten alone but used to flavor and garnish a huge variety of dishes and drinks. Both grow in warm climates on glossy-leaved evergreen shrubs, though the lemon's birthplace is thought to be eastern India, while the lime originated in Indonesia. Both spread ultimately to the Middle East, the lemon appearing in Italy by around A.D. 200. By A.D. 1000 both fruits were taking root throughout the Mediterranean region; a half-century later, they arrived in the Americas with the explorer Christopher Columbus.

Choose and Use
Choose fruit that are heavy for their size, barely soft to pressure, and thin skinned with great aroma when gently scratched. Use lemons and limes in place of vinegars on salads and instead of salt for savory dishes such as chicken. Flavor water with a twist of lemon or lime for flair. The zest of these fruits is particularly aromatic and flavorful, an excellent addition to baked goods, salads, and seafood dishes. Vitamin C helps the body absorb iron, so squeeze some lemon or lime onto an iron-rich protein (such as beans) or dark greens (spinach, collards, kale).

GIVES YOU

Vitamin C
Phytonutrients
(limonoids)

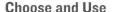

CONSIDER ✦ JUICING CITRUS

When a recipe calls for citrus juice, using fresh is worth the effort (and avoids packaging). Sometimes the fruit is particularly hard and doesn't feel juicy. Giving it a roll on your counter or popping it into the microwave for ten seconds will get the juices flowing.

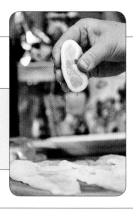

Vinaigrette is often made with oil and vinegar, as its name implies. But lemon or lime juice also makes a tasty salad dressing: a Greek dressing commonly uses lemon juice, for example, while a Mexican salad is perfect with lime.

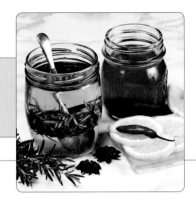

For Your Health

Laboratory studies have shown that limonoids, natural plant compounds found in citrus fruits, are toxic to certain types of cancer cells. But a more certain asset is this: A single ounce of lemon juice packs 20 percent of the day's recommended intake of vitamin C, and a scant 7 calories. That makes lemon (or lime) a great way to give food a satisfying dash without laying on the salt, sugars, and calories.

For Our Planet

Most of the lemons in U.S. grocery stores are grown in California or Arizona. By the end of the twentieth century, a bacterial disease called citrus canker helped dramatically shrink lime groves in Florida, once a major source. An outbreak that began in the 1990s has resulted in the burning of millions of citrus trees. Fortunately, this flavorful tangy green fruit is still readily available from Mexico.

✦ TAKE AWAY

Squeeze either of these citrus fruits into food or drink for a zesty flavor.

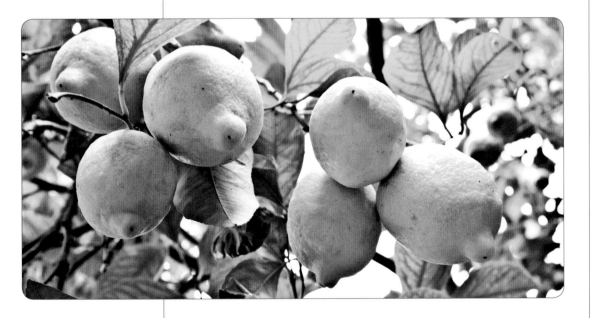

MANGO

Mangos have grown around the Sea of Bengal—in the area of present-day India, Bangladesh, and Myanmar (Burma)—for millions of years, though the first fruits were not nearly so large, sweet, and smooth-fleshed as today's mangoes, thanks to thousands of years of cultivation. The mango plays an important role in the cultural and religious traditions of its birthplace. The Buddha sought the refuge of a mango grove to meditate, and Buddhist monks are said to have carried the fruit east into Asia. Hindus hang garlands of bright green mango leaves in their homes to celebrate weddings and their autumn Festival of Lights, Diwali. It was in India that Portuguese colonialists first discovered the fruit in the 1500s, later carrying it to South America.

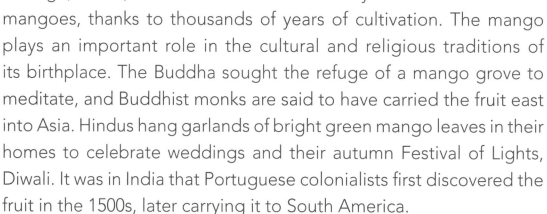

Choose and Use

Depending on the variety, a ripe mango may be yellow, green, or red. Choose a plump, slightly tender fruit that emits a sweet aroma at the stem. Mangoes add a velvety texture to fruit salads and a cool, mild flavor to the piquancy of many chutneys and salsas. Try this tropical fruit in a mango lassi, a traditional drink made of mango, yogurt, and milk popular in India and Pakistan, or combine it with chopped peppers and lime juice for a bright, summery fruit salsa.

GIVES YOU

Vitamin C
Pyridoxine
Vitamin E
Dietary fiber
Phytonutrients
  (carotenoids)

PREP TIP ✦ SNACKING ON MANGO, FRESH OR FROZEN

Mango's juicy, sweet flesh with its bright orange color is something most kids love. Carefully remove the peel with a sharp knife (it's bitter and inedible) and then cut into chunks for a healthy snack. Throwing long wedges into the freezer on a hot summer day is almost like stick-free ice pops.

Most people love salsa, and the most familiar version found in Mexican restaurants is chock full of chunky tomatoes, peppers, and onions. Many fresh fruits can also be made into salsas—no tomatoes needed—and make an excellent accompaniment to grilled fish, chicken, or tofu. Simply mix diced mango with a colorful red or green pepper and onions along with freshly squeezed lime juice and a bit of olive oil, and you're all set. Jalapenos are optional for heat!

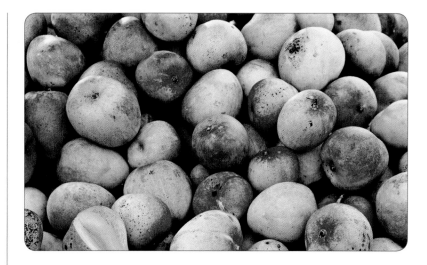

For Your Health

The rich, almost creamy orange flesh of a mango provides many of the same nutritional advantages as the similarly colored cantaloupe. Mango has a bit more calories but also more dietary fiber. Like cantaloupe it packs a hearty supply of vitamin C, required for tissue growth and repair, and carotenoids, which the body can convert to vitamin A, essential for healthy vision, especially in low light. Like cantaloupe, mango is also distinguished by the sheer variety of vitamins and minerals it contains in modest amounts—including folate and pyridoxine (vitamin B6), which help control blood levels of a key marker for heart disease (homocysteine); vitamin E, an antioxidant; and vitamin K, which helps the body use calcium to build bones.

For Our Planet

The U.S. is the world's leading importer of this tropical fruit. Most mangoes on U.S. shelves come from Mexico, Peru, Ecuador, and Brazil. A limited number are certified by the Rainforest Alliance or Fair Trade USA, which check that growers meet standards for treatment of workers and environmental stewardship. Testing in 2013 by the Environmental Working Group found mangoes to be low in pesticide residues.

✦ TAKE AWAY

Add vitamin- and fiber-rich mangos to your plate for a blend of savory flavors.

ORANGE

Beginning in the Renaissance, wealthy European families considered it most desirable to outfit their estates with an elegant, glass-enclosed greenhouse filled with orange trees—glossy-leaved evergreens that produce waxy, five-pointed white flowers and of course the coveted exotic fruit. The tree was a relative newcomer to the continent, having arrived with Portuguese sailors or perhaps Spanish traders before 1500. Christopher Columbus brought its seeds to the Caribbean in 1493. The orange's place of origin is Asia, probably China in particular, where it's been cultivated for millennia.

Choose and Use

Look for navel oranges in the winter months, choosing fruit that is neither hard nor spongy-soft. Simply peel and eat. So-called juice oranges, available late winter through fall, have a thinner skin and a few seeds, but their flesh is every bit as tasty. They are refreshing in seafood and poultry marinades, or joined in a sun-splashed salad with beets and spinach, good sources of iron. Mandarin oranges packed in their own juice make an easy, nutritious, and affordable alternative to keep handy on pantry shelves. The clementine, a variety of Mandarin orange

GIVES YOU

Vitamin K
Vitamin C
Folate
Dietary fiber
Manganese
Vitamin B6
Potassium
Phytonutrients
  (carotenoids,
  glucosinolates,
  phytosterols,
  flavonoids/phenolic
  acids, lignans)

PREP TIP ✦ KEEP IT WHOLE

It takes about a pound of oranges to make eight ounces of juice. You do get plenty of vitamins in that little drink, but you also get a lot more sugar and calories than you would in a whole orange—with almost none of the fiber. Juice is less satiating, and, like other sweet drinks (even those from naturally occurring, not added, sugars), OJ can raise your blood glucose and insulin sharply, a risk factor for type 2 diabetes and heart disease.

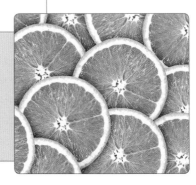

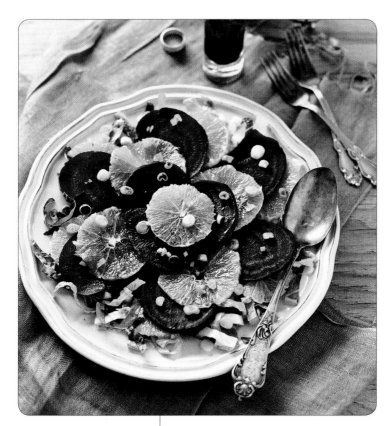

usually eaten fresh during its winter season, provides the same sweet, nutritious refreshment as its larger cousin in a natural snack-sized package.

For Your Health

Oranges and orange juice are a critical source of vitamin C in American diets, and it's not surprising—an extra-large orange provides more than the recommended daily intake, along with about 20 percent of an adult's daily fiber needs. A leading antioxidant, (vitamin C) may help the body ward off the cell damage that contributes to aging and disease.

Data from one large population study, published in 2010, showed that smokers who consumed more citrus fruits were less likely to develop the type of lung cancer most closely linked to smoking. In another population study, researchers found that women who consumed the most flavonones (a type of flavonoid) had almost 20 percent lower rates of clot-induced stroke compared with those who consumed the least amount of these phytonutrients. In the large American study, fully 82 percent of the flavonones consumed came from oranges and orange juice.

For Our Planet

Most of the fresh oranges available in supermarkets come not from the Sunshine State, but from California. Though Florida dominates orange production in the U.S., its fruit is mostly processed into juice—and that's how Americans consume the bulk of their oranges. Often "not from concentrate" juice mixes domestic juice with product imported from Brazil. Processing, long-term storage, and packaging also add to the carbon footprint.

✦ TAKE AWAY

Peel back an orange's dimpled skin to taste its sweet, fibrous flesh, highly nutritious in its raw form.

PAPAYA

The papaya "tree"—actually a large, shrub-like herb—is a tropical plant to the Americas. From somewhere in the region of southern Mexico it spread throughout Central America, into the Caribbean, and, in the 16th century, to India, landing in Europe in the 17th century. Today the major papaya-growing countries are India, Brazil, Indonesia, Nigeria, and Mexico.

Choose and Use

Papayas are yellow and sweet smelling when ripe but can be purchased green and allowed to ripen at room temperature. Slice the fruit lengthwise, scoop out its black seeds, and use it as a bowl for fruit salads or in a spicy fruit salsa. Roast it like butternut squash or grill it like a pepper for an interesting side dish. Add shredded green papaya to marinades to tenderize meat or poultry.

For Your Health

Rich and dense as this opulent fruit may seem, half a large papaya—an ample serving—has fewer calories than an apple or pear. It packs a one-two punch of vitamin C and carotenoids, which are supplied in part by the orange and yellow pigments and which the body converts to vitamin A. A diet high in these pigments has been associated with reduced risk of cardiovascular disease and some cancers.

GIVES YOU

Vitamin C
Folate
Vitamin E
Potassium
Dietary fiber
Phytonutrients
    (carotenoids,
    flavonoids)

PREP TIP ✦ CUT OR SCOOP

It's simple to cut a ripe papaya in half lengthwise with a sharp knife. (When working with harder green papaya be sure to hold the fruit firmly.) A large spoon will easily remove the seeds. Using a melon baller to remove circular chunks means you don't have to peel it!

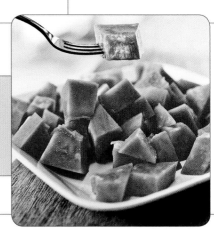

PAIRINGS ✦ ASIAN SALAD

Indigenous to many Asian countries, papaya is often used in flavorful Pan-Asian cooking. The less-familiar green papaya, an unripened version of the familiar orange-fleshed fruit, is often used in Thai salads when combined with red or yellow peppers, onions, sprouts, and chopped peanuts; a traditional dressing including fish sauce, lime juice, garlic, and a bit of sugar completes this colorful dish.

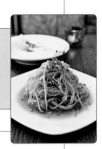

Ounce for ounce, the fruit has more than half the potassium of a banana, a key component of the low-sodium, high-fiber diet recommended to control blood pressure. Papaya also is the source of papain, a digestive enzyme used commercially as a meat tenderizer that may have pain-killing and anti-inflammatory effects, although studies looking at its use as a supplement have not uncovered definite benefits.

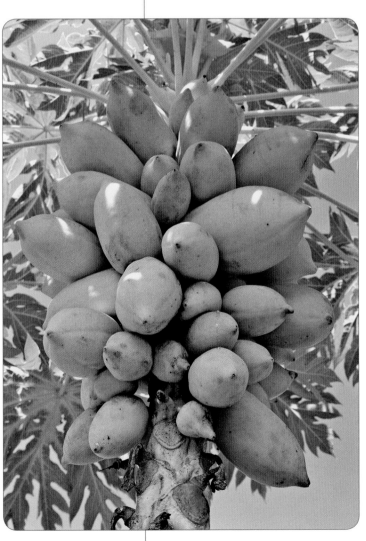

For Our Planet

Though Hawaii once was an important papaya producer, American grocers now get most of their papaya as fresh fruit from Mexico and Belize. Since a major outbreak of papaya ringspot virus in the 1990s devastated the Hawaiian papaya industry, growers there have bounced back by planting a variety genetically modified to resist the virus, thought to have saved the Hawaiian papaya industry. Hawaii's major buyer, Japan, approved the GM papaya after extensive safety testing. Few of these "Rainbow" and "SunUp" papayas are sold in the continental U.S.

PEACH

The ancient Chinese began cultivating their native peach tree some 4,000 years ago, nurturing a tradition that prizes both the wood and the fruit as symbols of long life and good fortune. Testament to the peach's continued popularity in China, the country still produces about a third of the world's peaches, mostly on small farms, and consumes nearly all of them domestically.

The Silk Road carried the peach west to Persia (present-day Iran) and into the Mediterranean region. In the 16th century, European explorers brought the peach to America—perhaps Florida—where it naturalized extensively and was cultivated and eaten by Native Americans.

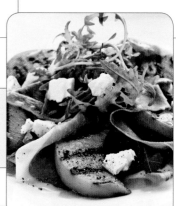

Choose and Use

A ripe peach may sport more or less blushing pink color depending on the variety. (There are also white peaches, as well as aptly named donut peaches.) But it won't be green, and it will give off a nectar-sweet aroma. A classic ingredient in desserts from cobbler to sorbet, peaches also make a fine poultry glaze or base for herbaceous salads using mint, cilantro, or ginger. Grilling or roasting peaches makes a terrific dessert, especially on an outdoor grill in the heart of summer. Canned (in juice), frozen, and dried peaches retain much of their nutritional value and are convenient, affordable alternatives to fresh.

CONSIDER ✦ FRESH, FROZEN, OR CANNED?

While nothing beats a juicy, fresh peach when in season, frozen and canned are fine alternatives to keep on hand. They are just as nutritious as fresh—as long as you choose brands with no added sugar or sodium—and make a great dessert or snack.

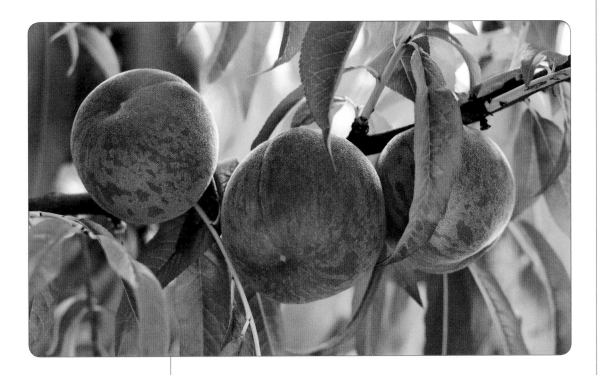

GIVES YOU

Vitamin C
Niacin (vitamin B3)
Dietary fiber
Potassium
Phytonutrients
(carotenoids)

✦ TAKE AWAY

Velvety, succulent peaches add color and flavor to many recipes, both savory and sweet.

For Your Health

Though not as packed with vitamins A and C as, say, papayas or cantaloupe, yellow peaches are a good source of both these essential vitamins. A large peach also contains about 10 percent of a day's recommended intake of potassium, which balances the sodium in your body, helping to maintain healthy fluid balance and blood pressure. Peaches are also one of the few fruits to contain a significant amount of niacin, a water-soluble vitamin that the body neither makes nor stores but which it needs to convert carbohydrates into glucose it can use as fuel.

For Our Planet

California supplies roughly half the country's fresh peaches, but this summer fruit grows in 28 states. This offers a great opportunity to go easy on the environment—and enjoy full-flavored, peak-season, tree-ripened peaches—by buying locally. In-season peaches sold not far from the orchard will taste delicious, and your dollars will be supporting local businesses and farmers. If it's a practical option, buying organic peaches is also an excellent way to support organic farming. In the Environmental Working Group's 2013 testing, peaches ranked fifth among fruits in pesticide residues.

PEAR

Pears appear to have grown wild in much of Europe and Asia for millennia, giving rise to two basic types: the European pear (Bosc, D'Anjou, Bartlett) common in American grocery stores, and the Asian pear, which is round and crisp like an apple. Both have ancient roots in the human diet. Burned remains of European pear have been discovered in Neolithic sites in Switzerland and elsewhere. The ancient Greeks and Romans cultivated pears; the fruit is mentioned with apples, figs, grapes, and other fruits in Homer's *Odyssey*.

Choose and Use

Pears are in season in fall and winter. A slightly yielding neck indicates ripeness. Pair them with apples and a tangy cheese, slice them onto a peanut butter sandwich, toss them into salads, or poach them with white wine, balsamic vinegar, and water, or red wine with a cinnamon stick and cloves. No need to remove the peel, which is full of fiber and phytonutrients and highly palatable. Eating the skins will reduce your food waste too.

For Your Health

A pear, though smooth as silk, provides more fiber than an apple, orange, or banana. Plenty of fiber helps prevent constipation, reduce "bad" LDL cholesterol, and regulate blood sugar (glucose). Pears are especially rich in phytonutrients. In 2012 data on more than 12,000 cases of diabetes among pooled populations from three separate studies showed that consuming large quantities of certain flavonoids called anthocyanins—and specifically a combination of apples and pears—reduced risk for type 2 diabetes.

A subclass of phenolic acids called cinnamic acids, abundant in pears, may have some activity against gastric cancer. A Mexico City study examined 257 cases of the cancer compared

GIVES YOU

Dietary fiber
Vitamin C
Phytonutrients
(flavonoids,
phenolic acids)

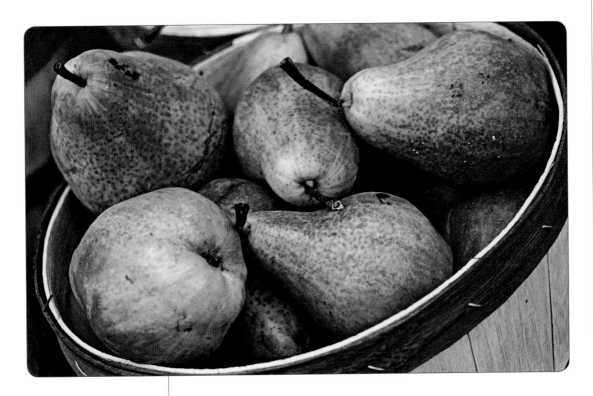

Complete your dish with slices of juicy pear, known for its flowery aroma and phytonutrients.

with age- and gender-matched healthy controls, and found that high intake of cinnamic acids reduced risk. The biggest dietary sources of these phytonutrients in the study were pears, mangoes, and beans.

For Our Planet

Most U.S. pears come from the West Coast states, with imports from Argentina and Chile available off season, from late winter to early summer. New York was once the leading pear-growing state, but a disease called fire blight that thrives in moist conditions, along with cold winters, led to the decline of East Coast commercial pear cultivation by around 1900.

PAIRINGS ✦ PEARS WITH BLUE CHEESE AND WALNUTS

A fall favorite, a gorgeous red pear is reminiscent of autumn leaves. Pears are classically paired with blue cheese and walnuts. Whether part of a cheese tray or tossed with your favorite lettuce for an elegant salad, keep the peel for color and fiber.

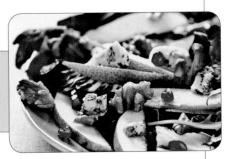

PINEAPPLE

In 1493, Christopher Columbus encountered pineapple on the island of Guadeloupe, becoming the first European to sample the strange, sweet-and-sour, prickly-skinned thing natives of the Caribbean called the "excellent fruit." Later, American colonists thought it excellent, too. Rare, expensive, and exotically sweet before the widespread availability of sugar, the pineapple became the ultimate dinner-party offering and a symbol of hospitality. In recent decades, fresh pineapple consumption has again shot up in America, partly on the strength of a new, super-sweet variety known as the MD2.

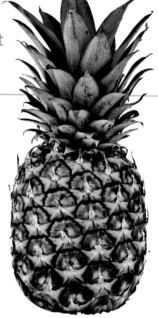

Choose and Use

Pineapples do not ripen after picking, so choose one that's ready to enjoy: a sweet-smelling fruit that weighs heavy in the hand. For much of the twentieth century, Americans ate a lot more canned pineapple than fresh, but fresh pineapples have become increasingly popular since the 1990s; they're more work to prepare, but typically deliver superior flavor and more vitamin C.

For Your Health

The pineapple is a bromeliad, but like a citrus fruit it's very acidic and has plenty of vitamin C—nearly as much as an orange. Unlike citrus fruits, though, a serving of pineapple contains three quarters of the recommended daily consumption of manganese, a mineral studied for its possible role in slowing bone loss in post-menopausal women and easing symptoms of premenstrual syndrome. Pineapple is the only food to contain a group of protein-digesting enzymes called bromelain, used in supplement form by Europeans to reduce inflammation after sinus and other surgeries. Natives of South and Central America used the fruit itself as a poultice to treat wounds.

GIVES YOU

Vitamin C
Manganese
Thiamin (vitamin B1)
Vitamin B6
Dietary fiber
Bromelain

CONSIDER
✦
IN PRAISE OF FROZEN

In the U.S., a local
pineapple is hard
to come by. So why
not buy frozen?
The fruit is picked
ripe and processed
soon after harvest,
locking in sweetness
and nutrients for
the journey to
your freezer. Or
use the thawed,
unsweetened chunks
in salad, as an accent
for savory seafood
dishes, or in an Asian
stir-fry.

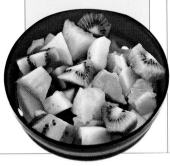

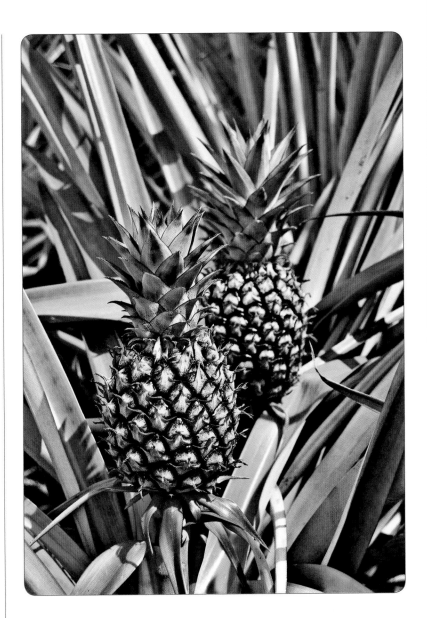

For Our Planet
Costa Rica is the largest exporter of pineapples to the U.S. and
Europe, having taken over the role from Hawaii toward the end
of the twentieth century. The product, perhaps thanks to its
tough skin, is relatively free of pesticide residues, according to
the Environmental Working Group. But environmental and labor
groups have complained that Costa Ricans face harsh working conditions and contamination of local soil and water from
pineapple-field runoff.

PLUM

There are many varieties of the plum tree, which are sprinkled with white blossoms in spring, followed by purplish, pitted fruit. More than two thousand years ago the ancient Chinese domesticated *Prunus salicina*, which came to be called Japanese plum after widespread cultivation there. The smaller and more oval-shaped European plum has its origins in the Caucasus. North America has its own wild plums, but Americans today generally eat Japanese plums.

Choose and Use

Look for a fruity aroma, deep color with a whitish blush, an unwrinkled skin, and slight give in the flesh. Though plums ripen after picking, if harvested too early they will remain sour. Eat them raw or stew them a few minutes with a little sugar and water for an intensely colored topping to pancakes, oatmeal, ice cream, or yogurt.

For Your Health

A juicy plum is a decent source of essential vitamins C and A as well as dietary fiber. But it's the diminutive fruit's ample supply of phytonutrients—plant compounds called phenolic acids and pigments known as flavonoids—that shoot plums up the charts when it comes to antioxidant power, at least as measured in the lab. Plums are particularly rich in a reddish-purple pigment

GIVES YOU

Vitamin C
Dietary fiber
Vitamin A
Vitamin K
Phytonutrients
(flavonoids,
phenolic acids)

PREP TIP + ENJOY THE VARIETY

You might not know it from the supermarket, but plums come in many colors and sizes. In addition to the common purple and red, there are almost-black, small Italian plums (used to make prunes) and you might also find green plums at your local farm stand.

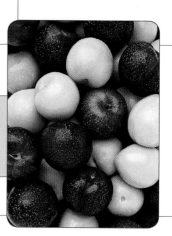

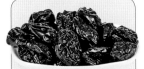
class called anthocyanins. Though cause and effect remain unclear, research suggests that people who eat lots of produce vividly colored with these pigments have a lower risk of cardio-vascular disease and cancer.

For Our Planet

Because plums are inexpensive and grow in many regions, they're a good fruit to purchase locally, in season, cutting down on the environmental costs of transportation. Domestic plums, mostly from California, are available June through December. Or you may be able to find them in season at a neighborhood farmers' market. In the off-season, most supermarket plums come from Chile.

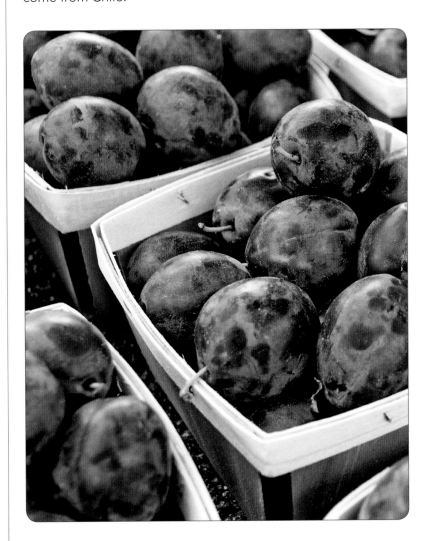

POMEGRANATE

Probably domesticated some 5,000 years ago in the area of present-day Iran, the pomegranate with its seeds like polished rubies spread west to Greece and along the Silk Road to China. It had an important place in ancient civilizations. In Greek mythology, Persephone, daughter of Zeus and the harvest goddess Demeter, ate four seeds of a pomegranate in the underworld. As a result she was forced to spend four months of each year there—the winter months when plants go dormant. Many of the world's religions hold it is an important symbol, and it's thought that the original tree fruit in the Garden of Eden was pomegranate, not apple, since the timing is otherwise anachronistic. In twenty-first-century America, U.S. consumers are now embracing the pomegranate as a potent antioxidant.

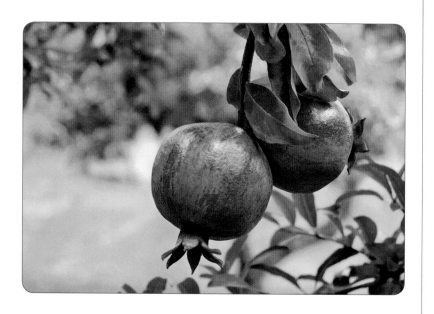

GIVES YOU

Vitamin C
Vitamin K
Folate
Potassium
Dietary fiber
Phytonutrients
    (ellagitannins,
    flavonoids)

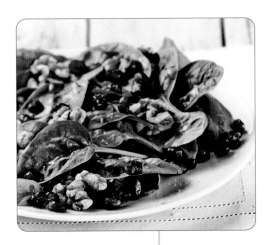

Choose and Use

Look for a fruit that's heavy for its size and has a rich red or reddish-brown color. Try it in Middle Eastern and Greek-style salads and savory dishes featuring couscous, quinoa, lamb, chicken, feta cheese, or mint. It also makes a tasty, nutritious snack all on its own.

For Your Health

Drinking pomegranate juice may reduce risk factors for cardiovascular disease and, in men with prostate cancer, slow increases in prostate-specific antigen levels, a marker for the disease. Scientists believe this may be attributable to the fruit's unusually high level of ellagitannins, phytonutrients with strong antioxidative effects. Pomegranates are also rich in flavonoids, including anthocyanins, which may reduce risk for cardiovascular disease. But so far research has been limited to the laboratory (looking at cultured cells and mice, for example) and small-scale human trials. The fruit itself has some advantages over juice. One pomegranate provides around half the vitamin C and dietary fiber you'll need in a day. Pomegranate juice, on the other hand, has no (vitamin C), very little fiber—and 50 percent more calories than orange juice.

For Our Planet

Most fresh pomegranates on U.S. shelves are grown in California and are in season from September through February. In warm-weather months the fruit is likely to have traveled far, including from India, which processes and packages the seeds (or arils) for sale in U.S. grocery stores.

✦ TAKE AWAY

Slice into a nutrient-packed pomegranate to discover a cache of ruby red seeds, ideal for salads or snacks.

PREP TIP ✦ **CLEANING THE JEWELED FRUIT**

Pomegranates are a little like crabs; it's not easy to get at the good bits. Cut the pomegranate in half around its equator. Hold one half of the fruit, cut side down in your hand over a bowl. Use the back of a spoon to lightly beat the skin and watch as the seeds fall out, perfectly clean of pith. Continue until all the seeds have been knocked loose. It's probably best to wear an apron for this task.

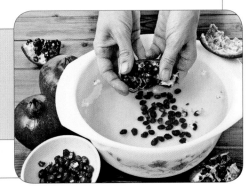

RASPBERRY

The Latin name for this delicate fruit, *Rubus idaeus*, comes from the Latin *ruber*, for red, and Mount Ida, near the ancient city of Troy in present-day Turkey, where the fruit may have originated. In fact the hardy plants are native to temperate zones throughout Europe, Asia, and North America, springing up in the semishade of forest floors and thriving especially in clearings. The ancient Romans spread the berry across their empire. Native Americans ate their own native raspberries and used the leaves as an astringent and to soothe diarrhea.

Choose and Use

In season during the summer months, raspberries have a sweet-tart flavor and layered texture that make them a wonderful base for salad dressings, jams, cobblers, and all kinds of baked goods. Try them with dark chocolate for an antioxidant-rich dessert. Toss them with summer greens, a mild, creamy goat cheese, and toasted walnuts or pecans for a tasty salad, or add them to a savory herbed whole grain pilaf or wild rice salad. Buy raspberries shortly before eating as they spoil quickly, and wash just before serving to preserve shelf life.

For Your Health

Raspberries are among the amplest sources of anthocyanins, the flavonoids that give them a crimson hue. Population studies have linked high consumption of these phytonutrients with lower risk of cardiovascular disease and cancer. In the lab, scientists have shown that ellagic acid (a product of ellagitannins) thwarts inflammation and the growth of cancer cells. The berries are also very high in manganese, a mineral important to maintaining strong bones, and fiber, which helps lower cholesterol and regulate bowel function. In fact, raspberries have more than twice the fiber of strawberries.

GIVES YOU

Vitamin C
Vitamin E
Vitamin K
Dietary fiber
Manganese
Magnesium
Phytonutrients
(flavonoids,
ellagitannins)

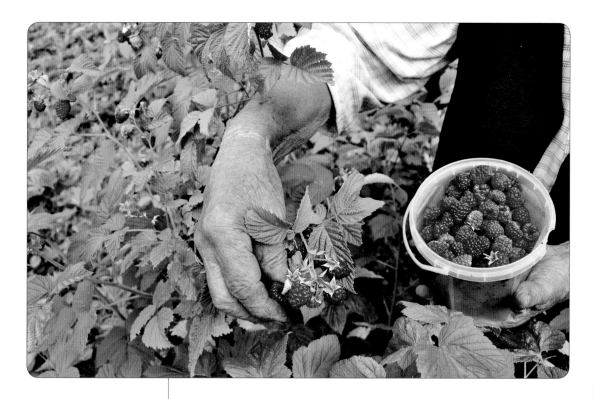

✦ TAKE AWAY

Snack on these brightly colored, vitamin-rich fruits or incorporate them as a tasty ingredient in a favorite dish.

For Our Planet

Though Washington, Oregon, and California are the major raspberry-growing states (supplemented by imports from Canada in summer and Mexico off season), the berries lend themselves to cultivation on small farms across the country. Fresh, local berries are generally the tastiest and most eco-friendly; look for them in season at farmers markets, roadside stands, or pick-your-own operations on nearby farms. Plucking these fragile berries from thorny canes is a highly labor-intensive process—one reason why raspberries tend to be expensive. Frozen raspberries are a practical, affordable, and nutritious option.

PREP TIP ✦ STORING

Many people wash fruit and vegetables right after food shopping so they're ready to go. Unfortunately, this step decreases shelf life. Berries in particular are highly perishable, so it's best to store them unwashed in a covered container then rinse gently in cold water right before consuming.

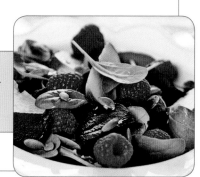

STRAWBERRY

Like so many fruits, today's familiar garden strawberry is a product of the Age of Exploration. It is a cross between two American wild strawberries—a small, flavorful one from eastern North America, and a larger though less tasty berry native to Chile—that took place in 18th century France, after Europeans carried the two American varieties home. In the last century, horticulturalists have bred garden-strawberry hybrids for size and durability in transit. Local berries commonly seen at farmers markets are often smaller, sweeter, darker, and more easily bruised than the larger, pink variety you commonly see in the supermarket.

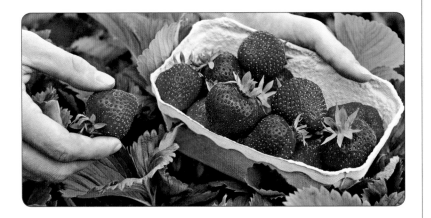

GIVES YOU

Vitamin C
Folate
Manganese
Dietary fiber
Phytonutrients
    (flavonoids,
    ellagitannins)

PAIRINGS ✦ HEALTHY ELEGANCE

Chocolate-covered strawberries are commonly served at weddings or garden parties, a sumptuous treat everyone loves. Easy to make at home—just dip the washed berries in a bowl of melted dark chocolate and set in the fridge—this is actually one the healthiest desserts out there.

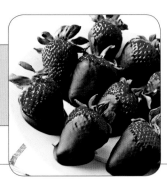

Strawberries are vulnerable to a variety of pests—and conventional growers combat them with an armamentarium of chemicals that are toxic to the environment and farmworkers. Fumigants that sterilize soil before planting have been particularly controversial. Long the fumigant of choice, methyl bromide is being phased out because it depletes the Earth's ozone layer. A proposed alternative, methyl iodide, was withdrawn from the U.S. market in 2012 after widespread alarm over its health risks to farm workers and consumers. For all of these reasons, selecting organic strawberries is better for the planet and for people.

Choose and Use

Look for deep and even coloration and a texture that is yielding to slight pressure. Berries should be red, not green- or white-tipped; they are nonclimacteric and will not ripen after picking. Smell is a false indicator of quality in strawberries. New varieties from California and Florida have been hybridized to be alluringly pungent, but they are barren of flavor. A dash of pepper or sprinkling of fresh basil can bring out the berries' sweetness in savory salads. Squeeze a little lemon or orange juice over berries that need a flavor lift. They're wonderful chopped in a homemade muesli with uncooked oats, other dried and fresh fruits, nuts, yogurt, and milk (cow's, soy, coconut, rice, or almond all work well).

For Your Health

Like raspberries, strawberries contain a plethora of natural plant compounds—including deep red colorants called anthocyanins (a type of flavonoid) and ellagitannins—that may have protective effects against heart disease and cancer. What's more, ounce for ounce, strawberries just about match up with oranges in vitamin C, a powerful antioxidant that's vital for tissue repair.

Several observational studies have linked high strawberry intake with lower risk for cardiovascular disease or death from cardiovascular disease, with one study showing that women who ate the most berries lowered their chance of heart attack by almost a third.

For Our Planet

Available year-round, strawberries are shipped mainly from California, Oregon, or, in winter, Florida. A few imports hail from Mexico. This is a good fruit to purchase in season, locally. Stem-ripened berries from your local market are far more flavorful than varieties bred to withstand long-distance shipment. You'll taste the difference.

PROTEINS

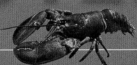

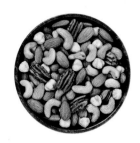

After water, protein is the most prevalent constituent of the human body. It is an important structural element of every cell, and the major component of muscles, eyes, skin, hair, and bone. Proteins also perform myriad jobs in the body. They act as antibodies, fighting off infection; enzymes, which speed chemical reactions; hormones, the body's chemical messengers; and transport devices that, for example, carry oxygen through the bloodstream.

Proteins are made up of 20 amino acids in different combinations. The body constantly breaks down its proteins into their constituent amino acids and "recycles" them into new proteins. We also replenish our supply of amino acids from the protein we eat in food. In fact, the body cannot make nine of the amino acids that form proteins, so these amino acids are only available through diet.

Like the other two macronutrients, carbohydrates (sugars) and fats, protein in the diet provides energy (or calories) that fuels the body. Fat is the most concentrated source of energy at approximately nine calories per gram; protein and carbohydrates each contain four calories per gram.

Fuel for Life

But the body uses these energy forms in very different ways. It draws immediately on carbohydrates, which break down in the digestive tract and enter the bloodstream as glucose. After this supply of carbohydrates is exhausted, the body can switch metabolic pathways, breaking down and burning stored fat instead. Only after both these energy stores are depleted does the body begin to break down stored protein, much of it found in muscles, and convert it to the body's major fuel source—glucose. While an adaptive response to provide the body energy, this may result in wasting and, ultimately, death if energy intake continues to be inadequate. On the other hand, when the body gets more dietary protein than it needs, along with ample calories, it will convert the excess protein to body fat.

The old-fashioned advice to build a strong body by eating plenty of protein-rich food is not altogether wrong. Everyone needs to consume protein, not so much for its calories but for the raw amino acids needed for growth, maintenance, and repair throughout the body. However, most Americans consume more protein than necessary: Americans get roughly 70 percent of their protein from animal products, the most protein-dense foods. Deficiency is rare even among vegans; they tend to eat more legumes, soy products, whole grains, and nuts, all of which provide protein. Though these plant-based proteins may lack a particular essential amino acid (grains are low in lysine, for example, and legumes are low in methionine), a diet rich in diverse foods generally allows those consuming plant-based diets to easily meet their protein needs.

Protein for a Hungry World

Inadequate dietary protein is a problem for many people in the developing world. They not only lack access to expensive, resource-intensive, nutrient-dense animal products but may also depend heavily on a single staple—such as sorghum, corn, or cassava—which compromises their ability to obtain all nine essential amino acids needed for optimum health.

According to UNICEF, about a third of child deaths under the age of five are attributable to undernourishment. In these cases, protein deficiency often takes place in the context of *energy* deficiency—too few calories—along with deficits in vitamins and minerals. One study examining the diets of

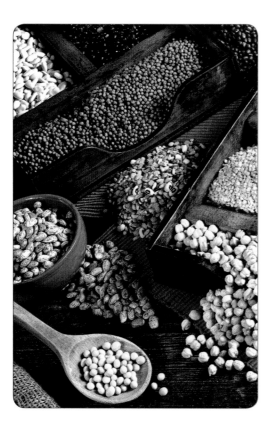

children in an Indian slum found their protein came mostly from plant foods, with animal products (including milk) consumed only once or twice a week. A scant 3 percent of the children had inadequate protein intake with sufficient calories overall, whereas the largest segment—41 percent—got enough protein but too few calories. As a result, their bodies may draw down fat and protein reserves for energy, perhaps stunting their growth.

Healthy Proteins

Meanwhile, wealthier folks' heavy reliance on animal proteins has its own consequences, in terms of health and the global environment. For one thing, full-fat dairy products and many meats are loaded with saturated fat and cholesterol and other stuff too (one ounce of cheddar cheese can have six grams of saturated fat for a third of the recommended daily intake, plus a tenth of your daily cholesterol). Replacing these fats with monounsaturated and polyunsaturated fats—fats found in alternative protein sources like nuts, seeds, and oily fish—significantly reduces blood cholesterol and risk for heart disease, America's number-one killer. Most Americans also don't get enough fiber, which pulls cholesterol from the blood, stabilizes blood sugar, and contributes to healthy bowel functioning. Unlike animal products, which contain no fiber, legumes, whole grains, and nuts are fiber powerhouses that also provide ample servings of protein (although some of these are not complete sources of the essential amino acids). Indeed, the U.S. Department of Agriculture (USDA) dietary guidelines recommend a shift to heart-healthier plant-based protein sources.

As poor nations achieve greater prosperity, their citizens often move away from heart-healthy, plant-based diets and eat more high-protein meat and dairy. This trend is

Heavy reliance on animal proteins has consequences, in terms of health and the global environment.

fueling a global boom in production of animal products—the United Nations Food and Agriculture Organization (UNFAO) projects a doubling of demand for meat in the first half of the 21st century—that the Earth can ill afford.

As it is, livestock production places a heavy burden on the natural world, taking up fully 30 percent of the world's land surface and generating some 18 percent of annual greenhouse gas emissions worldwide. Instead of eating plants ourselves, we grow them (often using fossil-fuel-intensive technologies) to feed animals, an inefficient system that drains the planet of precious natural resources, including land and water.

The rise of "factory" farming, which focuses on intensive production at low economic cost, means food animals are now raised in ways unknown to earlier generations. Use of growth-promoting hormones and antibiotics has increased dramatically in recent decades; 80 percent of all antibiotic use in the U.S. is in farm animals. These spread to water and soil through the animals' waste and agricultural run-off. And the drugs permit animals to grow in very confined, unhealthy conditions that many condemn as inhumane and unethical.

A Way Forward

Change, though, is afoot. People are eating more organic and free-range meat and dairy products, which slightly mitigates environmental impacts and may be more humane to animals. Americans are also eating significantly less meat, at least over the last several years. Schools, other institutions,

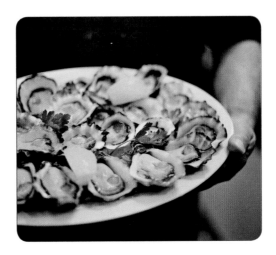

and individuals from around the world have joined the U.S. Meatless Monday campaign launched in 2003 by the Johns Hopkins Bloomberg School of Public Health. The aim is not necessarily to cut out these nutrient-dense foods altogether but to enjoy them in moderation and thereby reduce negative impacts on human health and world ecology. According to the Environmental Working Group, if everyone in America ate no meat or cheese one day a week this year, it would be equivalent to taking 7.6 million cars off the road—hardly a solution to the factors driving climate change, but a step in the right direction.

Turning less reflexively to ham and cheese may even open our eyes to wonderfully tasty plant-based proteins that have been with us for millennia—from the little black bean of South America, gleaming with antioxidant pigments, to rich, spreadable nut butters and sea-fresh, iron-dense oysters and clams.

ALMOND

The almond tree grows wild in parts of the Middle East, where it was probably domesticated a few thousand years ago. One of the first nut trees cultivated by people, the almond is mentioned in Genesis, the first book of the Bible. It is not a true nut but a seed—the pit of a plumlike fruit whose outer flesh is tough and green. Learning to grow the tree for food required people to select trees producing a sweet seed. In wild varieties, the "nut" is not only bitter but toxic, producing cyanide when crushed.

Choose and Use

Almonds can be purchased whole, sliced, or slivered, the latter two very nice for adding crunchy protein to Swiss chard, salads, green beans, or casseroles. Try them as a nutritious and more affordable alternative to pine nuts in pesto, or drink low-fat almond milk as a substitute for cow's milk. Blanching removes the almond's brown skin, along with antioxidant flavonoids and, to some tastes, pleasing texture and flavor. Roasting in itself does not appreciably change nutritional content, but look out for added salt, oils, and sugar—which mean extra calories to an already energy-dense food.

GIVES YOU

Protein
Dietary fiber
Riboflavin
Vitamin E
Manganese
Magnesium
Phosphorus
Copper
Calcium
Iron
Monounsaturated and
    polyunsaturated fats
Phytonutrients
    (flavonoids,
    phytosterols,
    phenolic acids)

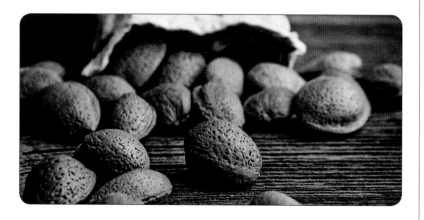

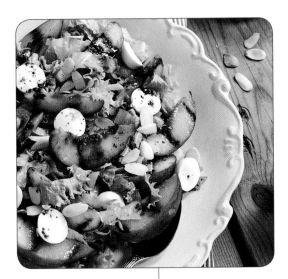

For Your Health

For the calories (about 160 in a small handful), almonds offer more protein and fiber than most other nuts. They're also high in healthy monounsaturated fats, which lower cholesterol, and have the highest concentration of any nut of alpha-tocopherol, a form of vitamin E. Vitamin E is a potent antioxidant; it prevents the damage that results from the natural process in which cells react with oxygen, producing volatile "free radical" molecules that injure other cells. Oxidation of cholesterol helps it stick to blood-vessel walls, one mechanism in the development of heart disease.

Because of these nutrients some studies show adding almonds to the diet helps lower "bad" low-density lipoprotein (LDL) or total cholesterol, although a 2009 review of studies concludes that they have a "neutral effect" on blood lipids.

For Our Planet

Around 80 percent of the world's almonds are grown in California orchards, and demand is growing. These orchards rely mainly on honeybees to pollinate trees so they can produce fruit (and seeds). In recent years sensitive bee populations have plunged due to a phenomenon known as colony collapse disorder. Scientists now believe pesticides play an important role in the problem. Water demand is also a major concern in California's Central Valley, where the bulk of the world's almond growing takes place. A major state plan to divert water to this valley from Northern California's Sacramento–San Joaquin Delta has been controversial, although the plan also includes restoration of the delta.

✦ TAKE AWAY

Try highly nutritious almond products in place of everyday items such as cow's milk and peanut butter.

PREP TIP ✦ ALMOND BUTTER

Almonds are lower in saturated fat and higher in calcium, iron, and fiber than peanuts. Their rich, ever so slightly bitter flavor makes a spread that stands up well to fruity jams and holds the interest of sophisticated palates. To be sure, almond butter is a little harder to find and more expensive than peanut butter, but, on occasion at least, well worth it. Added to soba noodles or whole-wheat spaghetti, it makes an easy sesame noodles-style dish.

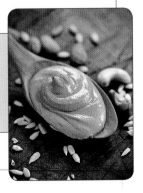

BEEF

Dating as far back as 20,000 years, cave paintings at Lascaux, France, depict enormous grass-eating beasts along with other wild animals. Aurochs, the prehistoric ancestors of domestic cattle, roamed across much of Asia, Europe, and North Africa for many thousands of years, playing an important part in the development of human societies. People managed to tame and keep aurochs beginning about 8,000 years ago in the Near East, with independent domestication also occurring on the Indian subcontinent. Long before domestication, the cattle best known in North America, *Bos taurus*, split from the humped cattle (or zebu) domesticated in Pakistan.

Choose and Use

Beef is a food best eaten in moderation or used as a flavoring (in broth, for example) for other foods. Lean cuts of beef—flank steak, New York strip steak, lean ground beef, eye round roast—are healthier but require careful cooking. Sear the meat, then cook it slowly on low heat; leaner meat cooks up to a third more quickly than fatty beef. A little cooking oil may be required for

GIVES YOU

Protein
Zinc
Iron
Selenium
Phosphorus
Vitamin B12
Vitamin B6
Riboflavin
Niacin
Vitamin B5

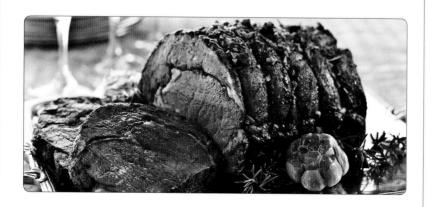

steaks and burgers. Try adding smoked paprika, oregano, fresh herbs, or Worcestershire sauce to lean burgers.

Look for grass-fed beef that is free of hormones and antibiotics. Cattle fed exclusively on pasture grasses (rather than corn and other grains) tend to be leaner in general, with a higher concentration of heart-healthy fatty acids (including polyunsaturated omega-3 fatty acids) than conventionally raised beef.

For Your Health

Beef, it's true, is chock full of saturated fat (and cholesterol). A six-ounce serving of prime rib can dish up more than half the government-recommended daily limit. Research shows that eating fewer saturated fats protects against cardiovascular disease—particularly if those fats are replaced not by refined carbohydrates like high-carbohydrate but nutrient-poor white bread and white pasta but by the healthy fats contained in nuts, seeds, oils, and fish, which have a positive effect on cholesterol levels.

But, to put things in perspective, whole-milk cheese, pizza, baked and dairy desserts, and even chicken contribute more than does beef to Americans' saturated fat intake. And beef is an excellent source of complete, readily absorbable protein, which the body requires to build many of its components and to serve as energy backup when carbohydrates and fats are low.

Beef also has more iron—which carries oxygen in the blood and helps muscles use it—than chicken, fish, or pork.

For Our Planet

High meat consumption, together with the industrialized production systems developed to meet demand, have extremely serious consequences for the environment. All beef is resource intensive; more than two-thirds of the world's agricultural land is devoted not to human food but to growing feed for livestock. It takes about 6.6 pounds of grain and roughly two thousand gallons of water to produce a single pound of beef. Cows are a major contributor to climate change as their distinctive digestive process produces the potent greenhouse gas methane; indeed livestock are responsible for 28 percent of methane generated by human activities, with beef being the principal source. Concentrated feedlot operations where cattle are fattened for slaughter pollute soil and water.

FOOD SCIENCE
✦
CONSIDER THE TRUE COST OF BEEF

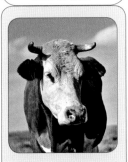

Putting cattle out to grow on natural pasture grasses is a slower, more expensive way to raise them. It's also more humane to the animals, less burdensome on the environment, and ultimately less costly to human health. Sure, the price tag on a pound of grass-fed beef is higher than on conventional beef, where the true costs are hidden from the consumer. Consider eating less, and paying more. Beef really shouldn't be a food of default, served up quick and cheap on every corner, but an occasional high-protein treat.

BLACK BEAN

Like the pinto bean and kidney bean, the black bean is a variety of the common bean, *Phaseolus vulgaris,* which comes in many shapes and colors. In prehistoric times wild beans grew in a large area from Mexico to Argentina and were domesticated in two locations—in Peru some 8,000 years ago, and in Mexico about 7,000 years ago. Both the Aztecs of Mexico and the Incas of Peru grew beans along with maize and squash in a combination known as "the three sisters." These plantings complemented one another horticulturally—beans provide nitrogen to the soil and squash plants retain moisture—and nutritionally, since beans and maize together provide all nine essential amino acids.

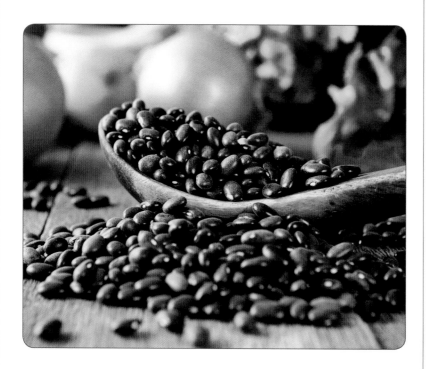

GIVES YOU
Dietary fiber
Protein
Manganese
Copper
Phosphorus
Magnesium
Iron
Potassium
Zinc
Folate
Thiamine
Phytonutrients
   (flavonoids,
   phenolic acids)

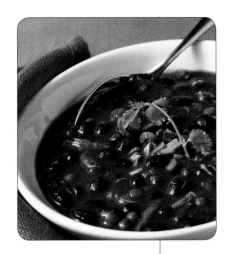

Choose and Use

Dried beans can be soaked overnight, but the quick-soak method is just as good: Rinse the beans and place in a pot with water added to about two inches above the beans. Boil for two minutes, then remove from heat, cover, and let stand for an hour. Cook the beans according to the direction or recipe. Salt beans only after cooking because it slows the process. Canned beans (with no added salt) are a cheap and convenient pantry staple for southwestern scrambles, black-bean hummus, Mexican salads, veggie burgers, soups, and chilis.

For Your Health

For your heart, you can't go wrong with a cup of black beans. It provides protein along with well over half the fiber you'll need in a day. That soluble fiber lowers cholesterol and keeps blood sugar in check, while ample quantities of magnesium (nearly a third of the daily recommended intake) and potassium help control blood pressure. A cup of black beans also provides more than half the daily recommended intake of folate, which helps curb blood levels of homocysteine, a marker for cardiovascular disease.

Like many berries, black beans get their deep color from anthocyanins, which have antioxidant and anti-inflammatory properties important for heart health and cancer prevention.

For Our Planet

Beans can essentially fertilize their own soil; their root systems harbor bacteria that convert atmospheric nitrogen to a form the plant can use. Small grains and corn, which have different nutrient demands, are often grown in rotation with beans, a form of polyculture that protects the soil and avoids the vulnerability to pests that results when a single crop is grown over the long term.

✦ TAKE AWAY

Black beans contain protein, fiber, and other nutrients essential for heart health.

PREP TIP ✦ THE FOUNDATION OF TEX MEX

Black beans are a common ingredient in a wide variety of Tex-Mex dishes, burritos, and beyond. Giving dried beans a quick soak overnight and simmering on the stovetop decreases packaging. They're cheaper than canned and cook very quickly, too.

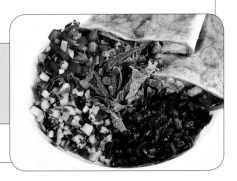

BLACK-EYED PEA

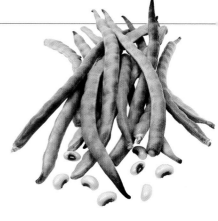

The black-eyed pea, an ivory-colored bean with a distinct black marking, was first cultivated about 5,000 years ago in West Africa. The beans were brought to the American colonies by way of the West Indies, along with enslaved Africans. Thus, in the New World, enslaved people, especially those of the Southern colonies where black-eyed peas took hold, were able to find ingredients for traditional African rice-and-bean dishes that, not incidentally, had provided a complete protein like the maize-squash-beans grouping cultivated by Native Americans. Black-eyed peas became a mainstay of soul food and Southern cuisine, often eaten for good luck on New Year's Day in a dish called "Hoppin' John."

Choose and Use

Though soaking is not strictly required for dried black-eyed peas due to their small size, a quick soak—boil them in water for a few minutes, then let stand, covered, for an hour or so—will reduce cooking time. Frozen are even easier to prepare. While traditionally seasoned with pork, the beans' fresh, earthy flavor can also be enhanced with onions, garlic, sweet and hot peppers, and salt; combine them with collard greens and corn bread for a classic Southern meal.

✦ TAKE AWAY

Black-eyed peas boast high protein, fiber, and vitamins.

FOOD SCIENCE ✦ PEA OR BEAN?

Unlike true peas like snow or sugar snap, black-eyed peas are botanically a legume that preserves soil quality by adding nitrogen; they require relatively little water and are extremely drought tolerant. Thought to bring good luck, black-eyed peas are popular at New Year's, but they're a great choice any time for sustaining our planet's precious natural resources.

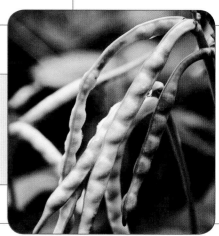

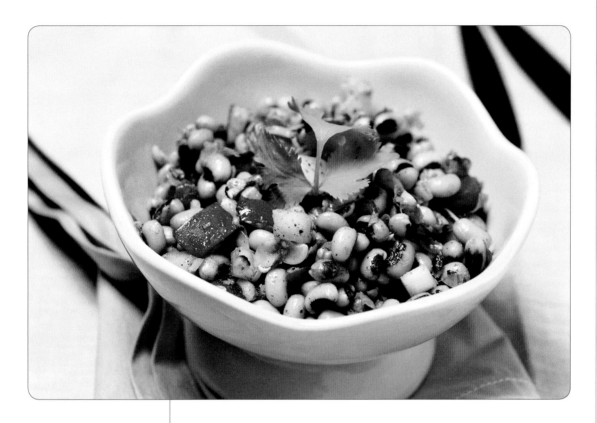

For Your Health

Black-eyed peas share the overwhelmingly positive nutritional profile of other beans—plenty of protein and fiber, and lots of B vitamins and minerals. Eating these and other beans regularly along with fruits, vegetables, and grains is a recipe for avoiding heart disease, diabetes, and excess weight. Their phenolic acid is a potent antioxidant.

Black-eyed peas are especially low in calories and high in folate; a cup has well over half the recommended daily intake. Folate is a water-soluble vitamin that may help prevent colorectal cancers from beginning.

For Our Planet

Nigeria and Niger are the biggest producers of black-eyed peas today, though they're also grown in the American South and California. The drought- and heat-tolerant plants are sometimes "double-cropped"—grown after wheat or another cash crop in the same season, which makes the land more productive. Their stalks are often saved for animal fodder, reducing food waste.

GIVES YOU

Dietary fiber
Protein
Manganese
Phosphorus
Copper
Iron
Magnesium
Potassium
Zinc
Folate
Thiamine
B6
Vitamin B5
Phytonutrients
 (phenolic acid)

CASHEW

The humidity-loving cashew tree bears a tasty but highly perishable fruit called the cashew apple. From the bottom of this fruit protrudes the kidney-shaped morsel we know as a cashew—not a nut, in fact, but a seed. The 40-foot evergreen cashew tree is native to coastal areas of Brazil and was an important food for indigenous peoples there. The tree traveled with 16-century Portuguese missionaries to India and East Africa, where it also thrived along the seacoasts. The nutritious nuts are often used in Chinese, Thai, and Indian cooking.

Choose and Use

Unsalted cashews add crunch to savory dishes and can be tossed onto salads or soups to boost the nutrition and texture. They can also be simmered into rice pilafs, soups, or vegetables to flavor the dish and release the nuts' nutrients. Their high oil content makes them subject to spoilage; store in the freezer or in an airtight container for up to six months. They should be crisp and sweet-tasting.

For Your Health

An ounce of cashews (a small handful) has nearly as much protein as an egg. Cashews are particularly high in oleic acid, a monounsaturated fatty acid also found in olive oil, which is heavily consumed in the vaunted Mediterranean diet.

It may well be due to the special fat composition of nuts that eating them very regularly, as opposed to rarely or not at all, seems to reduce rates of cardiovascular disease, and lower risk factors for diabetes and "metabolic syndrome," a very common collection of factors (excess abdominal fat and high blood sugar, cholesterol, and blood pressure) that together dramatically boost heart-disease risk. While quite

GIVES YOU

Protein
Monounsaturated and
   polyunsaturated fats
Thiamin
Vitamin K
Manganese
Copper
Phosphorus
Magnesium
Iron
Zinc
Selenium
Phytonutrients
   (flavonoids,
   phytosterols)

PAIRINGS ✦ STIR-FRY CRUNCH

Starchier than many other nuts and also a good source of fiber and minerals, cashews are a favorite for snacking out of hand. (Go for unsalted.) They are also a common ingredient in Chinese stir-frys, adding crunch and protein as well as heart-healthy fats and minerals. Select 3 to 4 vegetables that are in season and sauté in peanut oil. Add an Asian-inspired sauce along with sliced water chestnuts and cashews for a flavorful dinner served over brown rice or quinoa.

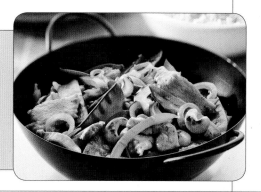

calorically dense, cashews and other nuts can even be part of a successful weight-loss diet as long as they are consumed in moderation.

For Our Planet

Cashew trees stabilize soil and generally do not require pesticides or herbicides. Major producers of cashews include Vietnam, Brazil, India, and parts of East and West Africa. Vietnam has sharply increased cashew production in recent years and is now the top exporter to the U.S.

✦ TAKE AWAY

For a healthy heart, eat a handful of cashews.

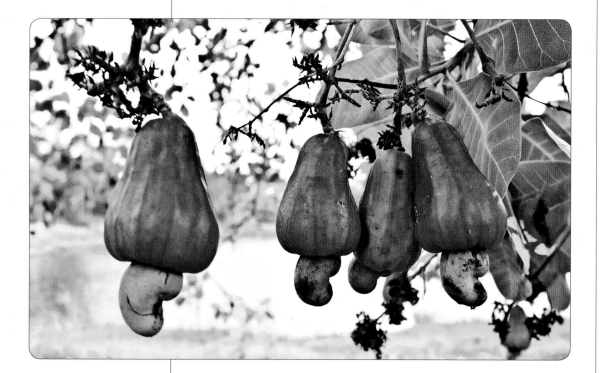

CHEESE: HARD, SOFT, COTTAGE

The most basic step in making cheese is fermenting milk with bacteria that convert its sugars to lactic acid. In fact, the craft of cheese making deploys a veritable menagerie of fermenting microorganisms—including a variety of bacteria, molds, and yeasts. The choice of organism is one of the most important elements in determining taste and consistency.

The so-called starter culture begins to curdle the milk, its liquid whey separating from the solid curds. Next comes rennet, a substance found in the stomach linings of young calves that helps them digest their mother's milk (although today most cheeses are produced with genetically engineered rennet). The enzymes in rennet further separate the solid curds from the watery whey. The product is salted, and other organisms such as mold may be introduced. The cheese is allowed to age over a period of days or even years.

Apart from the lightly acidified "fresh" cheeses, such as cottage cheese or ricotta, cheese is easier to store and carry than milk, and—thanks to acid, salt, and low moisture—keeps much longer.

This is one reason people have been making it for millennia. Though the origins of cheese making are obscure, the art apparently arose soon after the domestication of milk-giving beasts in the Near East and, subsequently, Europe. The earliest evidence, dating back 7,200 years, comes from milk-fat deposits in pottery found at sites in Poland.

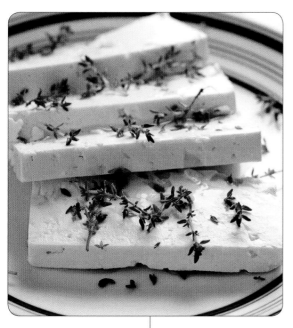

Choose and Use

The old adage holds true: All things in moderation. A little blue cheese crumbled over vegetables, slabs of creamy feta enjoyed in a Greek salad, or a slice of cheddar with fruit and a hearty bread all please the senses, feed the appetite, and nourish the body. Parmesan and Romano are relatively low in saturated fat compared to other cheeses, keep well, and are excellent grated fresh over pasta or mixed greens. Ricotta is low in salt and high in calcium and protein, a common ingredient in both savory and sweet Italian dishes that can also be spread on bread or fruit.

For Your Health

Cheeses vary a lot in their nutritional content. Most—including such diverse types as cottage cheese, Swiss cheese, mozzarella, and cheddar—are good sources of protein. Cheese also provides plenty of calcium and phosphorus, both important to building strong bones and teeth.

On the other hand, cheese is high in saturated fat, accounting for about 16 percent of Americans' overall consumption. Research shows replacing saturated fats with whole grains and unsaturated fats lowers cardiovascular risk. Cheese is also a salty food, which, especially when potassium intake is low, can contribute to high blood pressure.

GIVES YOU

Protein
Calcium
Phosphorus
Zinc
Vitamin A
Riboflavin
Vitamin B12

FOOD SCIENCE ✦ KEEP IT REAL

Whether you're moved by an interest in personal health, the environment, animal welfare, rich and subtle flavor, or all of the above, hold out for a real cheese that's carefully chosen and responsibly made. Why not eat a little less cheese rather than buy "low-fat" versions souped up with salt, sugar, and flavor additives in an unavailing effort to make up for the absence of fat? And why not pay more for an artisanal or farmstead cheese made with milk from pastured animals? Certified organic products mean no hormones or antibiotics, pesticide-free feed, and, in the case of some companies such as Organic Valley, a policy of humane animal treatment on small farms.

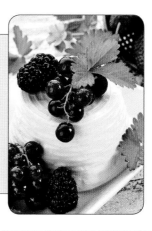

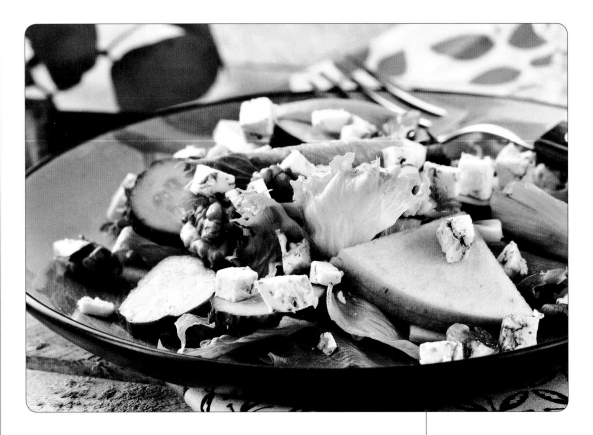

But studies examining whether eating cheese increases a person's risk of heart disease, stroke, and diabetes have produced equivocal results. This may be partly because cheese, like other foods, contains more than just saturated fats and salt and is consumed as part of an overall dietary pattern that will include a host of other foods.

Published in 2012, a review of studies concluded that most population studies fail to link dairy intake with heart disease or stroke, regardless of fat levels. The same review found that fat intake from cheese raises "bad" low-density lipoprotein (LDL)

PREP TIP ✦ LESS IS MORE

The big flavors of cheese mean a little goes a long way. Whether thinly shaving a hard Italian cheese or crumbling a soft chèvre or blue, cheese adds richness and depth to salads and other dishes.

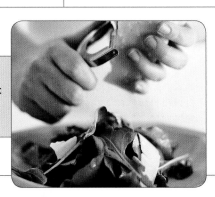

cholesterol less than the same amount of fat from butter. Meanwhile, there's some suggestion that people who eat more lowfat dairy products may have reduced blood pressure and lower risk for stroke and type 2 diabetes.

For Our Planet

The main reason to eat cheese sparingly isn't to save the body from disease but to spare the global environment from the impacts of livestock production. A 2011 report by the Environmental Working Group found that cheese is third only to lamb and beef in greenhouse gas emissions per edible pound. Indeed, the conventional dairy industry is all but indistinguishable from the beef industry. After a few years, dairy cattle are sold for slaughter, making up some 18 percent of U.S. ground-beef supply. Their calves are also sold for meat. All cattle produce methane and consume enormous quantities of feed and water (more than 800 gallons of water are required to make a pound of cheese). Concentrated operations pollute air, water, and soil. U.S. dairy cattle are often given antibiotics to stave off udder and other infections, and nearly one in five is given growth hormones to stimulate milk production, though studies show this tends to increase rates of mastitis and lameness.

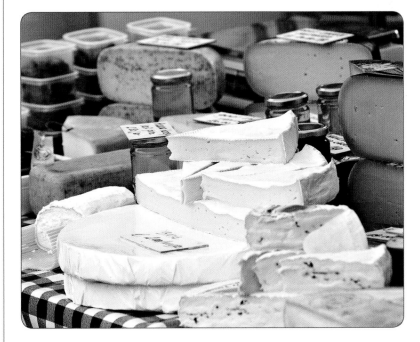

CONSIDER ✦ TERROIR

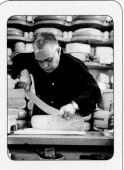

The word "terroir" is most often used when referring to wine, but it is true of many drinks and foods. Animals like cows, goats, and sheep who have dined on grasses where they live creates distinct flavors to their milk and artisans use unique enzymes when making cheese, further imparting terroir to the world's cheeses.

✦ **TAKE AWAY**

Cheese is a good source of protein and calcium, though many are high in saturated fat and salt.

CHICKEN

Now the most common bird in the world, the ubiquitous domestic chicken is most likely a descendant of the Red Junglefowl, which in the wild feeds on insects, seeds, and small animals, and flies only to reach its nest in a tree or other elevated site. Domestication probably took place in Southeast Asia more than 7,500 years ago. Chickens' inability to migrate far means their spread throughout the world was accomplished by people.

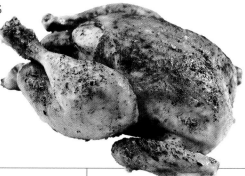

  In the 1990s, for the first time, Americans began eating more chicken than beef.

Choose and Use

No need to avoid dark meat; though a little higher in saturated fat than white, it's also got a tad more vitamins and, according to many, much more flavor. But going for skinless chicken is well worth it, since fat is heavily concentrated in the skin. Chicken can be grilled, oven roasted, lightly pan fried, or poached in low-sodium broth or wine. Marinate the meat in lemon with a dash of salt and pepper, or bake it with rosemary and other aromatic herbs. Breading and deep-frying, of course, add a great deal of saturated fat, and "nuggets" are often made of reconstituted meat along with corn-based fillers and other additives.

For Your Health

Chicken is an excellent source of animal protein. Compared with 85 percent lean ground beef, a portion of chicken breast has about the same amount of protein but fewer calories and, if you eat it without the fatty skin, about a third the total fat. And the fat is composed differently. Stacked up against beef, pork, and lamb, chicken fat has a significantly higher ratio of cholesterol-lowering monounsaturated and polyunsaturated fats to

GIVES YOU

Protein
Selenium
Phosphorus
Niacin
Vitamin B6

✦ TAKE AWAY

Chicken is low in saturated fat, as long as you remove the skin before cooking.

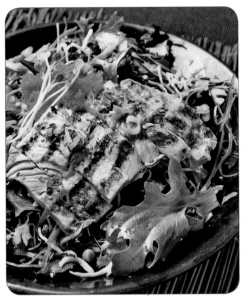

saturated fats, although fat composition changes based on animals' diets.

Half a roasted chicken breast confers more than half the suggested daily intake of niacin, one of the B vitamins that helps the body convert food to energy and play a basic role in nervous-system functioning. Published in 2004, a study examining the effects of diet in thousands of elderly Chicagoans found that those who consumed lots of niacin in their food had slower age-related mental decline and fewer cases of Alzheimer's disease.

For Our Planet

In its 2011 Meat Eater's Guide to Climate Change and Health, the Environmental Working Group ranked chicken as having the lowest overall greenhouse-gas emissions of any meat, with a higher percentage—about 25 percent—produced during processing rather than in raising the animals. To produce a pound of chicken takes about 468 gallons of water and 2 pounds of grain, a lot less than is required for a pound of beef, pork, or lamb. That said, EWG advises consumers to opt for chickens labeled organic, pasture-raised, or antibiotic-free.

CONSIDER ✦ THE REAL COST OF CHICKEN

Most broilers are raised amid their own droppings on the floors of dark barns that hold thousands of birds—and fed antibiotics to promote fast growth despite this unwholesome confinement. "Free-range" birds have continuous access to an outside space, but government regulations don't characterize the required space; in any event, since the birds are bred for heavy breasts and thighs, many do not avail themselves of the opportunity. The less common term "pasture-raised" has no legal definition but has been adopted by farmers to suggest the chickens are raised on actual pasture. "Organic" is probably the most meaningful term on chicken labels. The chickens must be free-range and raised on organic feed without antibiotics (which means they have to be kept healthy by other means). The higher price tag on organic or antibiotic-free chicken reflects lower costs for the environment, the animals, and human health.

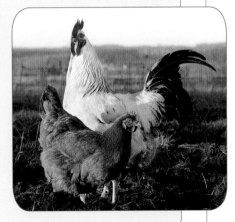

CRUSTACEANS: CRAB, SHRIMP, LOBSTER

Crustaceans, with their tough, jointed exoskeletons, proliferated during the Cretaceous period, 145 to 66 million years ago—long predating the rise of mammals, and certainly the emergence of anatomically modern humans some 200,000 years ago.

From available evidence, it seems that hunter-gatherers added shellfish and other marine resources to their diet of fruits, nuts, and meat as long as 164,000 years ago. This is the date attached to a site on the southern coast of Africa, where a group of *Homo sapiens* had migrated, perhaps driven by climate change that brought cold, dry conditions. They survived by exploiting the ocean's bounty, including whelks and the spiral-shaped giant periwinkle. Not much later, their relatives, the Neanderthals, were collecting shellfish at sites in Spain and Italy.

In ancient times, the Greeks and Romans drew shrimp, lobster, and crab from coastal waters, and ate all three, although their recourse to crab meat was apparently not enthusiastic. Native Americans who lived by coasts and bays also took advantage of protein-rich crustacean populations, catching shrimp and crab in weirs, and harvesting lobster by hand for use as both food and fertilizer.

American shrimp and crab fisheries are among the country's largest and most valuable; lobster is also a high-value U.S. fishery. These rich shellfish are favorites among American consumers, too—especially shrimp, now the most popular seafood in the U.S.

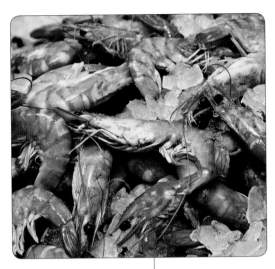

Choose and Use

Crustaceans should have bright, firm shells and give off a sea-fresh aroma, not a rank fishy smell. It's important to keep them cool and prepare or freeze them as soon as possible after purchase.

If buying lobster or crab live, here's how you kill it with compassion: freeze it for twenty minutes to render it insensible. Then, for the crab, stab through its head with a sharp, heavy knife. For the lobster, lay it on its back and swiftly split it along its midline, from the head to the tail. This will destroy its decentralized nervous system. Then steam, boil, or sauté.

Though traditionally eaten with plenty of butter, mayonnaise, and even steak and potatoes, the lightly chilled meat of these animals is so rich that it is happily paired with lighter fare—lemon, fresh herbs such as cilantro or dill, tomatoes, red peppers, avocado, corn, spring greens, or asparagus.

For Your Health

Shrimp, lobster, and crab pack a very generous portion of protein—nearly as much as tuna—with comparatively few calories.

Though known to past generations as high in cholesterol, the buttery flesh of our favorite crustaceans contains negligible amounts of saturated fat, a much bigger dietary contributor to high cholesterol in the blood than dietary cholesterol. In fact research conducted in the late 1990s suggests eating lots of shrimp has no ill effect on overall blood cholesterol. The nine-week study added ten ounces of shrimp a

GIVES YOU

Protein
Vitamin B12
Niacin
Selenium
Phosphorus
Zinc
Copper
Iron
Omega-3 fatty acids
Phytonutrients
   (carotenoids)

CONSIDER ✦ SEA BUGS, LAND BUGS

Crustaceans are arthropods, animals without spines that also include spiders, scorpions, and insects. As ubiquitous in aquatic environments as insects on the earth, crustaceans that crawl along the ocean's floor are often called "sea bugs." While unfamiliar to Americans, "land bugs"—in other words, insects—are consumed around the world and in many places are considered a delicacy. A 2013 report by the Food and Agricultural Organization of the United Nations touted the bright future of insect farming and consumption to address food insecurity and malnutrition.

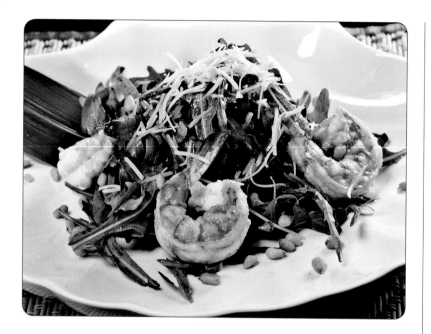

day to a low-fat diet and tested it against the baseline low-fat diet and the same diet plus two hard-boiled eggs daily. Both the high-cholesterol shrimp and egg diets raised "bad" low-density lipoprotein (LDL) cholesterol, but they also boosted high-density lipoprotein (HDL) cholesterol, an effect most pronounced in the shrimp eaters. HDL cholesterol collects excess cholesterol from the blood and returns it to the liver. It's when HDL levels are low and LDL levels are high that cholesterol builds up in blood vessels and compromises their functioning. The researchers suggested this effect of shrimp might be due to its high levels of healthy polyunsaturated (omega-3) fats.

Finally, these aquatic creatures are loaded with a highly absorbable form of the mineral selenium, as well as a carotenoid coloring called astaxanthin, both of which have demonstrated antioxidant and anti-inflammatory effects in laboratory studies.

For Our Planet

With so many kinds of seafood available from so many sources—not to mention produced and harvested by such diverse methods—finding the most environmentally responsible products is no mean feat. It's simplest to rely on seafood decision guides produced by groups like the Monterey Bay Aquarium, the New England Aquarium, and National Geographic.

PAIRINGS
✦
DITCH THE BUTTER

One of the best-loved seafood dishes in America is steamed lobster, classically served as part of a clambake with melted butter for dipping. Other shellfish (and finfish, too) are also commonly served in rich, buttery sauces. While a little butter can be fine once in a while, olive oil is a healthier choice and pairs beautifully with fishes of all kinds—including lobster—along with a squeeze of fresh lemon juice.

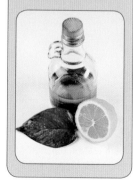

The shells from your crustaceans put you on your way to creating a broad array of soups from homemade stock, whether clam chowder using clam shells, lobster bisque using lobster shells, or bouillabaisse using the shells from a range of different fishes. It's also a super way to use all parts of the animal and save money: no need to buy store-bought stock.

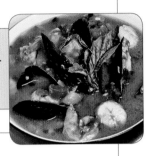

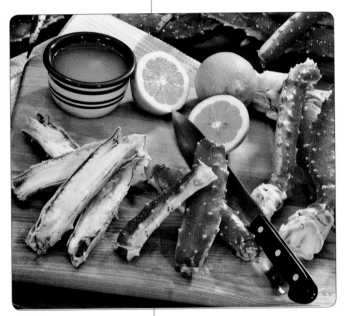

In 2013, for example, the Monterey Bay Aquarium guide lists 12 types of shrimp, three of which it labels as best avoided. It lists eight kinds of lobster, with only one, the Caribbean spiny lobster from Brazil, getting the thumbs-down. The nonprofit names 14 types of crab, discouraging consumption of one, king crabs trapped in Russia. Fishing and aquaculture practices can change over time, however, so it's important to keep updated when selecting any seafood.

Lobster and crab are generally sustainable choices; most of those that find their way onto a plate in the U.S. were wild-caught in U.S. waters. Shrimp, the most popular seafood in America, poses serious problems. The institute suggests avoiding imported shrimp that's farmed in open systems, which can smother adjacent water and soil with pesticides, waste, and other contaminants; often shrimp farms themselves have replaced mangrove swamps, valuable centers of biodiversity. The trouble is, this kind of shrimp constitutes the bulk of what Americans eat, with 90 percent of it imported, most often from Southeast Asia or Latin America. Systems are improving abroad; meantime, seek out U.S.-farmed or wild-caught shrimp. The information changes often; so it's best to visit the National Geographic Web site at www.nationalgeographic.com/seafood-decision-guide.

✦ **TAKE AWAY**

Pair crustaceans with lemon, herbs, or vegetables.

EGG

Since before recorded history, people have gathered eggs from birds' nests for a few mouthfuls of protein. The domestication of the chicken beginning some 7,500 years ago in Southeast Asia made that process much easier, although in ancient Egypt, Greece, Rome, and China its eggs were not necessarily more popular than those of the duck, goose, quail, and pigeon. By the Middle Ages, chickens were fully domesticated in western Europe; both the nobility and peasants ate eggs, which, along with fish, replaced meat on Christian fast days.

For much of U.S. history, egg production has been a domestic undertaking, with backyard chicken coops becoming especially popular in the 19th century. Providing eggs and, on occasion, meat, a brood of chickens often served as a complement to a home vegetable garden.

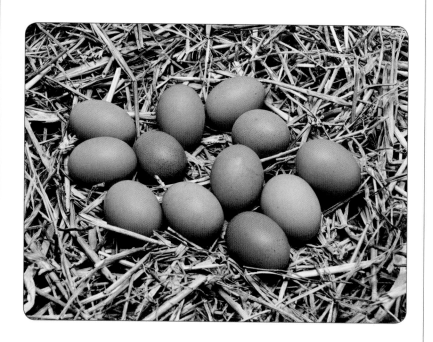

GIVES YOU

Protein
Vitamin A
Riboflavin
Vitamin B12
Choline
Selenium
Phosphorus
Iron
Phytonutrients
  (carotenoids)

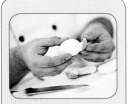

Hard-cooked eggs are used in many dishes, from egg salad to beloved stuffed eggs But have you ever noticed how sometimes they're especially difficult to peel? Nothing at all to do with color, fresher eggs are harder to peel than older eggs. Planning ahead and using older eggs will save you a bit of extra work.

Choose and Use

An egg with a piece of whole-grain toast and a bit of fruit is truly a great way to start the day—filling, relatively low-calorie, and nutritionally balanced.

Are some eggs healthier than others? Whether an egg is white or brown simply reflects the color of the hen. "Vegetarian" eggs come from hens not fed meat and bone meal, a common practice in conventional poultry farming. Eggs advertised as enriched with omega-3 fatty acids come from hens reared on flaxseed and other omega-3-rich foods. That's fine as far as it goes, but consuming the fatty acids directly in salmon and other oily fish (for example) will provide the most valuable fats in greater quantities.

For Your Health

In the 1980s, public health authorities raised the alarm over the sky-high cholesterol content of eggs: A single large egg serves up 70 percent of the recommended daily consumption. But since then scientists have realized that dietary cholesterol is not as important a factor in blood cholesterol as once believed. In fact, a 2013 analysis of eight published population studies concluded that eating up to an egg a day is not associated with a hike in risk for stroke, or, except perhaps in the case of diabetic patients, heart disease. Eggs are also rich in choline, which benefits cell structure and neurotransmitter synthesis.

For Our Planet

The most meaningful distinctions among egg products have to do not with personal dietary preferences or human health but with animal welfare and the environment. The vast majority of laying hens in the U.S. are confined their whole lives in cages (banned in Europe) that prevent natural behaviors or indeed much movement at all; the hens, according to the Humane Society of the United States, "endure constant suffering."

"Free-range" eggs come from hens that at least are permitted to roam in a barn and have continuous access to the outdoors. Certified organic eggs are even better; the birds must be free-range and raised on vegetarian feed (meaning no fish meal or ground-up animal protein) produced organically. They cannot be given antibiotics (another routine practice in conventional egg production). By law, no chickens are given hormones.

✦ TAKE AWAY

Choose eggs that have been produced ethically and sustainably.

FAVA BEAN

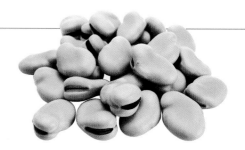

Thousands of years ago, while native peoples of Central and South America were cultivating the common bean (varieties include the black bean and kidney bean), across the Atlantic, groups in Eurasia were growing fava beans. This tender legume was domesticated more than 6,000 years ago, probably somewhere in the eastern Mediterranean. Still a favorite dish in parts of the Middle East and Europe, fava beans were the bean Europeans knew until the Age of Discovery, when explorers introduced the common bean, the highly variable *Phaseolus vulgaris*, from the Americas.

Choose and Use

Shelling and peeling the skin from fresh fava beans is a time-consuming chore unless you're ready to make a fun project of it; kids can help. A bag of frozen beans makes the enterprise simple as can be. Boil them for a few minutes, then eat them with Greek yogurt, olive oil, and fresh mint. Or whip up a chunky, rustic hummus in the blender, an enticing nutrient-rich alternative to mayonnaise on a sandwich.

For Your Health

Fava beans have a bit less fiber and protein but also fewer calories and carbohydrates than kidney or black beans. Like other beans they provide an ample quantity of folate, important for cell division, especially in pregnancy, and a smattering of other

GIVES YOU

Protein
Dietary fiber
Folate
Thiamine
Riboflavin
Niacin
Vitamin K
Manganese
Copper
Phosphorus
Magnesium
Iron
Potassium
Phytonutrients
(flavonoids,
phytosterols,
phenolic acids)

PREP TIP ✦ SPRINGTIME FAVORITE

Fava beans are a springtime favorite with a very short season. Preparing fresh favas is a labor of love, however, involving removing them from their pods, steaming, and peeling. Frozen are just as nutritious and can be enjoyed any time of year, without all the work.

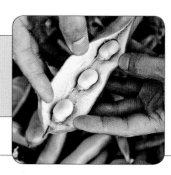

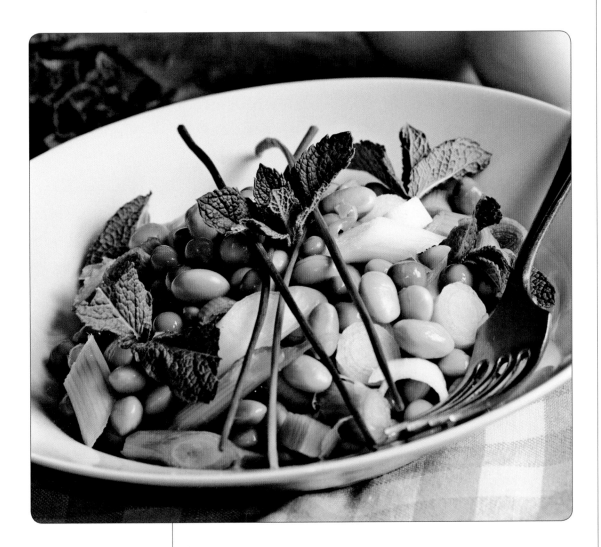

B-complex vitamins that are key to converting food into energy the body can use. And fava beans also provide minerals that are required for heart function and healthy bones.

For Our Planet
Canada grows a good deal of fava beans for export to the U.S., but major producers worldwide are China, Ethiopia, the U.K., Egypt, France, and Australia. Grown for animal feed as well as human consumption, like other beans the fava bean is sometimes used as a cover crop to protect soil and retain moisture, or rotated with grain crops to take advantage of the bean's ability to replenish soil with nitrogen. Beans are an environmentally friendly source of calories.

✦ TAKE AWAY

Fava beans have fewer calories and carbohydrates than other types of beans.

GARBANZO BEAN

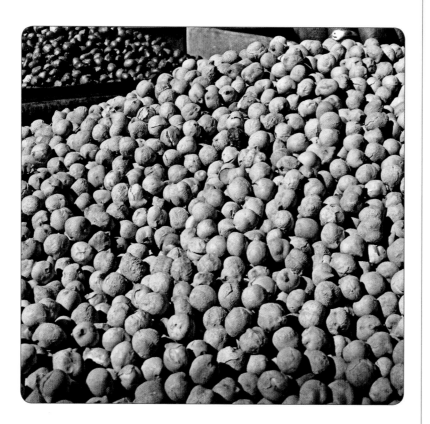

The garbanzo bean or chickpea is one of the first legumes people learned to cultivate along with grains during the advent of farming in the Neolithic period. The green-leafed annual plant with its trumpet-shaped blossoms and nutritious fleshy seeds was probably domesticated in the area of southeastern Turkey roughly 7,000 years ago, then spread southwest into the Middle East and northwest into southern Europe. Chickpeas are among the most beloved legumes in the world today, the principal ingredient of foods such as falafel and hummus enjoyed throughout the Middle East and beyond.

CONSIDER
✦
DRIED VERSUS CANNED

Buying dried garbanzos reduces packaging and costs less than canned. Preparation requires overnight soaking—or an hour-long soak in a hot water bath—before simmering on the stovetop. Takes time, but it's easy and the beans are firm and fresh tasting. If you keep cans on hand for convenience, make sure to select a no salt added brand.

PREP TIP ✦ CREAMY HUMMUS

Once enjoyed only by health food fanatics, hummus is now mainstream. A simple purée of garbanzos, tahini (sesame paste), olive oil, garlic, lemon juice, and water whizzed up in a food processor, homemade hummus is a cinch to make and fresher tasting than store-bought.

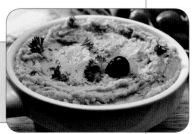

✦ TAKE AWAY

Take advantage of garbanzo beans' versatility—whole in salads, mixed into curries or soups, or blended into hummus.

GIVES YOU

Protein
Dietary fiber
Folate
Thiamine
Vitamin B6
Vitamin K
Manganese
Copper
Phosphorus
Iron
Magnesium
Potassium
Calcium
Zinc
Phytonutrients
  (phytosterols,
  phenolic acids)

Choose and Use

For a simple, cheap, and healthy dish, try chickpeas dressed with lemon, olive oil, and garlic. Including additional colorful vegetables makes a pretty and healthful chopped salad. Chickpeas are also great in Indian curries and vegetable dishes. Hummus, a chickpea spread made with tahini (sesame paste), olive oil, lemon, and garlic, is wonderful spread on whole grain bread or dark rye crisps along with tomatoes and sprouts. It's easy to make at home, and store-bought flavors like roasted red pepper or artichoke keep things interesting; be sure to check the ingredient label for sodium content. Frozen green garbanzos are excellent in sautés, minestrone soups, and salads.

For Your Health

Chickpeas share their most impressive assets with other beans: they are fiber-dense and a good source of protein. And that makes them a satisfying food that's healthy for the heart.

Squeeze a little lemon on your bean salad; the vitamin C in lemons aids the absorption of the iron in chickpeas. Magnesium supports nerves and muscles.

A cup of chickpeas provides half the dietary fiber recommended for the day. Most people don't get enough fiber, some of which helps pull cholesterol from the blood and regulate its uptake of sugars.

For Our Planet

U.S. per capita consumption of garbanzo beans has been slowly increasing in recent years, and that's all to the good. The plant is adaptable to weather and requires relatively little water. U.S. supplies come largely from the American West and Canada.

GREEN PEA

The pea plant grows wild in the Near East and Mediterranean basin, where it was likely domesticated some 9,000 years ago as foragers learned to cultivate its nutritious seed. For many centuries the seeds in their peapods were allowed to dry like other legumes and formed the basis of gruels somewhat like the modern split pea soup that helped stave off starvation. By the 19th century, "fresh" immature green peas consumed as a vegetable had become a popular side dish. In the U.S., peas were among the first vegetables to be commercially canned and frozen in the 1920s. Green or garden peas, snap peas, snow peas, and dried "split" peas are all varieties of the legume *Pisum sativum*.

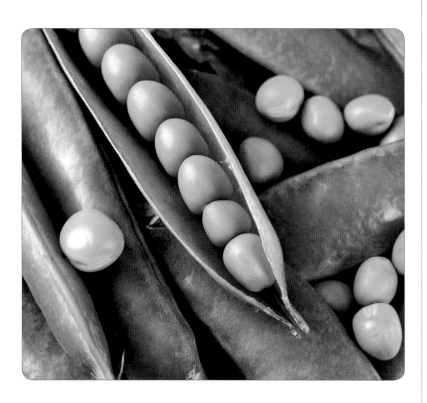

GIVES YOU

Protein
Dietary fiber
Vitamin C
Vitamin A
Vitamin K
Folate
Thiamine
Vitamin B6
Riboflavin
Niacin
Manganese
Magnesium
Phosphorus
Copper
Iron
Potassium
Zinc
Phytonutrients
   (phenolic acids,
   flavonoids,
   carotenoids)

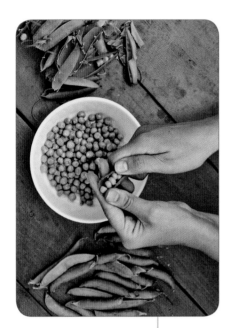

Choose and Use

Green peas, snow peas, snap peas, and split peas have similar nutritional profiles, although only two have edible pods, which are delicious and loaded with fiber. Fresh green peas are crisp and sweet, one of the first vegetables to come in season in the springtime, though often hard to find. Peas also freeze very well. Canned peas (and sometimes frozen) can come heavily salted; choose no-sodium products. For a delicious meal, toss fresh green peas with whole grain pasta and a bit of olive oil and Parmesan in spring and enjoy a split pea soup come winter.

For Your Health

Green peas combine some of the best qualities of beans with certain standout traits of fruits and vegetables. Like beans, they're a good source of fiber and protein (though their protein content is a bit lower) and are replete with B-complex vitamins and minerals. Like many fruits and vegetables, they're also loaded with vitamins C, A, and K, and plenty of phytonutrients, which together may act against cell damage from oxidation and inflammation, processes that accelerate many chronic diseases. Studies have also suggested that when diabetics eat more legumes, they achieve better blood-sugar control and are less likely to die from heart disease.

For Our Planet

Peas capture atmospheric nitrogen in the soil; eco-friendly, they are often used as cover crops to nourish and retain soil. Sustainably grown peas are raised in many states, particularly on the West Coast and in the upper Midwest, although imports from China and Latin America have increased in the last 20 years.

✦ TAKE AWAY

Choose peas for plant-friendly protein.

FOOD SCIENCE ✦ FROZEN PEAS

Green peas are at their sweetest in the heart of summer, and shelling them is a fun way to get kids involved in cooking. Quickly blanched peas can be frozen to enjoy in colder months.

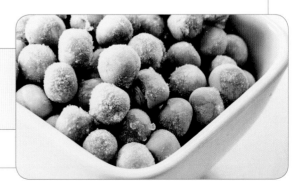

HAZELNUT

The hazel tree was probably domesticated in three separate locations: the Mediterranean (Italy and Spain), Turkey, and Iran, a region where the tree is widely cultivated today for its sweet and crunchy nut. Though it's not clear exactly when people first started growing rather than simply gathering hazelnuts, this transition certainly was accomplished by Roman times. Traditionally called filberts in the United States, hazelnuts are a more commonplace feature of European diets, especially in pastries and chocolate treats. The average Swiss person, for example, eats more than four times the amount of hazelnuts each year as the typical American.

Choose and Use

Familiar as an ingredient in praline candies and the chocolate spread Nutella, hazelnuts can also be toasted and sprinkled onto colorful salads, cooked into rice and vegetable dishes, or eaten out of hand as a filling, protein-rich snack. Check labels for added salt.

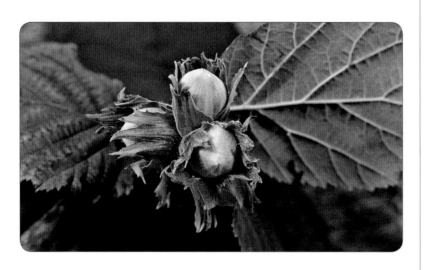

GIVES YOU

Protein
Dietary fiber
Monounsaturated and
     polyunsaturated fats
Vitamins E
Thiamine
Vitamin B6
Folate
Manganese
Copper
Magnesium
Iron
Phosphorus
Phytonutrients
     (flavonoids, phenolic
     acids, phytosterols)

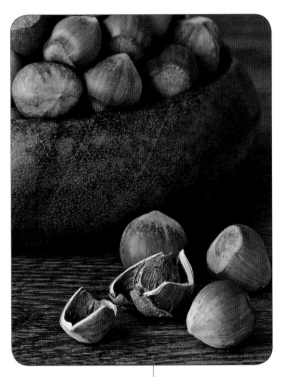

For Your Health

Based on a raft of studies, in 2003 the U.S. Food and Drug Administration approved a health claim for nuts saying that eating 1.5 ounces a day as part of a diet low in saturated fat and cholesterol can reduce the risk of heart disease. Like other nuts, hazelnuts are a high-fiber protein source; they also offer robust quantities of antioxidants such as vitamin E and flavonoids called flavanols (as well as anthocyanidins), which studies suggest may be beneficial to the heart. Perhaps the most important heart-protective feature of nuts is their high concentration of healthy unsaturated fats that lower low-density lipoprotein (LDL) cholesterol—and this feature is especially pronounced in hazelnuts. Hazelnuts provide mostly mono-unsaturated fats (like that found in olive oil)—12.8 grams in an ounce, versus 8.6 grams in almonds and 6.9 grams in peanuts.

For Our Planet

Hazel tree groves are long-lived, help prevent erosion, and require relatively little treatment with pesticides and fertilizers. Turkey is the world's biggest producer, followed by Italy and the U.S.; Oregon produces nearly all American-grown hazelnuts. A fungus called eastern filbert blight made cultivation of the nut impossible in the Northeast and devastated groves in the Northwest in the 1970s, requiring extensive use of fungicides. Today, varieties resistant to the fungus are helping to solve the problem.

✦ TAKE AWAY

High in essential fatty acids, hazelnuts promote heart health.

PAIRINGS ✦ NUTELLA

A chocolate shortage during World War II had confectioners turning to hazelnuts for inspiration, which were cheaper and more plentiful. Thus was born Nutella, the chocolate-filbert spread that's still popular today. Hazelnuts also became a filler for fine chocolates.

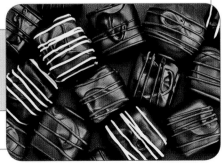

KIDNEY BEAN

Like the pinto and black beans so common in Latin American cooking, the red kidney bean is a variety of the common bean, *Phaseolus vulgaris*. The common bean was domesticated in two locations, Peru and Mexico, beginning some 8,000 years ago. Though native peoples of these regions did eat meat (the Aztecs, for example, dined on turkey and dog, while the Incas ate llamas), beans were an important source of protein among pre-Columbian peoples, whose agriculture did not include extensive domestication of food animals.

Choose and Use

Due to high quantities of a protein called phytohemagglutinin, raw kidney beans are toxic. As few as four or five beans may bring on symptoms including nausea and vomiting, and under-cooked beans may be as toxic as raw ones, so be sure to boil kidney beans briskly after soaking. Canned beans (with no salt added) are just about equal in nutritional quality to dried. They are delicious in a traditional chili or rinsed and tossed into a chopped salad or included in a mixed bean salad.

GIVES YOU

Dietary fiber
Protein
Manganese
Copper
Phosphorus
Magnesium
Iron
Potassium
Zinc
Folate
Thiamin
Vitamin B6
Vitamin K
Phytonutrients
(flavonoids,
phytosterols,
phenolic acids)

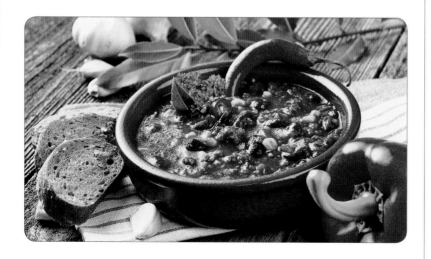

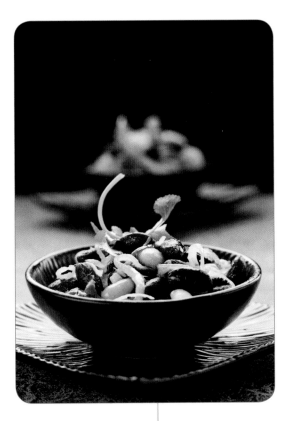

For Your Health

Kidney beans boast a nutritional profile very similar to their close relative, the black bean. A cup packs 15 grams of protein—more than you'd get in two large eggs. Whereas many protein sources common in Western diets are loaded with saturated fat and cholesterol but mostly devoid of fiber, kidney beans have neither saturated fat nor cholesterol, and they provide nearly half the fiber recommended for a day. Because fiber helps regulate the pace at which sugars are released into the bloodstream, eating plenty of kidney beans is likely to have a positive impact on cholesterol levels. Kidney beans are also a great source of the B-complex vitamin folate and provide a range of minerals in moderate supply. Unlike black beans, a cup of kidney beans contains nearly a fifth of the suggested daily intake of vitamin K, a nutrient that may help direct calcium to the bones where it's needed to build bone matrix, and out of the arteries, where deposits of calcium are a factor in vascular disease.

For Our Planet

Beans do not compete well with weeds and are not tolerant of waterlogged soils, so they may develop fungal diseases requiring application of fungicides. On the other hand, they fix nitrogen from the atmosphere, enriching the soil they grow in, and are often grown in rotation with other crops to replenish fields for replanting. As a low-cost source of plant protein, beans are gentle on the environment.

PREP TIP ✦ **BEANS AND RICE**

Rice and beans is a dish traditional to many Central and South American cuisines and can be prepared using many different beans seasoned with spices like cumin, garlic, and coriander. With their dark red hue, kidney beans are especially colorful. Don't forget to use brown rice!

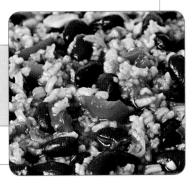

LAMB

All sheep are descended from an animal called the mouflon, which may be the first food animal ever domesticated, a process made easier by its relative docility and herding behavior. Humans first brought the animals under domestication for their meat and milk in the area of today's southwestern Iran some 9,000 years ago. A 6,000-year-old small statue of a woolly sheep recovered from a site in Iran suggests that, by then, people were breeding the creature for its fleece as well. New Zealand and Australia are the major producers of sheep meat, accounting for some 90 percent of exports.

Choose and Use
Lamb shank is the leanest cut of this meat, delicious slow-cooked in Mediterranean dishes including tomatoes, onions, garlic, wine, and plenty of spices. Grass-fed lambs will have higher amounts of healthy omega-3 and omega-6 fatty acids than those raised on corn. Organic lamb must meet the U.S. Department of Agriculture's requirement for grass feeding during the pasture season (at least 120 days a year) and will not have been treated with antibiotics.

For Your Health
A lamb chop and sirloin beefsteak provide a similar complex of B vitamins, minerals (including iron), and protein. But there's a big difference in their fat profiles. Lamb generally has even more saturated fat than beef. Unlike beef, it is also quite high in monounsaturated and polyunsaturated fats—"better fats"—as the American Heart Association puts it. A three-ounce serving of sirloin steak has 11.9 mg of polyunsaturated omega-3 fatty acids, whereas a similar portion of lamb chop contains 93.5 mg—not comparable to the prodigious amount of these heart-healthy fatty acids you get in salmon, but worth noting.

CONSIDER
+
CARBON FOOTPRINT

Among all foods, lamb has the highest carbon footprint. But don't be fooled: it's not because it's usually imported from the other side of the world. One U.K. study found that grass-fed lamb from New Zealand had fewer carbon emissions than factor-farmed lamb from England, highlighting the higher impact of meat production on climate change compared to food miles, or how far it's traveled.

PAIRINGS ✦ **MINTED LAMB**

One of the most energy-intense foods you can eat, lamb is best enjoyed in moderation, if at all. Although more frequently consumed in Mediterranean countries, lamb is often a favorite for Easter celebrations in the United States. With its big flavors, lamb pairs well with bright herbs like mint. While often in the form of thick jelly, a simpler preparation of olive oil, spices, and fresh mint is a lighter choice.

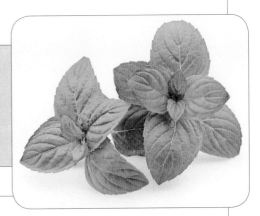

GIVES YOU

Protein
Vitamin B12
Niacin
Riboflavin
Selenium
Zinc
Phosphorus
Iron
Monounsaturated and
    polyunsaturated fats

Lamb is also higher than beef in polyunsaturated omega-6 fatty acids; though omega-6 fatty acids are controversial because they promote inflammation, research suggests that when they replace saturated and trans fats they help reduce risk for heart disease. The American Heart Association recommends getting at least 5 to 10 percent of calories from omega-6 fats.

For Our Planet

The Environmental Working Group's Meat Eater's Guide to Climate Change and Health lists lamb last on its roster of foods— "worst choice." Overall, beef has a much larger impact on the environment simply because it's produced in vastly larger quantities. However, sheep, like cows, are ruminants that produce methane, a potent greenhouse gas, in their digestive process, while yielding significantly less edible meat per pound of live weight. To produce a pound of lamb requires more than 700 gallons of water and about three pounds of grain. The Environmental Working Group recommends grass-fed lamb over lamb "finished" on grain or grain by-products.

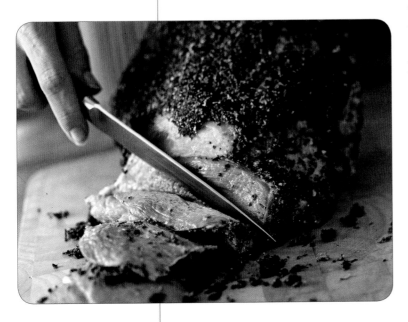

LENTIL

Among the crops that founded agriculture in the Fertile Crescent were wheat, barley, flax, and four legumes—chickpeas, green peas, bitter vetch, and lentils, domesticated at least 9,000 years ago. These crops spread east into Persia (ancient Iran) and India, and west into North Africa and eventually Europe. Protein-dense lentils form the basis of traditional dishes in these parts of the world today, from Indian dal to Middle Eastern mujaddara to hearty European soups that harken back to slow-cooked pottages eaten in medieval times.

Choose and Use

Lentils come in a variety of flavors, colors, and textures, from the yellow split lentil of Indian dal to the peppery French green lentil to the common red and brown lentils of soups and stews. They usually come dried but require no soaking and cook in about 30 minutes. Salt strengthens the structure of beans and will prevent softening, so don't salt until fully cooked. Rather mild-tasting themselves, lentils soak up the flavor of spices and broths. Red lentils break down quickly when cooking, creating an almost-creamy texture to a healthful, beautiful soup, delicious when spiced with cumin, cinnamon, and paprika.

For Your Health

If legumes generally are a very healthy food, it may be fair to say that lentils are the super-legume. A cup of kidney beans or chickpeas provides as much as half the dietary fiber recommended for a day; a cup of lentils provides even more at 63 percent. Most beans provide about 15 grams of protein per cup; lentils provide 18 grams. Lentils have more iron than many legumes, and a cup offers a whopping 90 percent of the day's recommended intake of folate.

GIVES YOU

Protein
Dietary fiber
Folate
Thiamine
B6
Vitamin B5
Niacin
Riboflavin
Manganese
Phosphorus
Iron
Copper
Potassium
Magnesium
Zinc
Phytonutrients
   (phenolic acids,
   flavonoids,
   phytosterols)

PREP TIP ✦ **THE DIVERSITY OF LENTILS**

Lentils come in assorted colors and textures, commonly enjoyed hot as a side dish or in a soup. Red lentils will break down during cooking, creating an almost creamy texture, whereas others retain their shape. Cooked lentils like green or brown make a delightful salad, warm or cold, when tossed with olive oil, lemon juice, and fresh herbs.

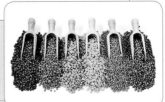

✦ TAKE AWAY

Lentils offer more protein, fiber, and folate than other legumes.

A review of ten human trials, published in 2011, found that diets enriched with plenty of legumes lowered "bad" low-density lipoprotein (LDL) cholesterol by an average of 8 mg/dL. In another study, published in 2012, diabetics who added a daily cup of legumes to their diets enjoyed better blood-sugar control and lower blood pressure than those who added whole-wheat products. All of the nutrients in lentils combined together probably play an important role in these benefits.

For Our Planet

Washington, Idaho, and Western Canada are major producers of lentils, though most are exported. The drought-tolerant crop is little bothered by pests or diseases, and contributes nitrogen to the soil; it is often rotated with wheat. Lentils are a very important food in India, which produces and consumes about a quarter of the world's crop.

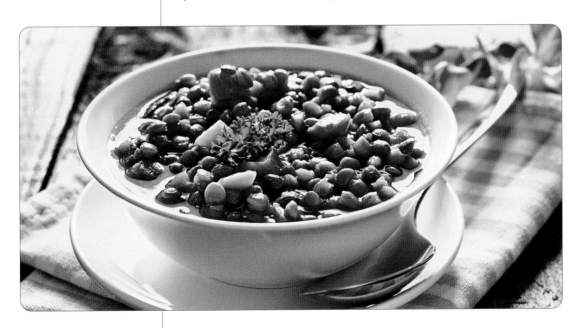

MOLLUSKS: CLAM, MUSSEL, OYSTER

All over the world, along coastlines and beside streams and rivers, thousands and tens of thousands of years ago, human groups left evidence of their feasting on mollusks. Called shell middens, these heaps of discarded shells are sometimes the leavings of a single meal. In other cases, they show evidence of long occupation, as in the 30-foot pile of oyster shells discovered in Damariscotta, Maine; Native Americans added to this heap for a thousand years, between about 2,200 and 1,000 years ago. The southern coast of South Africa is dotted with 3,500 shell middens, including the earliest known find, dating to 140,000 years ago.

Whether sought out as a marginal food in times of want or incorporated on a large scale into human economies, mollusks, those mouthfuls of protein, clearly played an important part in the diets of many hunter-gatherers as well as early farming peoples.

Clams, mussels, and oysters belong to a class of mollusks called bivalves. Two symmetrical shells joined by a hinge enclose a soft body that includes gills for breathing and sieving food, and a simple digestive tract.

PREP TIP ✦ **MAKE SURE THEY'RE ALIVE**

Don't wash mollusks until you are ready to use them; soaking them in a water bath with a little flour helps remove excess sand. Mollusks that are opened prior to cooking and do not close when tapped are dead and must be discarded.

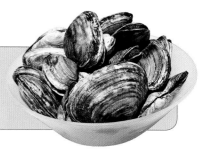

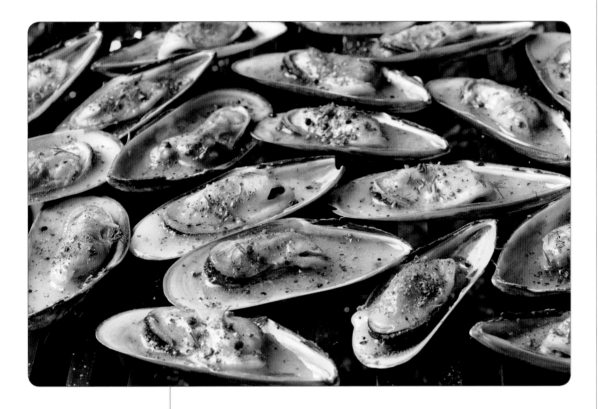

Choose and Use

Highly perishable bivalves should be purchased live and kept refrigerated. Expect a fresh sea smell and firmly closed shell; if slightly open, the shell should close when you tap it.

Rinse the shells thoroughly to eliminate sand and grit. Clams, oysters, and mussels can be steamed, baked, or grilled; or you can steam them open, remove the meat, and finish cooking in a soup, stir-fry, or sauté. When steaming, place the bivalves in a wide pot for maximum surface exposure and add liquid—wine and fresh herbs, beer and garlic, water, whatever your recipe calls for. Clams and mussels will open when done (about 6–10 minutes for clams, 3 to 5 for mussels), but oysters may not; tapping on the shell produces a hollow sound when they're cooked, usually after 5–10 minutes.

Of course, some people love nothing better than the delicate, briny taste of raw oysters "on the half shell." Buy them in the half shell, or shuck them yourself. Favorite accompaniments? Just a dash of lemon, or Tabasco, Worcestershire sauce, cocktail sauce, or mignonette made of vinegar, shallots, and lemon juice.

✦ TAKE AWAY

Clams provide high amounts of iron, mussels essential fatty acids, and oysters zinc.

For Your Health

It comes as a surprise to many that mollusks, which seem such delicate morsels, are chock full of protein and iron. Clams in particular pack nearly as much protein as ground beef or chicken, with scarcely any saturated fat. And a serving of clams—about ten small ones—provides all the iron you'll need in a day, and then some.

A tad less impressive than clams on the protein front, at 665 mg per ounce, oysters are among the best sources of the omega-3 fatty acids that promote a healthy heart and eyes and may lower the risk of dementia. Oysters also contain plenty of zinc, which the immune system needs to combat infection. Six steamed oysters have a paltry 60 calories.

Mussels are also a good source of omega-3s, and, like clams and oysters, are loaded with protein, iron, and B-complex vitamins, especially B12. The body can store this essential vitamin in small quantities, but because of reduced absorption many older people are at risk of deficiency, which can cause problems with balance, mood, and memory. A serving of clams provides 14 times the recommended daily intake, oysters about 5 times, and mussels more than 3 times the daily suggested intake. Although most sodium in the diet comes from processed foods, mollusks are naturally high in salt due to their seawater habitat.

GIVES YOU

Protein
Vitamin B12
Riboflavin
Niacin
Vitamin C
Vitamin D
Iron
Zinc
Copper
Manganese
Selenium
Phosphorus
Unsaturated fats

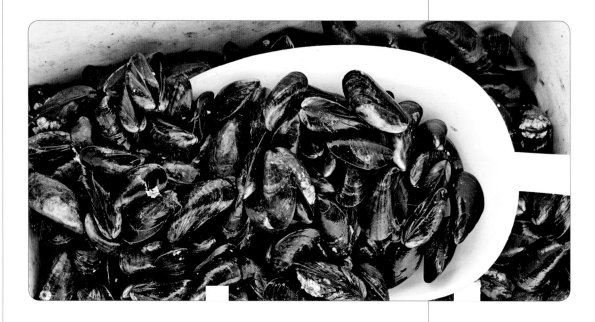

For Our Planet

More good news about mollusks: You can enjoy them knowing you're supporting hard-hit marine-based economies without breaking your own bank or harming the natural world in any way.

Most mussels are farmed, and oysters and clams are widely available both wild and farmed. But the distinction isn't quite as sharp for these shellfish as for other types of seafood. Farmed mollusks live in the ocean. They feed by filtering particles from water, which can actually help keep water it clean. Bivalves are often farmed in cages or on long ropes that hang from floating platforms. These methods have little to no environmental impact.

Wild oyster populations in particular have declined steeply since the 19th century, mostly due to overharvesting, although efforts are under way to restore populations in places such as the Chesapeake Bay and even the harbor of New York City, where fresh local oysters were once a favorite street and bar food. A potential long-term threat to all bivalves is the acidification of the world's oceans. The same human-generated carbon dioxide that is helping to warm the planet also settles into the ocean and makes seawater more corrosive. This seems to make it harder for marine creatures to build shells.

The Monterey Bay Aquarium lists all oysters and mussels as a "best choice"; clams are categorized as either a "best choice" or a "good alternative."

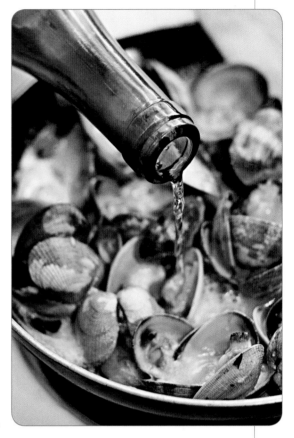

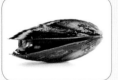

FOOD SCIENCE
✦
STORING MOLLUSKS

Buying mollusks from your local fishmonger is a treat, and simple preparations like olive oil, wine, and herbs, are the perfect accompaniment. Using them immediately is always the best bet, when they're freshest, but mollusks can be stored in the refrigerator for a few days. Place them in the coolest part of your fridge in a large bowl and cover loosely with a damp cloth.

PEANUT

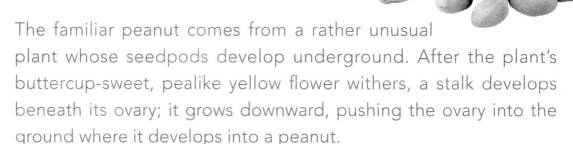

The familiar peanut comes from a rather unusual plant whose seedpods develop underground. After the plant's buttercup-sweet, pealike yellow flower withers, a stalk develops beneath its ovary; it grows downward, pushing the ovary into the ground where it develops into a peanut.

The oldest evidence of peanut consumption comes from Peru, where nut remains and peanut starch on human teeth date back as far as 8,000 years. But scientists believe the plant was domesticated even earlier in Paraguay or Bolivia, where it is native.

George Washington Carver, a botanist and educator born into slavery, promoted peanuts, a nitrogen-fixing crop to rotate with cotton, which had depleted the once-rich loam of the American South. Carver's popular 1916 bulletin on peanuts contained instructions for cultivation and 104 recipes. Peanut consumption took off in the U.S. in the early 1900s, when peanut butter first appeared in supermarkets.

Choose and Use

That little handful of peanuts, while nutritious, packs more than 160 calories. Sugary peanuts pack on nutrients you don't need. The same goes for peanut butter; look for no-salt, no-sugar-added brands that aren't made with trans fats. And skip low-fat peanut butter, which only replaces healthy fats with carbohydrates and sugar.

For Your Health

An ounce of these crunchy, mildly sweet nuts—a small handful—contains seven grams of protein, a little more than an egg. Cook them into a rice dish or spread peanut butter onto whole-wheat bread, and you'll have a meal with ample quantities of all the essential amino acids.

GIVES YOU

Protein
Dietary fiber
Niacin
Folate,
Vitamin E (alpha- and
  gamma-tocopherol)
Thiamine
Manganese
Magnesium
Phosphorus
Copper
Iron
Monounsaturated and
  polyunsaturated fats
Phytosterols (stilbenes)

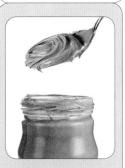

Peanuts are among the most popular nuts in America, from ballparks to lunch boxes. And just about everyone loves peanut butter, the creamy spread at its peanuttiest when made only with unsalted nuts and no added oils. Far more healthful than processed meats like bologna, a peanut butter sandwich on whole grain bread is a terrific lunch, whether for kids or adults.

✦ **TAKE AWAY**

Choose peanuts and peanut butters without added sugar and salt.

Peanuts also offer a modest amount of fiber and vitamin E, an antioxidant that, in the laboratory, has demonstrated activity against the oxidation of cholesterol (a factor in fatty buildup in the arteries) and formation of blood clots, which may cause heart attack or stroke.

In the late twentieth century, peanuts and peanut butter suffered from a reputation as food whose nutrient quality wasn't worth the calories and fat. It's true peanuts are about 50 percent oil, but the type of fat matters when it comes to health: peanuts are primarily unsaturated, heart-healthy fats. Of the 13.9 grams of fat in a small handful of peanuts, only 1.9 grams are saturated fat. Fully 6.9 grams are monounsaturated fat, which helps reduce low-density lipoprotein (LDL) cholesterol. Some research has also shown that peanuts consumed in moderation can also be included as part of a weight-loss diet.

For Our Planet

The U.S. is a major peanut grower, with production concentrated mainly in the Southeast and Southwest. Farmers often rotate the crop with corn and cotton because peanuts supply the soil with nitrogen. Peanut oil has shown potential as a biofuel, although demand for the crop as a food makes it more expensive than corn or soybean to produce.

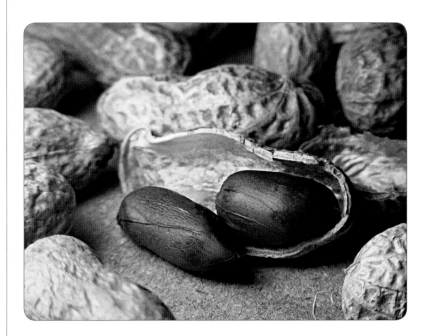

PECAN

The majestic pecan tree with its bright green pinnate leaves and long, twisting limbs is a native of the south-central United States, where it grows in the moist soil along streams and rivers. Native Americans gathered the hard-shelled nuts in autumn; indeed "pecan" is an Algonquin word that referred to all nuts requiring a stone to crack. Widespread cultivation of pecans did not take place until the 19th century. Even today, in its native range, about half of pecan production comes from wild-growing trees. U.S. production accounts for 80 percent of pecans grown worldwide.

Choose and Use

Smooth-textured and devoid of the slightly bitter nip of walnuts and almonds, pecans make great snacking when not coated with extra salt or sugar. They're also a nutritious addition to fruity quick breads and contribute earthy flavor to salads or cooked vegetables. As with all nuts, lightly toasting in the oven brings out their flavor and crunch. Native Americans use pecan meal to thicken stews.

GIVES YOU

Protein
Dietary fiber
Thiamine
Vitamin E
Manganese
Copper
Iron
Magnesium
Phosphorus
Monounsaturated and
    polyunsaturated fats

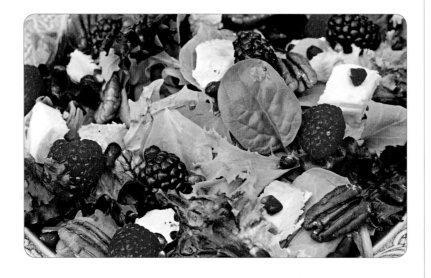

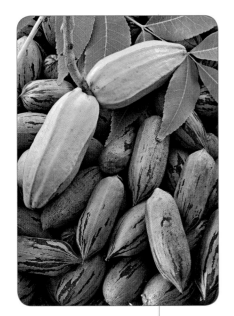

For Your Health

A little higher in calories and lower in protein than many nuts, pecans nevertheless are a good source of dietary fiber and especially of the heart-healthy fats that make nut oils more nutritious than animal fat.

A single ounce of pecans contain some 30 percent of recommended daily intake of fat. But well over half that fat is monounsaturated and another 30 percent is polyunsaturated—fats that bring a panoply of benefits, from cutting risk for breast cancer and dementia to improving blood cholesterol levels and perhaps assisting in controlling blood sugar.

One study adding pecans to a diet low in saturated fat and cholesterol found that the pecan-enriched diet delivered more calories as fat than the base diet, but lowered "bad" low-density lipoprotein (LDL) and total cholesterol more than the baseline low-fat diet. Pecans, like peanuts and walnuts, are also high in a form of vitamin E called gamma-tocopherol. Though its health effects are not well understood, some research suggests it may prevent cell damage from oxidation and inflammation.

For Our Planet

Gathering nuts from trees that can live a 100years or more is a sustainable practice, whether the trees are in cultivated orchards or natural stands thinned and nurtured by farmers. Farmers often plant legumes in the orchards to enrich the soil and attract insects that eat pecan aphids and other pests, contributing to a healthy ecosystem. Grazing livestock in pecan groves, where they nibble grasses and fertilize with their manure, is also common.

✦ TAKE AWAY

Pecans make an excellent snack and enliven salads and breads.

PAIRINGS ✦ **HEALTHY CRUNCH**

Pecans are sweeter than many other nuts and can even be a little chewy when raw. Toasting pecans, like other nuts, really brings out their flavor. Whether you prefer them raw or roasted, make sure to select unsalted. Pecans are a terrific addition to a green salad for crunch and nutrition. A handful of pecans alongside fresh fruits like strawberries, peaches, or plums makes a healthy snack. Or serve with a few pieces of good cheese for a French-inspired dessert.

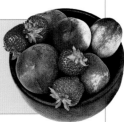

PINTO BEAN

Pinto beans are one of many varieties of the common bean, *Phaseolus vulgaris*, a major food of pre-Columbian native peoples in South and Central America domesticated in two locations—Peru, some 8,000 years ago, and Mexico, about 7,000 years ago.

These mottled legume seeds are the most popular bean in America and second only to black beans in Mexico. They are a frequent accompaniment to rice and the basis for refried beans, in which the beans are cooked, then mashed into a paste and fried or baked with seasonings like cumin, garlic, and chili power.

Choose and Use

Pinto beans take more time to cook than most—at least two and a half hours, after soaking overnight or using the quick-soak method. Salt and acids such as vinegar or lemon juice delay cooking, so add them late. But cooking with onion or garlic will impart a rich flavor to these mild, creamy beans. For more spur-of-the-moment meals, canned beans retain most of their nutritional value; canning adds sodium, so look for beans labeled no-salt and rinse the beans in cold water for good measure. Serve with seasoned brown rice for a wholesome meal. Spike with lemon juice, extra virgin olive oil, and hot sauce for a satisfying lunch. Peppery greens, beans, and a can of tuna make a great and easy salad or a pasta sauce when gently warmed.

✦ TAKE AWAY

Pair pinto beans with spices or garlic for a creamy, protein-rich dish.

PREP TIP ✦ **REFRIED BEANS**

Pinto beans are the traditional choice for refried beans. Fry smashed beans in vegetable oil and season with cumin, chili powder, garlic, and onion—add cayenne for kick—for a tasty side. Or stuff into burritos or tacos with salsa for a meatless Mexican meal.

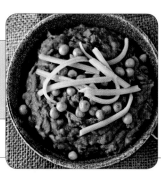

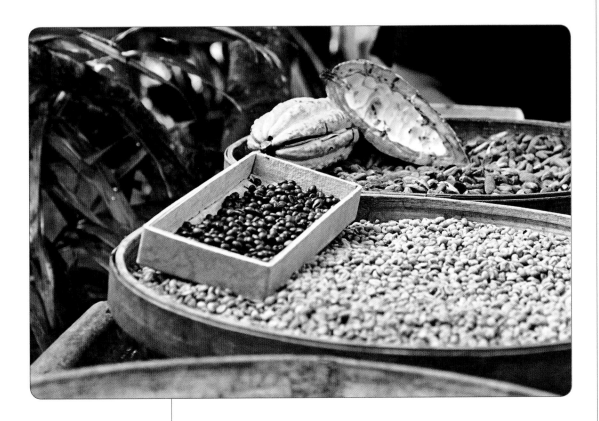

GIVES YOU

Protein
Dietary fiber
Folate
Thiamine
Vitamin B6
Vitamin E
Vitamin K
Manganese
Phosphorus
Magnesium
Potassium
Iron
Calcium
Zinc
Copper
Selenium
Phytonutrients
(phenolic acids)

For Your Health

A cup of pinto beans provides a good serving of protein—15 grams—along with well over half the dietary fiber intake recommended for a day, 74 percent of the folate, and 21 percent of minerals potassium and magnesium. All these, in different ways, are good for the cardiovascular system.

Population studies have shown that people who eat lots of legumes (including beans) are less likely to develop heart disease, diabetes, and colon cancer.

For Our Planet

Pintos account for nearly half of all U.S. dry-bean production, concentrated in the northern Great Plains. Though intolerant of moist soils and subject to fungal diseases, beans are relatively untroubled by insects. They are usually planted in rotation with cereal crops that have different nutrient requirements and disease susceptibility. Eating beans, an efficient plant-based source of nutrients, energy, and protein, is a good move for the environment as well as your own health.

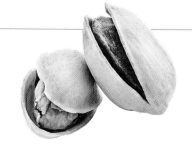

PISTACHIO

The pistachio is a comely little tree with a dense, bowl-shaped crown and reddish-brown bark. Ten thousand years ago, when hunter-gatherers of the Near East first began the transition to agriculture, pistachio trees mingled with oaks in forests reaching from the eastern Mediterranean to the Zagros Mountains of Iraq and Iran. People had gathered the nuts for thousands of years already, and would combine these foraged nuts with cultivated foods for millennia to come.

Movements associated with Alexander the Great, the Roman Empire, the Muslim expansion, and the Crusades all helped spread pistachios throughout the Mediterranean world. U.S. commercial production of pistachios came much later, in the 1970s. Today's California pistachios are a bit larger and easier to shell than the Turkish (Antep) variety, but some connoisseurs swear by the Turkish nut's sweet crunchiness. Sicilian pistachios are very green and often found slivered onto pastries and other desserts.

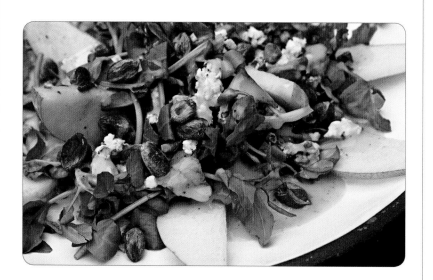

✦ TAKE AWAY
Add pistachios to salads and stuffings.

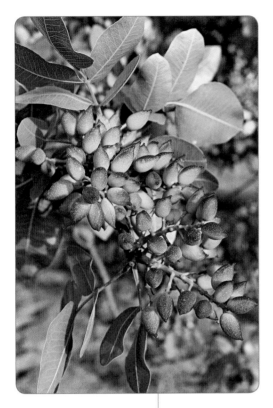

Choose and Use

The most common presentation of this green-tinted nut is as a snack food so heavily salted as to mask its delicate flavor. Try them instead sprinkled in a fruit salad, or with orange slices over peppery greens. Pistachios make terrific pestos, pilafs, stuffings, and crunchy crusts for fish or poultry. Because pistachio growing and processing require a lot of time and labor, the nuts are pricey; try buying them in bulk.

For Your Health

Along with protein, pistachios bring a great deal of fat to the table, but more than half that fat is unsaturated, predominantly monounsaturated fats that, when they replace less healthy fats, might help reduce a person's chances of getting breast cancer, developing age-related macular degeneration or cognitive decline, and suffering flair-ups of arthritis pain. These fats are considered to have salutary effects on cardiovascular health as well.

Indeed, one 2007 study that instructed subjects to take fully 15 percent of their calories from pistachios found they ended up consuming less of their energy in the form of saturated fat and saw small improvements in blood cholesterol. In another study, eating three ounces per day of pistachios over four weeks reduced blood levels of oxidized low-density lipoprotein (LDL) cholesterol—cholesterol that has reacted with oxygen and become, essentially, rancid, a process that promotes buildup on artery walls. This effect might have been in part due to the nuts' lutein, an antioxidant carotenoid that increased in the blood of subjects on the pistachio diet.

For Our Planet

In just 30 years the U.S. has become the world's second-biggest producer of pistachios, after Iran. Growing is centered in California. Each tree requires considerable investment and won't bear until after about 7 years but may continue producing for another 75. Water use is fairly high in pistachio orchards.

GIVES YOU

Protein
Dietary fiber
Vitamin E
 (gamma-tocopherol)
Vitamin B6
Thiamine
Iron
Magnesium
Potassium
Copper
Manganese
Phosphorus
Monounsaturated and
 polyunsaturated fats
Phytonutrients
 (carotenoids
 phytosterols,
 stilbenes, flavonoids)

PORK

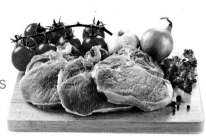

Wild boar were among the earliest animals to be domesticated, a process that in their case occurred on multiple occasions and in several locations in Asia and Europe roughly ten thousand years ago. Omnivorous, adaptable, and equipped with a sensitive snout that doubles as a digging instrument, for centuries pigs have been an inexpensive animal to raise, being turned out to forage in the forest, clear crop residues, or indeed gobble the waste from city streets. Pig varieties have diminished sharply as breeders select hogs that perform well in today's intensive production system.

Choose and Use

Add flavor to lean pork by marinating it in lemon juice, vinegar, wine—any acidic liquid—seasoned with plenty of spices and herbs. Then broil, grill, bake, or sear it in a pan using a little olive oil. Lean cuts are best for grilling, whereas fattier cuts lend themselves to barbecuing, slow cooking, and braising.

  With the rise of factory farming, old "heritage" hog breeds such as the Berkshire, Hereford, Tamworth, and Red Wattle are harder to find, but repay the effort and expense with juicy, layered flavor.

For Your Health

When it comes to health, all cuts of pork are not created equal. Lean cuts—tenderloin, chops, sirloin or top loin roasts—are comparable to chicken in levels of saturated fat and cholesterol, with both serving up a hefty portion of protein. They also provide iron, B-complex vitamins that help the body break down carbohydrates for energy, and minerals like selenium, which has antioxidant and anti-inflammatory properties.

  But processed meats—for example, ham, bacon, and

GIVES YOU

Protein
Thiamine
Niacin
Vitamin B6
Vitamin B12
Selenium
Phosphorus
Zinc
Iron

✦ TAKE AWAY

Choose lean, unprocessed cuts, and avoid processed products high in fat, sodium, and nitrates.

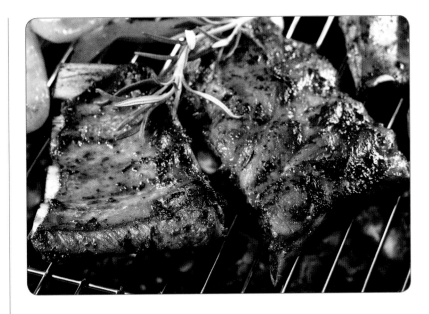

The growing awareness of the problems with confined animal feed operations (CAFOs) have led many to choose meat raised from free-range animals who live in more humane environments. Pastured pigs have room to roam and consume grass, which creates more nutritious pork. Even so, the amount of land, food, energy, and water needed to produce animal products like pork creates far more carbon emissions.

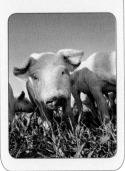

sausage—tend to have a lot more saturated fat and bucketsful of sodium (they're often cured). A single slice of bacon has 43 calories, 30 of which come from fat, a third of which is saturated fat.

In addition, whether because of their saturated fat and salt, nitrate preservatives, chemicals produced during cooking, or a combination of these factors, processed meat consumption has been linked to higher rates of heart disease, diabetes, stroke, and cancer in population studies.

For Our Planet

Once upon a time, pigs were a common and key element in traditional mixed farming, foraging and consuming all manner of farm waste while providing fertilizer as well as meat. Today, most hogs in the U.S. are raised in intensive "factory" farms with thousands of animals. Concentrated in the Midwest and Southeast, these farms may emit hydrogen sulfide, a gas that can cause flulike symptoms in humans, and their enormous waste lagoons pollute soil, air, and water. Crowding and extreme indoor confinement raise serious animal-welfare concerns.

Look for organic, pasture-raised, or free-range pork. Only the organic label is regulated; it means hogs will have organic feed and no antibiotics. Pork labeled "Animal Welfare Approved" will come from pastured animals.

PUMPKIN SEED

In the 1960s, archaeologists discovered seeds and rind from the squash species *Cucurbita pepo*, which includes the pumpkin, in a cave in Oaxaca, Mexico. In the 1990s advanced radiocarbon dating confirmed the astonishing age of the find: 10,000 years old. That made a pumpkin-like squash and its seeds (called *pepita* in Spanish) the first domesticated plant in the New World. Earliest farming in the Americas traces to around the same time that agriculture dawned in the Fertile Crescent and central China.

Pepitas are still popular in Mexico and Latin America as a snack and ingredient, ground into mole sauces, for example. Nutty-flavored pumpkin seed oil is widely enjoyed in central European countries as a dressing for potato or bean salads.

Choose and Use
Look for unsalted pumpkin seeds, raw or roasted. To roast them straight from the pumpkin, rinse off any flesh and let them dry thoroughly if you can. Then toss them with a little olive oil and your favorite seasoning—sea salt, garlic, cayenne

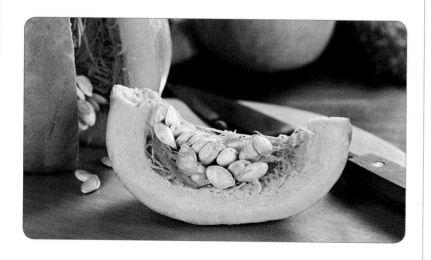

GIVES YOU
Protein
Monounsaturated and
   polyunsaturated fats
Vitamin E
Vitamin K
Zinc
Magnesium
Copper
Manganese
Iron
Phosphorus)
Phytonutrients
   (phenolic acids
   and phytosterols
   [lignans])

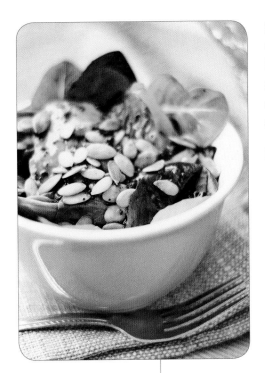

pepper, paprika, cumin. Roast in a 400-degree oven for at least 20 minutes, tossing occasionally. For crispier seeds, start by boiling them for 10 minutes in lightly salted water or bake longer at a lower temperature. Note that butternut squash seeds can be roasted in the same fashion.

For Your Health

Pumpkin seeds have about as much protein as almonds. Though short on fiber and rather high in calories due to their fat content, most of the fat is polyunsaturated, which, especially when they replace saturated fats in the diet, may protect healthy brain functioning and stave off type 2 diabetes, heart disease, and macular degeneration.

Pumpkin seeds are a good source of zinc, with a small handful providing a fifth of the recommended daily intake of this mineral. Zinc is critical to healthy immune functioning, and deficiencies have been linked to pneumonia in the elderly and diarrhea among children in the developing world.

Pumpkin seeds also contain various forms of vitamin E, including gamma-tocopherol, which may protect cells from oxidation and inflammation.

For Our Planet

Probably the most sustainable way to consume pumpkin seeds is to support a local farmer by buying a fresh pumpkin from August through early winter—and let the gourd do double duty as ornament and food. Though most of the canned pumpkin in the U.S. is grown in Illinois, packaged pumpkin seeds may well be imported. For more on winter squash seeds, see pages 96–99.

✦ TAKE AWAY

Roast pumpkin seeds yourself or purchase unsalted ones.

PAIRINGS ✦ AUTUMN TRAIL MIX

A special Halloween time treat is toasted pumpkin seeds eaten simply out of hand. These tasty, crunchy seeds can also be thrown onto a salad or combined with a selection of other nuts and dried fruits for an autumn-themed trail mix.

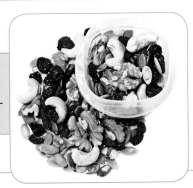

SALMON

There's something almost mythical about the life cycle of salmon. They hatch in inland freshwater streams and rivers. There the tiny fry mature into smolts ready to take on salt water before they head for the open ocean. Salmon reach maturity at sea, then return to their very place of beginning with an unerring homing device thought to involve both light sensing and smell. It is thought that geomagnetic imprinting plays a role. They spawn in these natal waters, and quickly die. Some salmon cover astounding distances in their journeys. One chinook salmon was tagged in the Aleutian Islands of the Pacific Ocean and recovered a year later in Idaho's Salmon River, having traveled some 3,500 miles.

For millions of years, these returning silver-colored fish have fed the land and its creatures with nutrients from the sea. The earliest evidence of people eating salmon comes from caves on the north coast of Spain and dates back as far as 16,000 years. Salmon bones some 7,000 years old have been recovered at a site on the Columbia River in Oregon.

PREP TIP ✦ CANNED SALMON

Many people think of canned salmon as an inferior food, or overlook it altogether. In fact it's highly nutritious and environmentally sound. Canned pink or sockeye salmon, which is labeled red salmon, is affordable and available on grocery shelves everywhere. It makes a wonderful sandwich melt. Toss it with a little mayonnaise, spoon it onto whole-grain bread topped with a thin slice of cheese, and put it under the broiler for a minute or two. Red salmon is canned with skin and bones cooked so they melt in your mouth, a highly bioaccessible source of magnesium, selenium, and calcium. Form it into patties with bread crumbs, mayonnaise, and mustard; broil for about ten minutes for a cheap, heart-healthy, protein-rich meal.

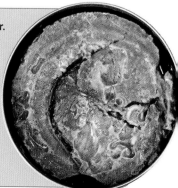

GIVES YOU

Protein
Niacin
Vitamin B12
Vitamin B6
Riboflavin
Vitamin D
Thiamine
Selenium
Phosphorus
Polyunsaturated fats

Choose and Use

Salmon is so rich and flavorful that common preparation methods tend to be light and healthy. Steaks can be pan-fried in a little olive oil, slow roasted, or grilled. Fillets are lovely poached, steamed in a foil pouch with lemon and garlic, fried in the skillet, or broiled.

For Your Health

On the question of protein quality and quantity, this silken, orange-fleshed fish stacks up well against beef. On the question of healthy fats? Salmon wins, hands down.

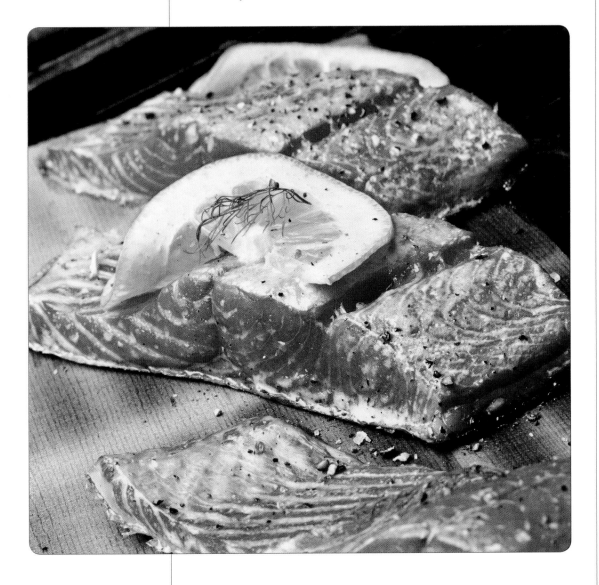

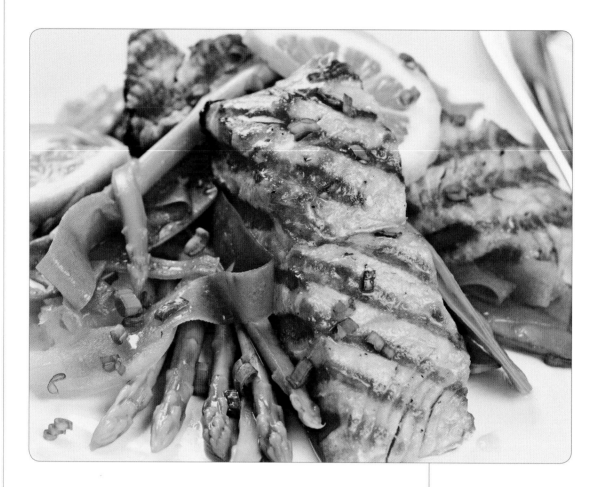

Salmon is one of the most bountiful sources of omega-3 fatty acids, polyunsaturated fats that may reduce a person's risk of heart disease, sudden cardiac death, stroke, and even arthritis and Alzheimer's disease. The particular omega-3s found in fish are especially beneficial. A review published in 2006 concluded that eating one or two weekly servings of fish, especially fatty fish like salmon that are high in marine omega-3s, reduces a person's chances of cardiac death by more than a third.

There are many possible mechanisms for this effect. The properties of omega-3s include effects on blood lipids called triglycerides, blood pressure, blood clotting, and heart rhythm.

For Our Planet
Go for wild Pacific salmon if possible—king (or Chinook), sock-eye (red), coho (silver), or pink (also called humpback)—and avoid farmed Atlantic salmon.

✦ TAKE AWAY

Salmon provides a wealth of fatty acids essential for cardiovascular health.

Lake trout and Arctic char are in the same family as salmon, have similarly lustrous pink flesh, and like salmon are rich in protein and omega-3 fatty acids. They're also environmentally responsible choices, for the most part. According to the Monterey Bay Aquarium, spotted seatrout wild-caught in Florida and Louisiana is a "best choice" from the standpoint of sustainability. It is advised, however, to limit consumption due to elevated mercury levels. Arctic char, generally farmed in closed, recirculating systems, is a "best choice" for marine sustainability.

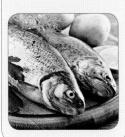

Pacific salmon are plentiful in waters off Alaska, Washington, and Oregon and are harvested in relatively sustainable ways. These were generally ranked as environmentally friendly choices as of 2013. But make sure to check these guides regularly; they change as fishing and aquaculture practices evolve.

The Atlantic salmon, which before the 19th century spawned in nearly every river of the American Northeast, now hangs on in small numbers at fewer than a dozen sites. Dams blocking major river systems and destruction of spawning habitat by development and agriculture are largely to blame.

Today, almost all Atlantic salmon sold in the U.S. is farm-raised, and most of it is imported from Canada, Norway, Chile, or the U.K. Unfortunately, farming has not been an eco-friendly alternative. Raised in pens in the ocean, millions of fish escape each year and can spread disease or breed with wild fish, perhaps making wild salmon populations less hardy. Salmon farms also release organic and chemical wastes into the ocean.

Though coho salmon farmed in inland tanks in the U.S. are an exception—and the industry is working to improve its methods—major environmental groups currently discourage the purchase of imported farmed salmon.

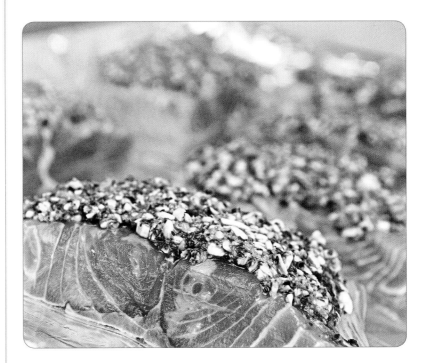

SESAME SEED

This tiny seed used for its oil and as a food was likely domesticated in the Indus Valley of northwestern India by 2500 B.C., spreading west to Mesopotamia by 2000 B.C. Still further west in ancient Egypt, the pharaoh Tutankhamun was entombed in 1323 B.C. with a variety of seeds, including sesame. An alabaster lamp in the shape of a lotus flower held traces of sesame oil.

The plant is an annual that stands a few feet high, with narrow deep-green leaves and a pale yellow trumpet-shaped flower. The sesame seed and its oil are common in Asian, Middle Eastern, African, and Indian dishes. Europeans and Americans favor the seed as a crunchy addition to bread and its crusts.

Choose and Use

Breads sprinkled with sesame seeds make a tasty, nutty complete protein, as does the popular Middle Eastern sesame paste tahini mixed with mashed chickpeas in hummus. The ancients used sesame seeds as a condiment mixed with herbs and salt to give flavor to foods. Tahini combined with olive oil, lemon juice, and spices makes a delightfully refreshing salad dressing. And sesame

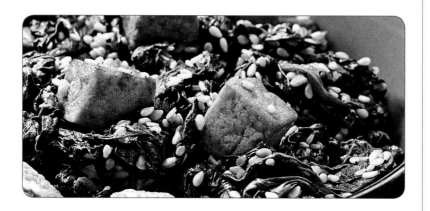

GIVES YOU

Protein
Dietary fiber
Thiamine
Niacin
Vitamin B6
Monounsaturated and
    polyunsaturated fats
Copper
Manganese
Calcium
Magnesium
Iron
Phosphorus
Zinc
Phytonutrients
    (phytosterols
    [lignans])

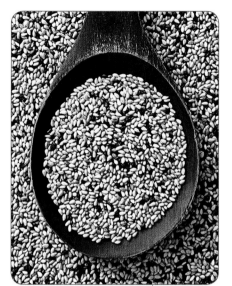

oil is great for stir-frying in a piping-hot wok, as it has a high smoke point. Sesame seeds come in a variety of colors, including brown, red, and black; darker seeds tend to have a stronger nut flavor and contain pigments with antioxidant properties. The antioxidants in sesame oil make it unusually slow to spoil.

For Your Health

An ounce of sesame seeds has almost five grams of protein and a sixth of your daily fiber. It is a powerhouse of minerals, providing more than a quarter of the daily requirement for calcium and nearly as much phosphorus, both important for building strong bones. Sesame seeds also provide ample supplies of zinc, critical to the immune system; antioxidants selenium and copper, which help the body absorb iron; and potassium and magnesium, which, when present in sufficient quantities in the diet, have been associated with lower blood pressure.

A good source of both mono- and polyunsaturated fats, sesame seeds are also replete with phytosterols, plant steroids that are similar to cholesterol and can block its absorption in the intestine. Consuming lots of phytosterol-dense foods has been shown to lower blood cholesterol. There's some evidence to suggest that phytosterols may also help prevent some forms of cancer.

For Our Planet

In the U.S., sesame growing occurs mostly in the Southwest, but the country imports more sesame than it grows. India and Guatemala are the top two sources. The drought-tolerant plant does well in poor climatic conditions and is an important cash crop in Nigeria, Sudan, and Ethiopia.

✦ TAKE AWAY

Sesame seeds add minerals and a tasty crunch to your dishes.

PREP TIP ✦ **TOASTING**

Sesame seeds are a favorite when it comes to Pan-Asian cooking. Toasting really brings out their flavor, and it's simple in a hot pan on the stovetop. Black and white sesame seeds create a pretty crust for seared fish like tuna.

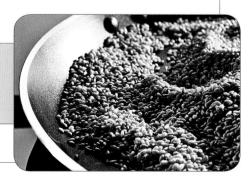

SMALL SILVER FISH: ANCHOVY, HERRING, MACKEREL, SARDINE

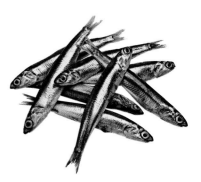

Anchovy, herring, mackerel, and sardine each comprise a number of species. The U.S. Food and Drug Administration lists 19 species that may be sold as anchovy, and 13 for which the marketing label "sardine" is permitted.

All these fish swim in schools near the surface of the ocean, and, at least when they are small, feed on plankton while themselves providing nourishment to sea birds, marine mammals, and larger fish.

People have enjoyed these fatty, protein-rich fish for thousands of years, inventing methods for smoking, pickling, fermenting, and packaging them to protect against rapid spoilage, a problem because of their highly unsaturated, very long chain fatty acid content.

Ancient Greeks and Romans used small fatty fish such as anchovies in a sauce called *garum*, salting them and allowing them to ferment in the sun for weeks or months. The fish paste itself fed the poor, whereas the liquid it exuded went to the upper classes.

"Kippers," the split and cold-smoked herring dish, was developed in the 19th century and is beloved by the English.

CONSIDER ✦ CHOOSE CANNED

Sardines, anchovies, and the like can be found fresh at your fishmonger's counter, but far easier is finding them on supermarket shelves. Inexpensive, they're a great ingredient to keep on hand in the pantry and are a sustainable choice because they are low on the food chain.

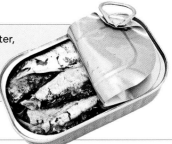

PREP TIP ✦ **PAIR WITH AROMATICS**

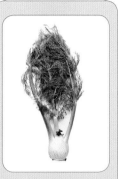

Most people have little experience with silver fishes, such as anchovies, other than as part of a classic Caesar salad or an occasional pizza topping. Pairing anchovies and other richly flavored, oily fish with fresh, crisp vegetables like fennel or celery provides balance and texture. For a special hors d'oeuvre or light lunch, serve on whole grain crackers or crispbread.

✦ **TAKE AWAY**

Try canned fish on crackers for a heart-healthy snack.

During the Napoleonic wars of the early 19th century, the French government offered a prize for a method of food preservation it could use to supply soldiers in the field; this resulted in canning, and, by 1820, the first canned sardines. Canned sardines became enormously popular among Americans during World War I, leading to the rise and eventual fall of Cannery Row, a concentration of sardine canneries in Monterey, California, made famous by John Steinbeck's 1945 novel by the same name. Scientists now believe naturally occurring climatic fluctuations may have contributed to the collapse of the Monterey sardine fishery, long attributed to overfishing.

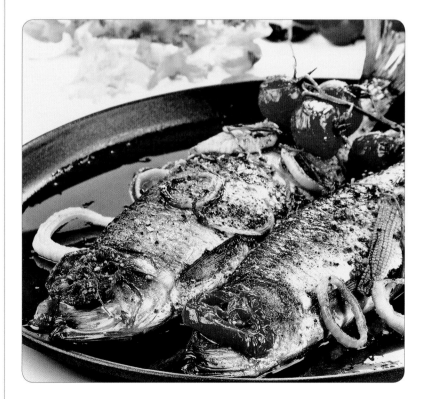

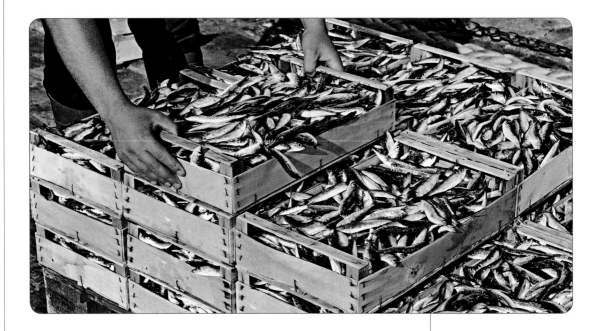

Choose and Use

With the occasional exception of mackerel and herring, these fish generally come to us heavily salted and canned or jarred in oil. Rinsing in water will somewhat reduce sodium content. Though all oil packaging boosts calories, many of these small fish are packaged in olive oil or other unsaturated fats, which are often heart-healthy monounsaturates. As with tuna, water-packed alternatives are usually available; some prefer their more delicate consistency. If you're fortunate enough to find any of these small, oily fish fresh, try grilling or lightly pan frying them; canned are delicious on crackers or in Mediterranean pasta and salad dishes.

For Your Health

Like the prized salmon and trout, these humbler oily fish are rich in omega-3 fatty acids, the polyunsaturated fats that may reduce a person's risk of heart disease, sudden cardiac death, stroke, arthritis, Alzheimer's disease, and age-related macular degeneration. Herring and mackerel also provide some mono-unsaturated fats, which lower blood cholesterol among other health benefits.

A 2013 study following 2,700 people age 65 and older over 16 years found that those with the highest blood levels of marine omega-3s (levels attainable by eating about five ounces of

GIVES YOU

Protein
Polyunsaturated fats
Vitamin D
Niacin
Vitamin B12
Vitamin B6
Riboflavin
Selenium
Magnesium
Phosphorus
Calcium
Iron

Puttanesca is common in Italy, a simple variation on tomato sauce featuring chopped anchovies and black olives. It's also a great way to boost the nutrition of pasta and get healthful omega-3s into finicky palates: your kids probably won't notice, and you'll enjoy the additional richness and flavor.

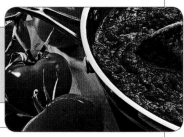

anchovy or herring a week) lived, on average, more than two years longer than those with lower levels.

Eating the soft bones of small mackerel, anchovies, and sardines also provides a concentrated source of calcium. Sardines, meanwhile, are an excellent source of vitamin D, needed to help the bones absorb calcium. Most people living in the northern hemisphere are deficient in vitamin D due to inadequate sun exposure; individuals who are older or obese are especially at risk.

For Our Planet

These little fish occupy the bottom of the food chain, feeding on tiny organisms and bits of algae. That makes them a more environmentally efficient source of food energy than larger fish. Indeed small oily fish are frequent ingredients in the fishmeal fed to livestock as well as farmed fish; it takes more than three pounds of these wild ocean fish to produce a single pound of farm-raised salmon—a concerning drawback of salmon aquaculture.

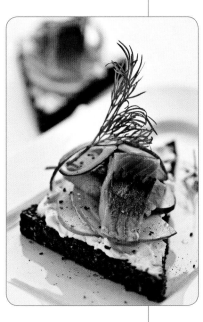

Fish lower on the food chain are also less likely to contain dangerous levels of mercury than larger fish such as tuna, due to their short lifespans and the fact that they don't eat other fish whose flesh may contain the pollutant. The larger king mackerel is an important exception; the U.S. Food and Drug Administration (FDA) advises pregnant and nursing women and young children to avoid it, although moderate consumption is fine for healthy adults.

It's also a good idea to check the Monterey Bay Aquarium or another seafood sustainability guide for up-to-date information on vulnerable fisheries. As of 2013, Monterey Bay advised avoiding sardines from the Mediterranean (Atlantic sardines) because of overfishing.

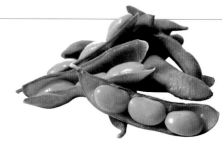

SOYBEAN

Some scientists are questioning the long-held theory that the Chinese alone domesticated the soybean some three thousand years ago. Analyses of charred remains from China, Japan, and Korea suggest that the small wild legume may have been eaten in China as long as nine thousand years ago, and domesticated there perhaps 5,000 years ago. Larger, domesticated types of soybean appear in Japan around the same time, and in Korea about 2,000 years later; it's possible people in these locations domesticated soybeans independently from the Chinese.

In any event, this nutritious legume has formed the basis of traditional foods prepared in these Asian societies for over a thousand years, including soy sauce (made from fermented soybeans), miso (a fermented soybean paste), and tofu (made from soymilk much as cheese is produced from animal milk).

Choose and Use

Texturized soy protein, the ingredient in many "fake" meats, retains much of the original soybean's fiber and other nutrients, as do roasted soy nuts and edamame, the soybean harvested and eaten while still green. Plain soybeans, dry or canned, can be used as you would any beans, in burritos, salads, soups, or stews, for example.

For Your Health

Soybeans get into Western diets in many ways, most often with their oil—which accounts for nearly 80 percent of edible oil consumed in the U.S. Soy protein, which goes into all sorts of processed foods, soy-based frozen desserts, nutrition bars, and (rehydrated into texturized soy protein) meat extenders and substitutes.

PREP TIP ✦ EDAMAME

Edamame is a Japanese favorite, common in sushi restaurants. Grab a bag of soybeans from the freezer and steam briefly, then serve in a bowl lightly salted for a different kind of snack.

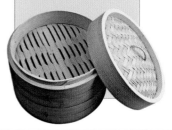

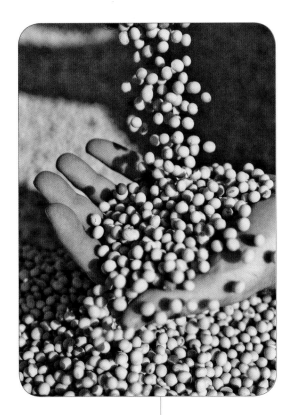

Taken whole—cooked like any other legume—the soybean provides protein comparable to that of an egg, with lots of fiber (40 percent of suggested daily intake in a cup), and plenty of iron. Its oil, quite low in saturated fat, is more than 50 percent linoleic acid, a polyunsaturated fat that lowers cholesterol when replacing unhealthy fats in the diet.

A great deal of research has focused on possible benefits from soy isoflavones, a type of flavonoid that binds (weakly) to estrogen receptors and thus has been proposed as a possible mechanism important in the prevention of heart disease, osteoporosis, and cancers of the breast, uterus, and prostate. However, a 2006 research review by an American Heart Association scientific committee concluded that the cardiovascular benefit of soy protein or isoflavones is "minimal at best," and evidence for benefits in bone loss and cancer is meager. On the other hand, the committee endorsed the notion that, because of their fiber, protein, favorable fat profile, and vitamins and minerals, soy products are a heart-healthy replacement for animal products high in saturated fat. For more on tofu, see pages 216–217.

For Our Planet

In the U.S., about 90 percent of the soybean crop consists of the "Roundup Ready" variety, genetically modified to survive applications of the commonly used weed killer. This has increased yields and cut down on the need for deep plowing with heavy equipment, which, proponents argue, maintains soil. But genetically modified crops are highly controversial, not least because of concerns about how they will affect the surrounding ecosystem. A study published in 2012 found that, rather than reducing the overall use of herbicides as claimed, Roundup Ready crops led to the development of herbicide-resistant weeds—something that also occurs with non-genetically modified crops—which actually led to increased herbicide use.

GIVES YOU

Protein
Dietary fiber
Polyunsaturated fats
Vitamin K
Riboflavin
Folate
Vitamin B6
Thiamine
Manganese
Iron
Phosphorus
Magnesium
Copper
Potassium
Selenium
Calcium
Zinc
Phytonutrients
   (flavonoids,
   phytosterols)

TOFU

The first step in making tofu is to cook ground soybeans in water, then strain out the fibrous solids. To the resulting soy milk the preparer adds a coagulant that causes the milk to separate into liquid whey and firmer lumps called curds. Pressed into cakes, these curds make the smooth, mild food popular in many Asian countries, especially China and Japan.

Tofu probably originated in ancient China well before its earliest documentation in A.D. 950. People may have stumbled on the process accidentally, perhaps by adding unrefined salt to a soybean stew or allowing it to coagulate under the influence of lactic-acid bacteria. Or maybe they learned the technique from migrating Mongolian herders, who had experience making a fermented-milk product.

Choose and Use

The harder the tofu, the more fat, calories, and protein it contains. Tofu processed with calcium sulfate as a coagulant will provide more calcium.

Tofu is a very versatile food that takes up cooking flavors. Silken tofu adds protein to smoothies and a creamy mayonnaise-like texture to sandwich spreads, salad dressings, pasta sauces, and sweet puddings; it's great chunked in soup, too. Firm or extra-firm tofu is excellent sautéed, stir-fried, or marinated and grilled; try it in a sandwich.

A light and zesty Japanese summertime dish is cubed silken tofu topped with fresh ginger, soy sauce, scallions, and other flavorings.

For Your Health

Though lower in fiber than other soy products, tofu offers ample quantities of protein as well as calcium, a real plus, especially for people who avoid dairy foods.

GIVES YOU

Protein
Manganese
Calcium
Iron
Phosphorus
Polyunsaturated fats
Phytonutrients
  (flavonoids)

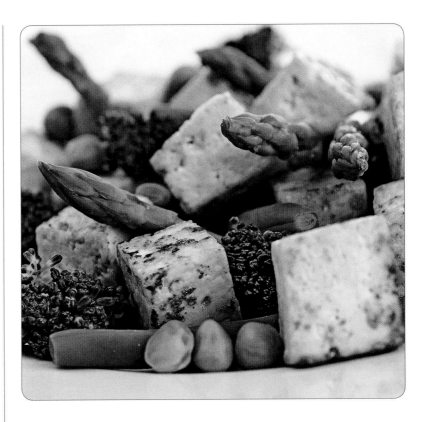

Miso, an ancient Japanese food, is a thick paste made by fermenting soybeans with salt and a special fungus. It's used as a flavoring for the familiar miso soup, as well as meat, fish, and tofu dishes, Miso has protein, fiber, and minerals (including calcium) but is also very high in sodium. Tempeh looks a bit like tofu, but it's made with whole soybeans instead of soymilk, contains more protein and fiber than tofu, and has a stronger, "meatier" texture. It comes from Indonesia, and is made by fermenting soybeans with fungus. You can slice or crumble tempeh and use it as a meat substitute in just about any dish, from burgers to stir-fries.

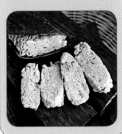

Some claims about the benefits of soy protein—that it offers important protection against heart disease and may prevent a host of cancers—have not been established unequivocally, according to a 2006 review by the American Heart Association. On the other hand, studies show that eating soy protein modestly improves cholesterol levels, so replacing saturated-fat-laden animal proteins such as cheese and meat with soy foods like tofu is likely to be a healthy change, for both you and the planet. A 2008 review concludes that soy protein also appears to slow bone loss in postmenopausal women.

For Our Planet

Eating plant-based proteins almost always has a gentler impact on the natural world than consuming animal products, and tofu is no exception. It's a cruelty-free, resource-efficient food whose production requires no animal feed and only a fraction of the water (about 244 gallons per pound) required to produce the same amount of chicken (about 815 gallons). The waste pulp of the soybean is often fed to animals.

TUNA

With its powerful tail and sleek body, the tuna plies the world's open oceans, a predator built for speed. Tuna spines discovered in a cave in East Timor, an island south of Indonesia, represent the earliest evidence of humans eating tuna, and indeed of advanced fishing techniques, since to harvest the meaty fish requires taking to the sea. The find dates to 42,000 years ago.

There are 15 species of tuna, a subgroup of the mackerel family, but 4 species make up the bulk of those caught for food: skipjack (roughly 60 percent of the catch), yellowfin (24 percent), bigeye (10 percent), and albacore (5 percent). The highly prized bluefin tuna fishery has been drastically overexploited and is subject to international quotas.

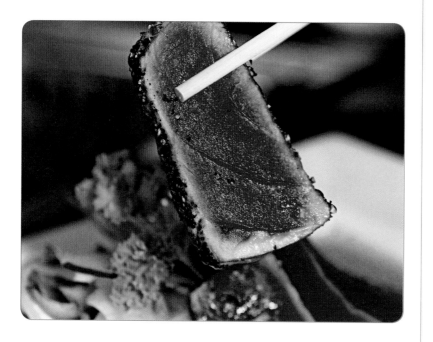

GIVES YOU

Protein
Thiamine
Niacin
Vitamin B6
Vitamin B12
Vitamin D
Selenium
Phosphorous
Potassium
Magnesium
Polyunsaturated fats

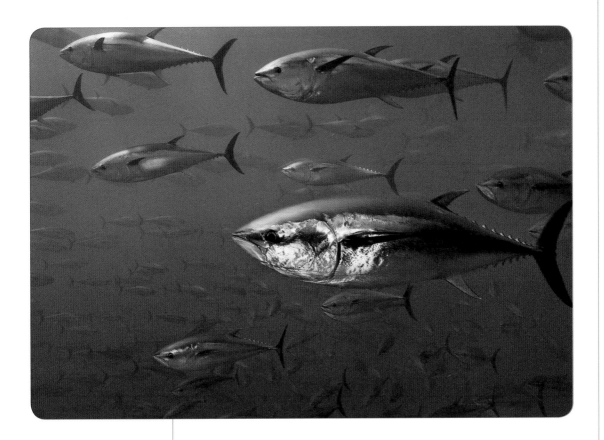

Choose and Use

Long-lived tuna tend to absorb mercury, the pollutant generated by industrial activities that settles into the ocean. For that reason, the U.S. Environmental Protection Agency (EPA) advises childbearing women and young children to limit consumption of "white" albacore tuna (which is higher in mercury) to six ounces a week, and canned "light" tuna to two meals (12 ounces) per week. Albacore (the only species canned as white tuna) along with bluefin tuna (found most often in sushi) are the species highest in omega-3 fatty acids. Frozen or fresh tuna steaks are most often yellowfin.

For Your Health

Tuna is a great protein source that's also high in healthy fish oil, with albacore tuna being comparable to some salmon species in marine omega-3 fatty acids. This type of polyunsaturated fat, population studies suggest, lowers the risk for heart disease, stroke, heart arrhythmias, as well as arthritis and Alzheimer's

✦ TAKE AWAY

Tuna is high in essential fatty acids, but it also absorbs mercury, so enjoy it in moderation.

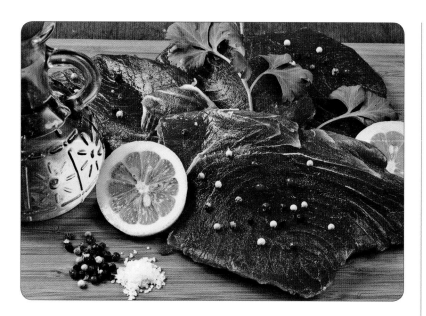

disease. Polyunsaturated fat is especially important in fetal development during pregnancy for brain and eye health. Some types of tuna are rich in potassium and magnesium, both important for maintaining healthy blood pressure and heart rhythm. A three-ounce serving of canned white (albacore) tuna offers 80 percent of a day's recommended intake of selenium, an antioxidant mineral that's vital to immune functioning and possibly cancer prevention.

For Our Planet

Tuna presents even the most environmentally responsible consumer with a confusing picture. Whether or not a particular tuna product can be considered sustainably caught depends on the species of tuna, how it was caught, and where. For example, most environmental groups caution against the use of the purse seine with a "fish aggregating device" (a large net similar to a bag with a drawstring encloses schools attracted by a floating object) as well as the longline (a very extensive line set at intervals with baited hooks) because of unacceptably high bycatch; these methods may snag and kill other fish, sharks, dolphins, sea birds, and sea turtles.

The Monterey Bay Aquarium discourages eating the massively overfished bluefin tuna in any context. Meanwhile, there are six stocks of albacore tuna in the world's oceans; most albacore are

PAIRINGS
✦
TUNA NIÇOISE

Tuna Niçoise is a popular salad in France and includes tuna, black olives, hard-cooked egg, green beans, and potatoes with Dijon or anchovy dressing. The traditional dish uses canned tuna, an economical choice that works perfectly for this dinner salad; a special version might substitute a seared tuna steak.

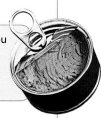

CONSIDER ✦ CHOOSING CANNED TUNA

Convenient and nutritious, no pantry should be without canned tuna. Selecting the best choice for you and the planet begins by reading the labels. Choose cans with no added sodium, which your body doesn't need. "Oil-packed" tuna can provide additional flavor, and most are healthy unsaturates, but "water-packed" is lower in calories. And don't forget to consult a sustainable seafood guide.

harvested from the Pacific, but one stock—North Atlantic albacore—is overfished, and its products are best avoided.

Here's the rub: At the fishmonger or in the grocery aisle, you usually cannot discover the provenance of a particular tuna product. Canned "chunk light" tuna is mostly skipjack, but how was it caught? Where did that *particular* albacore (steak or canned) come from—and was it harvested by minimal-bycatch pole and line?

The only practical approach is to go with marketers that have vetted their seafood sources. Find a fishmonger you trust. Or look online for products certified by the Marine Stewardship Council. Greenpeace endorses boutique brands like Wild Planet, as well as Safeway's "Safeway Select" canned tuna, caught by purse seine without fish aggregating devices, and Whole Foods "365" brand tuna, caught by pole and line.

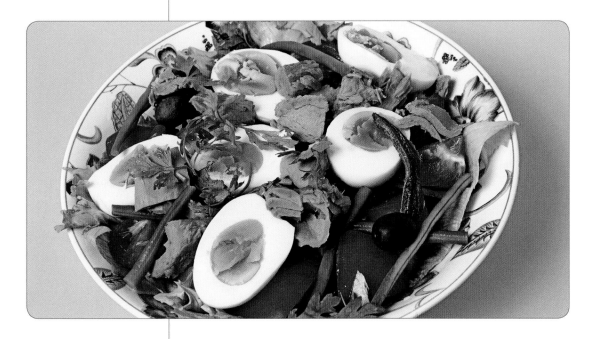

TURKEY

Several native species of turkey inhabited the Americas in the millennia before Columbus arrived on New World shores. Scientists believe the Aztecs of Mexico were the first to domesticate turkey. New research suggests this same domesticated turkey may have reached Mayan people in Guatemala by 2,000 years ago, and that the Anasazi of the U.S. Southwest domesticated their own turkey around 200 B.C.—not for food, but for feathers to use in rituals and to adorn blankets and robes. The Wampanoag, who took part in a harvest festival with the pilgrims of Massachusetts in 1621 (commemorated today as Thanksgiving) hunted but did not keep turkeys.

Choose and Use
When watching saturated fat and calories, skip the skin. Ground turkey breast made into patties with seasonings makes a tasty and nutritious, planet-friendlier alternative to beef burgers. Like other poultry, turkey carries bacteria such as *Salmonella* that can cause food poisoning; safe handling means washing hands, surfaces, and utensils after contact with raw turkey, and cooking it thoroughly to kill any bacteria.

For Your Health
Turkey is a lean, low-calorie protein source—with a whole lot less saturated fat than pork and beef.
   It's also comparatively high in iron and potassium, especially the dark meat. Like other meats, turkey is a good source of B-complex vitamins, which help the body produce energy from food and support normal nerve functioning.

For Our Planet
The Environmental Working Group lists turkey as a "good" meat choice, based on associated greenhouse gas emissions.

GIVES YOU

Protein
Niacin
Vitamin B6
Riboflavin)
Potassium
Selenium
Phosphorus
Zinc
Iron

✦ TAKE AWAY

Turkey is a naturally lean meat, but remove the fatty skin.

PAIRINGS
✦
**GROUND BEEF
SUBSTITUTE**

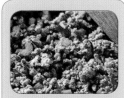

Ground beef is a common ingredient in dishes ranging from hamburgers and tacos to stews and casseroles. Any recipe that calls for beef can easily swap in turkey or chicken with similar results. While not the exact same flavor as beef, the seasonings and spices used in your recipe will no doubt keep your tastebuds happy. Selecting poultry over beef is a greener choice given the lower amount of resources needed to produce it.

But in conventional husbandry, the birds are often raised in enormous, densely packed barns and given antibiotics routinely to accelerate growth and control infection; this can promote the development of antibiotic-resistant germs. Bred for quick-growing and very large breasts, the Broad-Breasted White turkey sold by nearly all commercial producers cannot mate naturally and often ends up painfully overweight and lame.

There are also a lot of smaller-scale turkey farms in the U.S., including a few farms that raise heritage breeds like the Bourbon Red or Narragansett; these are more expensive than grocery-store turkeys, but in taste tests they win hands-down. Other good options are organic and/or free-range or "pasture-raised" turkeys; they're more humanely treated than conventionally raised birds and may be leaner and healthier, too.

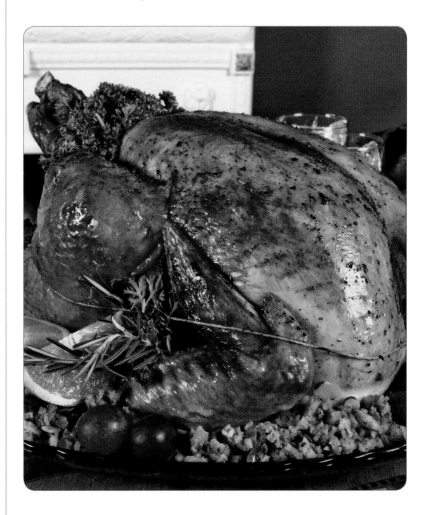

WALNUT

People probably first began to cultivate the walnut tree in the Caucasus 7,000 years ago. It's likely they gathered them even earlier in the nut tree's native range from the Balkans to the Himalayas. Enjoyed along with fruit after a meal, the large, protein-rich walnut was a favorite of the ancient Romans, and it spread throughout the empire. Whole walnuts lay on a table in the Temple of Isis at Pompei when the town was destroyed by the eruption of Mount Vesuvius in A.D. 79.

Though the peanut (which is actually a legume, not a tree nut) accounts for more than half of Americans' overall nut consumption today, the walnut's chewy texture and slightly bitter flavor make it the most popular nut for baking.

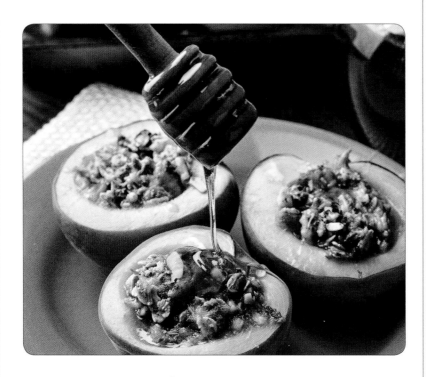

GIVES YOU

Protein
Dietary fiber
Vitamin E
Vitamin B6
Folate
Thiamine
Manganese
Copper
Magnesium
Phosphorus
Iron
Zinc
Monounsaturated and
    polyunsaturated fats
Phytonutrients (phenolic
    acids, flavonoids,
    phytosterols)

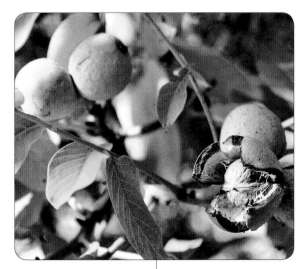

Choose and Use

Walnuts are extremely versatile, suited to savory and sweet foods alike. Sprinkle them into oatmeal, on salads—try spinach and spring greens, fruit such as pear, and a little blue cheese—or sauté them into pasta, rice, or cooked vegetables. They give breads and pastries a nutritional lift and heartier flavor. When looking to snack, watch out for products that have added sodium.

For Your Health

Among nuts, walnuts are uniquely high in phytonutrients. A 2007 study reviewing the chemical composition of ten nuts found they are number one in total phenols, a class of phytonutrients that includes phenolic acids and flavonoids, and ranked second in antioxidant capacity.

In a 2009 review of 13 small trials, researchers concluded that diets enriched with walnuts lowered total and "bad" low-density lipoprotein (LDL) cholesterol. Other small studies of walnut-enriched diets have shown reduced markers of inflammation, lower blood pressure, and improved function of the lining of blood vessels (which helps regulate blood pressure and clotting). And a 2013 study following 135,000 women over 10 years found those who ate the most walnuts lowered the risk of type 2 diabetes.

A little goes a long way, though; like all nuts, they are energy-dense and just an ounce of walnuts packs more than 180 calories.

For Our Planet

The U.S. is the second-largest grower of walnuts in the world, after China, and the world's biggest exporter. The vast bulk of this crop is grown in California, on thousands of farms averaging about 50 acres in size. Young trees don't bear for several years, but they typically live 75 years. Cash crops such as corn are sometimes grown between the tree rows while a walnut grove matures. Walnut trees put down very deep roots that help them survive drought and retain soil. The very hard hulls of the walnut are used commercially in various products, including plastics and glues, abrasive cleaners, and insulation.

PAIRINGS
◆
WALNUT PAIRINGS

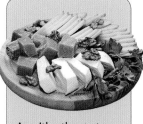

As with other nuts, toasting brings out the flavor of walnuts. Their slightly bitter taste pairs well with rich cheeses and are a terrific addition to green salads including citrus or berries; a vinaigrette made using walnut oil is the perfect dressing.

WHITE FISH: HAKE, HADDOCK, HALIBUT, FLOUNDER, COD, SOLE, POLLACK

Whereas oily fish are pelagic—they swim in the open water column—white fish are often demersal species, meaning they live near the sea floor where it's dark and food is relatively scarce. They eat mollusks, crustaceans, small fish, worms, and sea squirts.

The oil in white fish is concentrated in the liver. This tiny organ is dense with nutrients; indeed, discovery of the properties of cod liver oil in the 1930s led to the conquest of rickets, a severe vitamin D deficiency. However, processing the fish for food removes the liver, leaving flesh that is very lean and rather delicate of flavor.

By around A.D. 1000, the seagoing Vikings fished for cod from their longships, establishing an early international trade in cod, salted and dried for long-distance travel, between the Nordic countries and western Europe.

CONSIDER ✦ CHOOSING FISH

How is a person to know what to make for dinner considering the wide variety of fish at the seafood counter? While there are some minor differences in flavor and texture, the similarities make them equally good choices when it comes to simple seafood suppers. Chatting with your fishmonger about which is fish is freshest and in season is a good place to start. You'll also want to consult a sustainable seafood guide to understand which choices are the greenest.

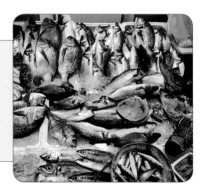

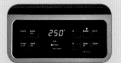

Many people are intimidated by cooking fish, but it's actually one of the simplest things you can prepare for dinner. Like other animal proteins, however, fish can dry out and become tough and flavorless if overcooked. A sure-proof way to ensure perfectly cooked and moist fish is by slow roasting at low heat for 30 to 45 minutes. (Time varies by thickness.)

GIVES YOU

Protein
Niacin
Vitamin B6
Vitamin B12
Vitamin D
Phosphorus
Selenium
Magnesium

Choose and Use

Rounder fish such as cod may be cut into steaks (across the bone), which grill nicely. Flat fish such as sole and flounders you'll find in fillets. These tender cuts do better with gentle treatments such as steaming (or baking in foil), poaching, broiling, or pan-frying. Halibut, cod, and pollack are fairly firm. Flounder and sole are delicate and easily overcooked; the fish is done as soon as it turns opaque throughout, about 10 minutes for each inch of thickness.

In general, any of these mild white fishes can be substituted for another. Cod is the traditional basis for the not-so-healthy, deep-fried fish and chips, but any white fish can be coated in egg, seasoning, and flour or cornmeal and pan-fried for a somewhat healthier approach that locks in flavor and moisture. Marinating

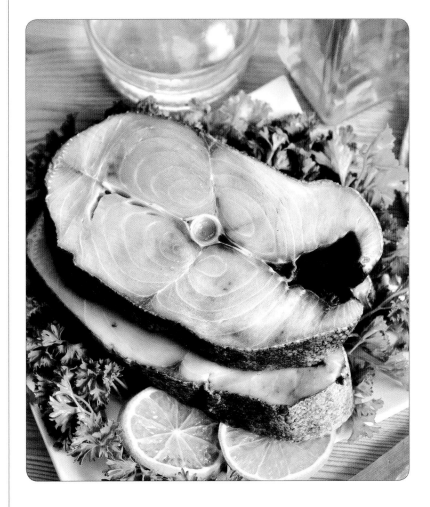

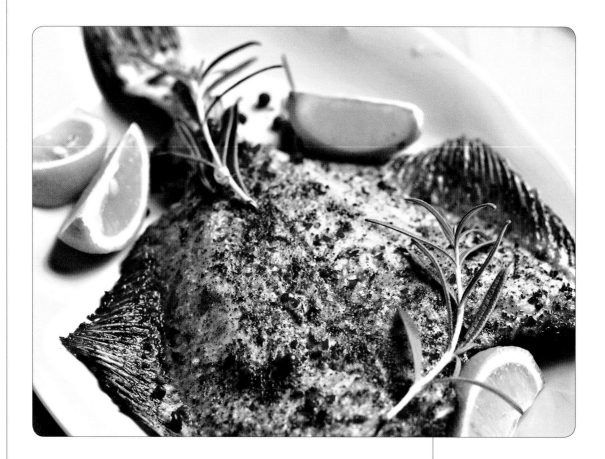

also helps keep these mild fish juicy, although some people find their subtle flavor is best accented with just a drizzle of olive oil or a little garlic, some herbs, and a squeeze of lemon.

For Your Health

The American Heart Association recommends eating at least two servings of fish—preferably fatty fish—each week, and that's largely due to the benefits of fish oil to the heart.

White fish are very low in oil, so they're much lower in omega-3 fatty acids than oily fish such as salmon or herring. Even so, the fat they do contain is largely healthy. And as a lean, low-calorie, low-sodium source of protein, white fish are an eminently healthy food in their own right.

White fish are particularly good sources of B-complex vitamins. Deficiencies of B6 and B12 are not uncommon among the elderly and heavy drinkers, among other groups. These vitamins are important regulators of homocysteine, a marker

✦ **TAKE AWAY**

These mild fishes taste divine with seasoning— olive oil, lemon, pepper, and parsley.

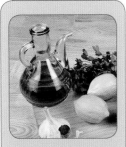

Because white fishes are so mild-flavored, they're a great way to get children eating more seafood. Those newer to eating fish may help their tastebuds adjust by serving it with simple sauces; ingredients like mustard and dill or lemon and parsley are wonderful complements. Far simpler, seasoning the fish with a bit of salt and pepper and a drizzle of olive oil is a lighter dish that's perfect for a weeknight meal.

for cardiovascular disease; they help the body metabolize food for energy and are vital to normal nerve function and the production of hemoglobin (a red protein that carries oxygen in the blood).

For Our Planet

Whether a white fish is sustainable depends on the particular species and how and where it's harvested. The Monterey Bay Aquarium's Seafood Watch program lists Pacific flat fish such as sole, flounder, and halibut as "good alternatives"—meaning there are concerns, but the negative environmental impacts associated are less extensive than those for items on the "avoid" list.

Cod and pollack are more problematic. According to Seafood Watch, most Atlantic cod available in the U.S. comes from well-managed fisheries of Iceland and the northeast Arctic; but only a small proportion of these cod are caught with hook and line, a technique with minimal environmental impact. Some cod fisheries are depleted by overfishing, and both cod and pollack are often gathered by bottom trawlers that scrape the ocean floor, destroying precious habitat.

The simplest approach may be to shop grocery chains with sustainable-seafood policies. Greenpeace conducts an annual CATO (Carting Away the Oceans) study, ranking major supermarket chains on their concern for sustainable seafood. See the most recent report at www.greenpeace.org/seafood.

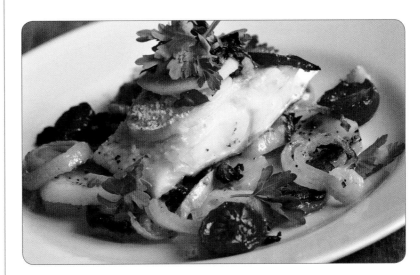

YOGURT

Early yogurt making has left little trace in the archaeological record. One theory about the origins of this tangy fermented food holds that, some 7,000 years ago, goat herders of Central Asia learned the process after noticing that milk carried in skins thickened and soured into an edible and longer-lasting food. The bacteria required to make yogurt might have come from plants or from the animal-skin sacs. The food then moved across Iran to Turkey ("yogurt" is a Turkish word whose root means "to condense") and the Balkans, as well as south to India.

The Nobel prize–winning Russian microbiologist Ilya Mechnikov first popularized yogurt as a health food in 1908 with a paper attributing the astonishing longevity of Bulgarian peasants to benign bacteria in yogurt that crowded out disease-causing germs.

Choose and Use

Greek-style yogurts tend to be significantly higher in protein and lower in sugar, but also higher in saturated fat. Choose non- or low-fat varieties of any yogurt (low-fat dairy consumption may be associated with reductions in blood pressure). Also check labels for sugar and calories, as they vary dramatically by flavor and type of yogurt.

Mixing yogurt with oats or other grains and fruit is a familiar favorite, but try cooking with it, too—in dips, salad dressings, sauces for savory dishes, and soups.

For Your Health

Yogurt's felicitous effects on the bowel are related to its "friendly" bacteria—two organisms specifically approved for this use by the U.S. Food and Drug Administration (FDA),

GIVES YOU

Protein
Calcium
Phosphorus)
Riboflavin
Vitamin B12
Probiotics

✦ **TAKE AWAY**

Enjoy yogurt's plentiful probiotics, but avoid flavored yogurts high in fat and sugar.

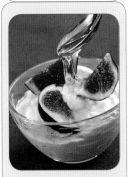

Fruit yogurt may sound healthy, but often, fruity additives contribute little nutritionally, while turning yogurt into a confection along the lines of ice cream or pudding. Select nonfat to retain the nutrients while keep the calorie and sugar at bay. And for a healthier dessert alternative, add chopped fruit or berries of your choice and drizzle with a bit of honey or agave.

Lactobacillus bulgaris and *Streptococcus thermophiles.* They convert milk sugars to lactic acid. Sometimes manufacturers add other bacteria such as *Lactobacillus acidophilus* for enhanced "probiotic" effect, establishing helpful organisms that will out-compete pathogenic bacteria in the digestive tract.

Research on probiotics is evolving, but studies have shown that consuming live-bacteria yogurts can help ease digestive troubles associated with irritable bowel syndrome, and stem the diarrhea that can result from taking antibiotics. Plain, low-fat yogurt tops the list of calcium-rich foods, which makes it a great snack for children age 9 to 13, teenage girls, middle-aged women, and the elderly, all at risk for inadequate intake of the bone-building mineral.

For Our Planet

Nonorganic yogurt raises all the environmental and animal-welfare issues associated with the conventional dairy industry. Animals are often treated with antibiotics, as well as growth hormones that increase their milk production but raise the animals' risk of lameness and painful udder infections. Dairy cattle produce methane, an important greenhouse gas, and waste ponds associated with large concentrated feeding operations can pollute the air with ammonia.

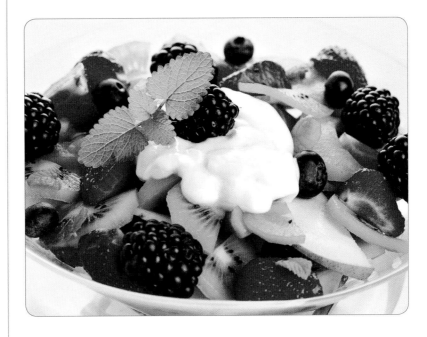

WHOLE GRAINS

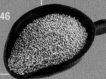

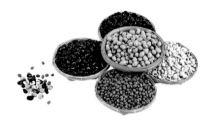

Beginning some 12,000 years ago, during the Neolithic agricultural revolution, humans learned to cultivate the cereals that grew naturally in their environments—wheat in the Near East, rice in China, maize in Central and South America, sorghum in Africa—and settled down in the first permanent villages to reap their increasingly ample harvests. As agriculture emerged and spread around the globe, cereal grains took up a central place in the human diet.

The ability to produce large quantities of carbohydrate-rich food led to population explosions, which in turn gave rise to more complex and stratified societies. But scientists believe that early farmers may actually have been less healthy than their hunter-gatherer predecessors. Reliance on a few staples—principally cereal grains—meant nutritional gaps, intermittent famine, and, eventually, smaller bodies, weaker bones and teeth, and shorter lives.

Today, cereal grains are still the very stuff of life for humanity, with eight cereals—wheat, maize, rice, barley, sorghum, oats, rye, and millet—accounting for more than half the calories and about half the protein consumed around the world. Without these staples, the planet would never have come to support seven billion human beings; deprived of grains today, many would starve. The cereal grains provide energy in the form of carbohydrates, some protein, and unsaturated fats; they fortify the body with B-complex vitamins, minerals, fiber, and an array of phytonutrients that may have anti-inflammatory and other salubrious effects. Cutting out grains to avoid carbohydrates or gluten (to which a growing number of people are sensitive, although frank celiac disease is relatively rare) doesn't necessarily yield a healthier diet, and often requires careful planning to provide fiber and other valuable phytonutrients grains provide.

Grain Values

Grains don't give the body everything it needs, of course. For example, they tend to lack vitamins A and C (ascorbic acid), calcium, and some of the essential amino acids that together make a nutritionally "complete" protein. (Quinoa is a notable example of a grain that includes all the essential amino acids humans need, which is partly why the United Nations named 2013 the International Year of Quinoa.) In some parts of the developing world, reliance on a cereal-based diet leads to iron or zinc deficiency. Unlike other cereals, corn contains a form of niacin (a metabolite of nicotine also called vitamin B3) that's not absorbable;

some Africans whose diets are dominated by this staple suffer from the skin sores, diarrhea, and mental impairment of pellagra, a deficiency disease 18th-century Europeans called corn sickness.

While over-reliance on a single cheap staple can lead to nutritional deficiencies, an additional problem is that oftentimes grains have been processed to remove coarse outer layers containing the valuable germ and bran—and along with them much of the food's nutritional value.

Grain Components

Until the 19th century, when the Industrial Revolution brought mechanization to the milling process, most people ate whole grains—whole wheat, brown rice, whole rye, and barley. But people soon came to prefer the soft texture and mild flavor of refined grain products, in part because they came to see "brown bread" and other traditional whole-grain foods as the province of a countrified lower class.

A cereal grain has three basic components. Enclosing the kernel are protective bran layers, which contain fiber, minerals, vitamins, and phytonutrients. Inside, at the base of the seed, is the germ. This is the plant's embryo, ready to sprout under the right conditions; it's replete with vitamins, unsaturated fats, and phytonutrients. Nestled beside the germ, accounting for most of the kernel's bulk, is the endosperm; this is the germ's starchy food source, and it's full of carbohydrates, along with protein and a small quantity of vitamins and minerals.

Refined grains are processed to eliminate most or all of the bran and germ, leaving only the carbohydrate-rich yet relatively nutrient-poor endosperm. This provides energy but is low in nutritional quality. In response to outbreaks of pellagra and other problems related to malnutrition, in the 1940s the U.S. government required refined grain products to be enriched with iron as well as B-complex vitamins niacin, riboflavin, and niacin; folate was added in the 1990s after studies showed that the babies of pregnant women who consume plenty of this B-complex vitamin are less likely to be born with spina bifida and other neural tube defects.

But even enriched white wheat flour has 25 percent less protein than whole wheat flour, as well as lower levels of vitamin E, some B-complex vitamins, and the minerals magnesium, manganese, potassium, and zinc. White flour contains less than one-quarter of the fiber of whole-wheat flour.

Healthy Whole Grains

The bottom line: Despite the current dietary fads focused on the low-grain diets of the Paleolithic period, people who eat diets high in whole grains tend to have lower rates of largely preventable diseases such as heart disease, stroke, type 2 diabetes, and perhaps colorectal cancer. The fiber in whole grains helps the digestive system function well and also helps people eating a plant-based diet maintain a healthy weight.

A survey in 2000 by the market-research firm NDP Group suggests people are eating more whole grains, but they still account for only 11 percent of grains consumed, indicating a persistent and marked preference for refined-grain breads, pastas, rice, and baked goods.

Part of the problem is that it takes some investigation to figure out just which foods really are whole grain. Breakfast accounts for

When you eat whole grains, you minimize waste by using the entire food source.

well over half the whole grains Americans eat, when shopping for cereals, check for the word "whole"—as in the whole wheat that is the principal ingredient in Wheaties, and the whole oats that go into Cheerios. Some will include multiple whole grains, with added bran.

The whole-grain contents of breads can be particularly obscured. "Enriched wheat flour" means white flour—and you'll find it even in many breads and snacks that contain some whole grain and are advertised as such. "Multigrain" means only that more than one grain is included; they may not be whole grains, so read the ingredient list for the word "whole." Color is not a very helpful indicator either; traditional pumpernickel bread is made with course whole-grain rye flour (called rye meal), but many commercial versions contain plenty of refined flour, wheat gluten to make it fluffier, and colorants to achieve the dark hue that comes from coarser flour and slow baking. Look for the label "100 percent whole grain."

Planet-Friendly Choices

To achieve a diet that's nutritious and enjoyable often means marrying healthy mainstays with dishes that provide a bit of novelty and variety. This certainly holds true for grains. If you enjoy a bowl of oatmeal every morning, you might sit down to a whole-wheat roll—or perhaps a side of quinoa—at dinner. For most people, an adjustment to the nuttier and more complex flavors of whole grains can be acquired with repeated exposure and delectable dishes.

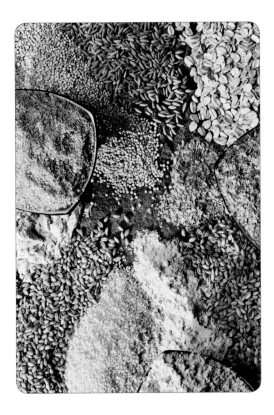

Most likely, you'll eventually come to prefer the taste and texture of whole grains—and your health will thank you for it. You will be making a planet-friendly choice too. Though animal products are far more resource intensive than plant foods generally, grains such as wheat and rice do demand a great deal of land and especially water. But by eating whole grains you are minimizing waste by using the entire food source. In addition, the nutrients that we lose by processing grains must then be added through another dietary source, thus requiring yet more resources to keep us healthy when we eat processed rather than whole grains.

AMARANTH

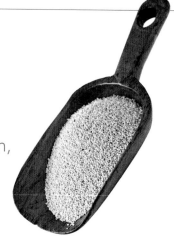

Amaranth grains are nestled in feathery crimson, purple, or gold flower clusters that adorn the tops of six-foot stalks. Not technically a cereal—the plant belongs to a different family than wheat and barley—amaranth has been consumed like a grain for thousands of years by Native American peoples, from the southeastern U.S. to South America. The Aztecs prized it as a staple food and the basis for religious ceremonies. After the Spanish conquest in 1521, Cortés and his people evangelized the Aztecs—and banned amaranth. Today, people in various parts of the world—from Mexico, to India and Nepal, to Greece—eat the seeds or greens of amaranth.

Choose and Use

Amaranth flour and seeds are available in health food and specialty grocery stores and are becoming increasingly available in super-markets. Cook the seeds in water like rice, and combine them with fresh vegetables, tofu, and savory herbs, or go sweet with a break-fast porridge loaded with raisins and nuts for a rice-like pudding. Amaranth seed can also be popped in a hot, dry pan, like popcorn. The flour is a common ingredient in gluten-free breads and cakes.

✦ TAKE AWAY

This protein-rich whole grain is vegan-friendly and gluten-free.

PREP TIP ✦ **PORRIDGE TO POPPED**

Amaranth is a highly versatile ingredient in the kitchen. The small grain absorbs water easily and thus makes an excellent gluten-free thickener substitute for wheat flour when making sauces. It also creates a fine hot cereal on a cold winter's morning. Amaranth can also be popped for a crunchy alternative to popcorn and, when combined with other flours, it provides great texture in gluten-free baking.

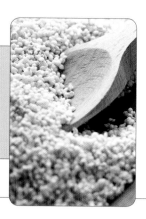

FOOD SCIENCE
✦
GLUTEN-FREE
POWERHOUSE

If you're going gluten-free, amaranth is a whole grain you'll want to meet. Not only does it have the highest protein content of any gluten-free grain, it has more protein than wheat. It's also a powerhouse when it comes to the minerals iron, calcium, and magnesium. Importantly, it also contains more lysine than other gluten-free grains, an amino acid many grains lack.

GIVES YOU

Protein
Dietary fiber
Manganese
Magnesium
Phosphorus
Iron
Copper
Selenium
Calcium
Pyridoxine (vitamin B6)
Folate
Zinc
Phytonutrients
  (phytosterols)

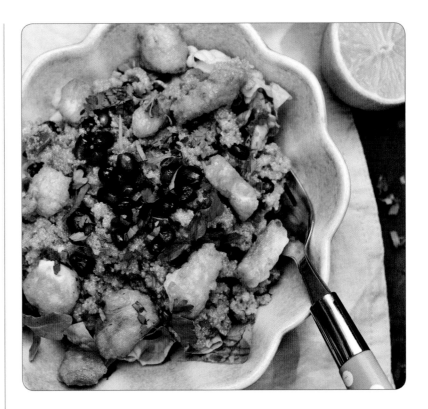

For Your Health

Amaranth has about as much protein as oats, and more than wheat, rice, or cornmeal. Unlike the protein in most grains, amaranth protein contains the essential amino acid lysine. Its high lysine content makes it a great addition to vegan diets, replacing the animal products that are the main source of lysine for most people. And its protein is gluten free, a plus for those with an intolerance or allergy. In addition to being high in cholesterol-lowering soluble fiber, amaranth is rich in phytosterols, plant compounds that resemble cholesterol and block its absorption into the bloodstream.

For Our Planet

No more than a few thousand acres of amaranth grow in the Midwest and Great Plains. A relative of pigweed, the plant is naturally drought and weed resistant. According to the Thomas Jefferson Agricultural Institute, the key cost in producing this grain is trucking it to one of the three main food companies that buy amaranth for redistribution or use in products.

BARLEY

Some 10,000 years ago, in the area of modern-day Jordan and Israel, the world's first farmers learned to sow this spiky grass for the nutrient-rich seeds clustered at its head. Archaeologists believe a second, independent domestication may have occurred about a thousand miles to the east. Over the next several millennia, the cereal spread along with agriculture itself into Europe. Today barley is grown around the world, and it enters the human diet mainly by way of animal feed and beer, the latter a tradition that reaches back several thousand years to the ancient Sumerians of Mesopotamia.

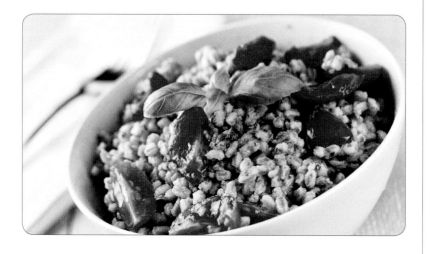

GIVES YOU

Dietary fiber
Protein
Manganese
Magnesium (if hulled)
Iron
Niacin (vitamin B3)
Riboflavin (vitamin B2)
Thiamine (vitamin B1)

PAIRINGS ✦ BEEF UP YOUR SOUP

Most people know barley from adding it to soups, and that's a great place to use it. A chewy grain that won't dissolve in your stock, barley adds texture and fiber that make soup a meal. It also makes a hearty pilaf when combined with mushrooms, onions, and sage.

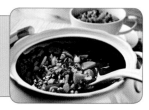

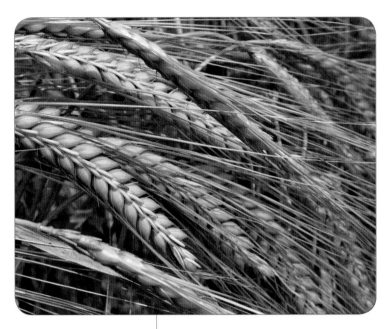

Choose and Use

Terrific in soups and stews or Middle Eastern–style salads, barley is cooked in water much like rice. It can be soaked to reduce cooking time. Barley bread is a dense, nutty accompaniment to tomatoes, olives, onions, and feta cheese. Or spread it with honey, jam, or protein-rich nut butter. It is an excellent substitute for beef in vegetarian chili.

For Your Health

The headline on barley: plenty of fiber (as long as it's pearled, not hulled). Ounce for ounce it has more fiber than just about any other whole grain. Dietary fiber, and in particular complex sugars called beta-glucans that are especially prevalent in barley fiber, are soluble fibers that help lower cholesterol by attaching to bile acids in the intestine and sweeping them out with waste. The resulting dearth of bile acids stimulates the liver to make more; to do that, it must draw down the bloodstream's supply of cholesterol, a component of bile acids. Published in 2010, a review of 11 randomized, controlled, clinical trials found that consuming barley and beta-glucans derived from the grain reduces cholesterol significantly

Based on this and other research, the U.S. Food and Drug Administration (FDA) allows whole-grain barley to carry a label saying it may play a role in reducing risk for heart disease.

For Our Planet

Barley is an adaptable, "high-residue" crop that helps prevent soil erosion and retain moisture. Most of the U.S. crop goes to malt (a key ingredient in beer) and livestock feed. Barley acreage has declined in recent years as farmers devote more land to high-priced corn—in growing demand for ethanol production—although commodity prices fluctuate, and corn is no different.

FOOD SCIENCE
✦
PEARLED OR HULLED

Barley is usually either "pearled" or "hulled," referring to the degree to which the grain has been processed. Not a "whole grain," pearled barley is polished and has most of its bran layer removed; hulled retains all of the fiber and nutrients and is the better choice for your body.

BROWN RICE

Prehistoric hunter-gatherers of Central China gathered rice grains growing wild in flood plains and rain-filled puddles. By 4,600 B.C. the very long transition to full-scale rice cultivation was well advanced. Today, 90 percent of rice is still grown in Asia, and many people worldwide depend on polished white rice as a staple food.

"Brown" rice describes not a particular variety of rice but a minimally processed form of rice considered whole grain in which only the husk has been milled away. For white rice, milling also removes the inner bran layers and tiny germ (from which a sprout would arise), leaving only the starchy endosperm (in the life cycle of the plant, the germ's food).

Choose and Use

You can choose brown rice whether you're eating sticky rice in sushi, a fluffy Basmati rice in an Indian dish, or a medium-grained rice in a Tex-Mex burrito. Cook rice in a heavy pot to avoid burning; no need to add oil or salt. The oil in its bran makes brown rice go bad faster than white, but refrigeration can extend its six-month shelf life.

For Your Health

Though enrichment of white rice restores thiamine and niacin stripped away in milling, and adds iron and folate, brown rice is

GIVES YOU

Dietary fiber
Manganese
Selenium
Magnesium
Niacin
Thiamine
Pantothenic acid
  (vitamin B5)
Pyridoxine

PREP TIP ✦ A BETTER-FOR-YOU RICE PUDDING

Leftover brown rice makes a rich but healthy pudding when combined with almond or coconut milk: simply boil on the stovetop and simmer until thickened. Season with cinnamon and vanilla for a tasty dessert. Fresh berries, golden raisins, or toasted almonds provide a further flavor boost.

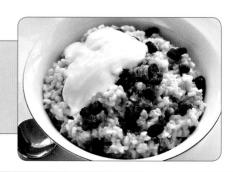

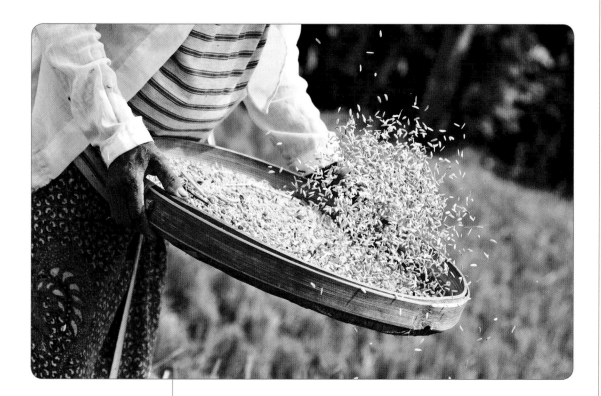

still a better source of fiber and minerals, especially manganese. Some lab studies suggest rice bran or the oil in rice bran can reduce LDL cholesterol and blood pressure, both risk factors for heart disease. A study published in 2010 looked at women in the large Nurses' Health Study and found that eating two or more servings of brown rice per week was associated with a lower risk of type 2 diabetes—whereas eating at least five servings a week of white rice boosted risk. That may be related to how fiber slows the absorption of sugars.

For Our Planet

Microbes feeding on organic matter submerged in flooded rice fields emit methane—an important heat-trapping greenhouse gas 21 times more potent than carbon dioxide. In fact, rice production accounts for about a fifth of human-generated methane. But farmers in both China (where rice production is a top source of methane) and the U.S. (where landfills and livestock operations are top sources) have made big improvements in the last decades by draining paddies mid-season—good news for the environment.

✦ TAKE AWAY
Introduce brown rice to your diet for greater fiber and nutritional value than highly processed white rice.

BUCKWHEAT

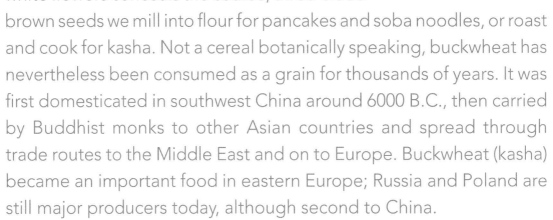

Buckwheat is a rather diminutive green plant with heart-shaped leaves. A profusion of delicate white flowers conceals the course, three-sided brown seeds we mill into flour for pancakes and soba noodles, or roast and cook for kasha. Not a cereal botanically speaking, buckwheat has nevertheless been consumed as a grain for thousands of years. It was first domesticated in southwest China around 6000 B.C., then carried by Buddhist monks to other Asian countries and spread through trade routes to the Middle East and on to Europe. Buckwheat (kasha) became an important food in eastern Europe; Russia and Poland are still major producers today, although second to China.

In the U.S., buckwheat is a minor crop, grown primarily for human food; when U.S. production peaked around the time of the Civil War it was a common livestock and poultry feed.

Choose and Use

Ground with its bran layers, buckwheat flour is a hearty, robustly flavored, high-fiber addition to griddle cakes, crepes, and baked goods, usually in combination with other grains because of its strong flavor. Toasting buckwheat groats (hulled grain kernels) before cooking in water or stock enhances their flavor and texture. Or you may buy them already roasted (often labeled

✦ TAKE AWAY

Enjoy buckwheat's lively flavor in flour or other dishes—this grain also supports probiotic health.

FOOD SCIENCE ✦ IT'S NOT WHEAT

Buckwheat is in no way related botanically to wheat, though it was given the name due to its similar properties. Technically a seed, most people recognize gluten-free buckwheat as a popular pancake ingredient in America. Buckwheat noodles are quite common in Japanese and Korean cuisine.

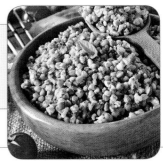

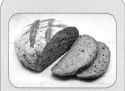
GIVES YOU

Dietary fiber
Protein
Copper
Magnesium
Potassium
Niacin
Pantothenic acid
Phytonutrients
  (flavonoids)

as kasha). Join them with mushrooms and onions, and add to bowtie pasta for a traditional eastern European dish—or create a hot breakfast cereal with fruit and a touch of honey.

For Your Health

Buckwheat is high in protein and relatively high in the essential amino acid lysine, lacking in most plant foods. It's high in both insoluble and soluble fiber, which together help regulate cholesterol and blood glucose, as well as maintain a healthy bowel, in part by providing fuel for "friendly" bacteria (probiotics) that crowd out pathogens. Buckwheat protein may also have an unusual ability to attach to cholesterol, limiting its absorption into the bloodstream. Buckwheat is the only grain that contains a phytochemical called rutin; in laboratory studies this flavonoid has demonstrated activity against blood clumping and inflammation. Buckwheat is gluten-free.

For Our Planet

Buckwheat grows quickly and thrives in poor soil. It's sometimes used as a cover crop to crowd out weeds and retain moisture and soil between cash-crop plantings. It can then be plowed under as a natural fertilizer (so-called green manure) and be allowed to decompose, thereby releasing its stored nutrients into the soil to feed the next crop.

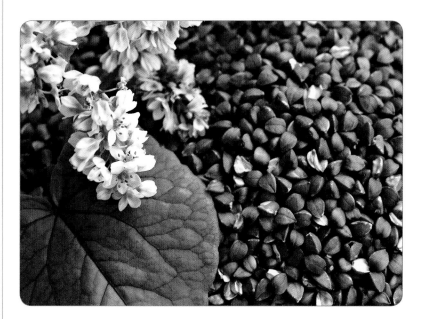

OATS

Early human foragers ate wild oats, but evidence of deliberate cultivation dates only to about four thousand years ago in central Europe; the grain head of the domesticated oat did not shatter and disperse, making it easier to harvest.

Choose and Use

Oats are one of the few grains typically eaten whole. In rolled oats, the groats, or hulled kernels, are simply flattened by heavy rollers and steamed. Thus they retain their full nutritional value: the inedible husk is removed but the bran and germ remain. Steel-cut oats have basically the same nutritional profile as whole rolled oats. Oat flour used to make breads and other baked goods also incorporates the whole grain. Everyday breakfast doesn't get much healthier than a classic porridge made from oats and the addition of dried or fresh fruit and nuts with nonfat milk—or almond, soy, and rice milks are also delicious. This makes for a hearty meal that will stabilize blood sugar and keep you feeling full throughout the morning.

For Your Health

When it comes to protein, whole oats pack both quantity—the highest of any cereal (not counting quinoa)—and quality, offering a well-balanced amino acid profile resembling that of soy, peas, and other legumes. Rice protein has a similar makeup but

GIVES YOU

Dietary fiber
Protein
Pantothenic acid
Thiamin
Manganese
Magnesium
Phosphorus
Zinc
Iron
Unsaturated fat
Phytonutrients
   (avenanthramides)

PREP TIP ✦ HOT BREAKFAST IN FIVE MINUTES

While many grains can be made into porridge, oatmeal is a classic that kids and adults have been enjoying for centuries. Steel cut oats have more "bite" than rolled oats, but whole rolled oats have just as much nutrition and cook in a fraction of the time. Combining oats with water and a touch of cinnamon makes a quick, healthy, and inexpensive breakfast that's especially delightful in colder months.

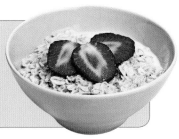

For years rice has been the popular favorite when it comes to an easy side dish. Today, many other grains are coming into their own as alternatives to keep dinner interesting. Oat groats have an almost nutty texture that are cooked similarly to rice and can be added to salads, made into pilafs, or served on their own to add healthy variety to meal time.

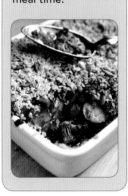

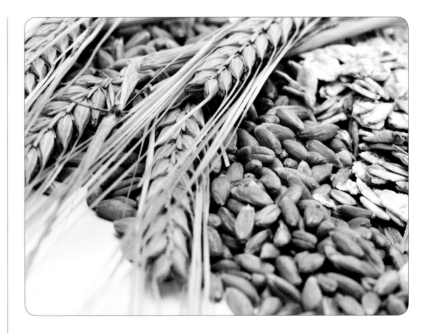

is low in quantity. (Both are gluten free, though some oat products in stores may be contaminated with gluten.)

Oats are high in soluble fiber, notably beta-glucan, that's especially helpful in lowering cholesterol; their polyunsaturated fats also reduce cholesterol levels. Research on the cholesterol-lowering effects of oats is solid enough that the U.S. Food and Drug Administration (FDA) and American Heart Association endorse a health claim for oats and oat products.

Oats are the sole source of a phytonutrient class called avenanthramides. Though it's not well understood, lab studies have shown antioxidant, anti-inflammatory, and anti-itch properties.

For Our Planet

Oats grow quickly and retain nutrients and moisture in soil, so farmers sometimes grow them to nourish or protect other crops. Though the U.S. is still a major producer, total acreage has been in decline since the 1920s, partly due to decreased need for horse feed.

QUINOA

Quinoa (pronounced KEEN-wah) is not a true cereal grain, but the dense, nutritious seeds clustered at the head of the goosefoot plant, a relative of beets, spinach, and chard. It originates from South America, and indeed was both a staple and a sacred food—the mother grain—of the Incas. Seduced by its delicate flavor and impressive nutrient profile, Americans have created growing demand for quinoa in recent years, but it is still grown chiefly in Peru, Bolivia, Ecuador, and Chile.

Choose and Use

Quinoa seeds are coated with a bitter-tasting resin that's usually rinsed off before marketing, but some prefer to rinse it again under cold running water for good measure. It cooks quickly, in about 15 minutes; avoid turning its pleasantly rustic texture to mush by overcooking. Quinoa of any color is excellent with iron-rich sautéed greens, in any kind of soup or stew, and as a nutritious alternative to rice in any dish; it makes a wonderful pilaf. It can also be added to green salads for a boost of protein, flavor, and texture. Mixed with nuts, fruit, and maple syrup, it makes an excellent breakfast as well.

For Your Health

When it comes to protein, quinoa is the mother of all grainlike foods, providing nearly twice the protein of most whole grains,

GIVES YOU

Protein
Dietary fiber
Manganese
Magnesium
Phosphorus
Iron
Calcium
Zinc
Copper
Potassium
Thiamin
Riboflavin
Folate
Vitamin E
Phytonutrients
  (flavonoids)

FOOD SCIENCE ✦ A GLUTEN-FREE GRAIN

Variety is incredibly important when it comes to diet, and there are lots of great grains from which to choose when making dinner. Quinoa's fluffy texture can be enjoyed the same way as rice—in pilafs or as a bed for stir-fry—and it's gluten free.

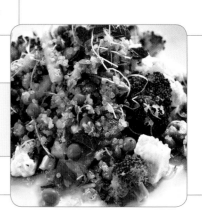

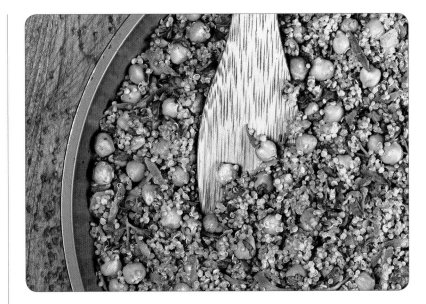

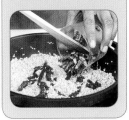

and a better-quality protein that includes all the essential amino acids. It is also a richer source of vitamin E than most other grains.

This mild-flavored pseudograin also packs a varied mix of nutrients unusual in grains, including calcium, healthy unsaturated fats, and an array of phytonutrients that may have antioxidant and anti-inflammatory effects.

Though little studied in humans, quinoa fed to rats on a high-fructose diet helped limit the animals' cholesterol and regulate blood glucose. People with celiac disease who add quinoa or oats, or foods made from their flours, to a "standard" gluten-free diet (that limits grains and relies heavily on rice) experience substantially improved intake of protein, iron, calcium, and fiber, according to a celiac specialist dietitian's retrospective review of diet history records that was published in 2009.

For Our Planet

Quinoa's surging popularity has dramatically increased its price both in wealthy nations and in its place of origin. South American growers and their communities reap substantial rewards, but locals are also being priced out of their nutritious staple and are substituting inferior foods such as white rice. The abrupt move to intensive cultivation for export has depleted the soil in some areas.

WHOLE WHEAT

Agriculture began with the domestication of wild wheat grasses some 12,000 years ago in the Fertile Crescent. Today wheat is second only to rice as a human food crop, providing the world's population with more than 20 percent of its total calories. A staple for roughly 40 percent of humanity—in Europe, North America, and parts of Asia—wheat is the key ingredient of bread in all its local varieties, as well as pasta, crackers, pastries, breakfast cereals, and noodles.

Choose and Use

Finding whole-grain wheat products can be trickier than it sounds. The label "wheat bread" or "multigrain bread" means next to nothing. Look for the term whole wheat, then check the list of ingredients to see whether whole grains predominate. Wheat-bran cereals may be full of fiber and nutrients, but they can lack some of the nutrients of cereals that also include the whole grain (whole wheat).

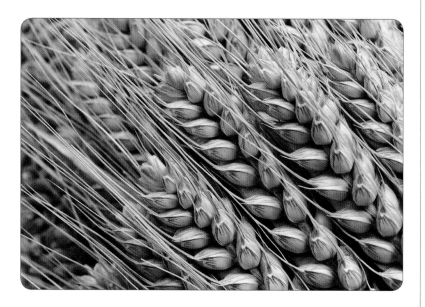

GIVES YOU

Dietary fiber
Protein
Iron
Phosphorus
Zinc
Copper
Thiamine
Niacin
Folate
Phytonutrients (lignans)

✦ TAKE AWAY

Ensure that mineral- and nutrient-rich whole grains are truly present in food by carefully reading labels.

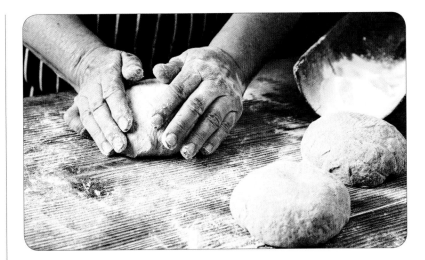

For Your Health

Americans consume plenty of wheat, but it's mostly refined, with the nutritious germ and bran layers milled away. The whole grain includes a host of components that contribute to health, including fiber, minerals, heart-healthy unsaturated fats, and phytonutrients such as lignans, which, by occupying hormone receptors, block hormones that may promote cancer.

Whereas refined-wheat products (like white bread) are a mainstay of diets that contribute to diabetes and other diseases through their deleterious effects on blood glucose and insulin, consumption of whole grains and foods that contain them help lower risk of heart disease and several cancers.

For Our Planet

Though not an especially resource-intensive crop compared with other staple foods, wheat is the most widely grown crop in the world. The big environmental challenge is the sheer demand for this grain, expected to climb 60 percent by 2050 due to population growth and increasing consumption of wheat products in the developing world. This will require increased yields; one controversial approach to meeting the demand is genetically modified wheat, under development by Monsanto and others. Wheat and other grains are most environmentally friendly when planted as part of a rotation of crops that helps to reduce fertilizer and pesticide use as well as to promote soil health and resiliency.

PREP TIP
✦
BULGUR WHEAT

A common way to encounter the whole wheat grain itself, known as bulgur, is with tomato, cucumbers, mint, parsley, and olive oil in the Middle Eastern salad called tabouleh. Bulgur has all the healthy pluses of whole grain, and it can be enjoyed much like rice, as a side dish to fish or poultry, in soups, or tossed into salads. It's also a terrific meat substitute in vegetarian chili.

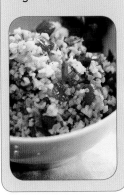

WILD RICE

Like some of the other "grains," wild rice is a wetland seed-bearing grass and not technically a cereal (grain). Native Americans may have gathered it from shallow streams and lakes since prehistoric times. Natives of the Great Lakes region where wild rice grows abundantly—the Ojibwe, Cree, and Menominee ("wild rice people," so named by the Ojibwe)—long enjoyed it as a staple. Today it is still collected from wild stands in Minnesota and other Great Lakes states, although most of the wild rice sold commercially is farmed in California, where the crop was introduced in the 1970s.

Choose and Use

Wild-gathered rice is more expensive than the farm-grown variety, although some find its varying flavor more stimulating to the palate. Both kinds add an earthy taste and texture to casseroles, pilafs, and traditional stuffings. Try it with sautéed mushrooms and onions or on salads of greens or citrus fruits.

For Your Health

Though brown rice is a little higher in fiber, wild rice provides more protein, with somewhat higher levels of lysine and methionine, essential amino acids that are typically lacking in grains. Wild rice is lower in carbohydrates than brown rice, which may

GIVES YOU

Dietary fiber
Protein
Zinc
Copper
Niacin
Riboflavin
Pyridoxine
Folate

CONSIDER ✦ THINK BEYOND HOT

Like some other "grains," wild rice isn't botanically a grain at all. Unique in taste, wild rice is often combined with rice or other grains to provide a balance of flavors. While often served hot as a side dish or poultry dressing, cold or warm rice makes a toothsome salad when tossed with salad greens, herbs, nuts, and fresh fruit. Toasted walnuts and orange segments go especially well.

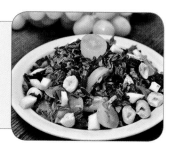

✦ TAKE AWAY
Treat yourself to wild rice, high in protein and omega-3 fatty acids.

be helpful in stabilizing blood glucose. Very low in total fat overall, wild rice is relatively rich in omega-3 fatty acids, a polyunsaturated fat that reduces inflammation and may thwart the development of heart disease and ameliorate ailments such as arthritis and depression.

For Our Planet

The development of cultivated "paddy" rice made the food more widely available, drove down its price, and, some argue, relieved pressure on wild strands. But some Native American and environmental groups have been concerned that the development of cultivated varieties robs Ojibwe of their treaty-granted rights to the wild rice and could lead to the contamination of wild strands. Several companies sell wild-grown "lake and river" wild rice, including Ojibwe-owned Native Harvest, whose product is traditionally hand harvested.

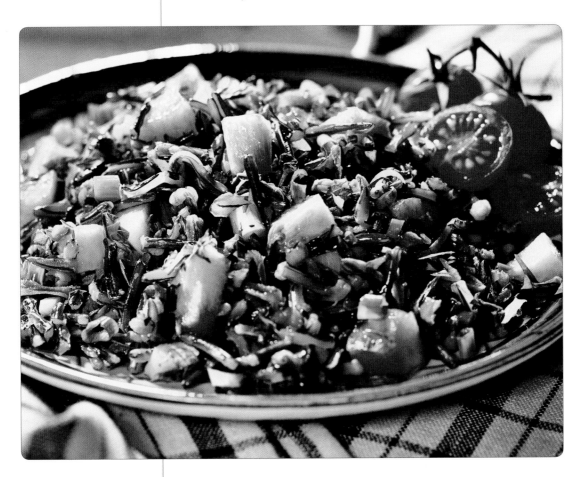

CHAPTER FIVE

FATS and OILS

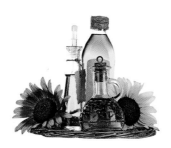

Fat gets a bad rap sometimes, but like protein and carbohydrates, it is a macronutrient essential to life. It is also the most energy-dense of the three, with more than twice the calories: about 9 per gram in fat compared to 4 per gram in protein or carbohydrates. Not only do fats and oils add flavors and textures to a wide range of foods, both savory and sweet, they are also important for preventing disease and staying healthy. Knowing which forms of fat and how much to eat is a key first step; knowing how to choose and use them is equally important.

Chemically speaking, fats and oils are characterized by their component fatty acids, 25 different naturally occurring combinations of carbon, hydrogen, and oxygen atoms. Fatty acids are differentiated by their atomic structures, particularly their "saturation," a term in chemistry referring to whether the fatty acid can absorb more hydrogen or not. An unsaturated fat will bond with more hydrogen molecules; a saturated fat will not.

Both saturated and unsaturated fats occur in nature. Animal fats such as suet, lard, and butter are *saturated fats*. They are solid at room temperature, have a greasy or waxy texture, and spoil more slowly than unsaturated fats.

By contrast, most plant-derived fats are *unsaturated fats*. Concentrated mainly in seeds or nuts, these fats are extracted by pressing or grinding, and they are liquid at room temperature. Unsaturated fats can be either monounsaturated or polyunsaturated, referring to the number of double bonds of hydrogen in the molecule. Double bonds make these oils more perishable and more sensitive to oxygen, heat, and light than saturated fats.

Two important classes of polyunsaturated fatty acids are available only from food: omega-6 and omega-3. Both occur in plant oils—omega-6 particularly in corn, safflower, and sunflower oil—and omega-3 fatty acids also occur in fatty fish like sardines, mackerel, and salmon. Western diets tend to be high in omega-6 fatty acids and low in omega-3 fatty acids. A typical American diet has a 20:1 ratio of omega-6 to omega-3, while some research suggests that a ratio of 3:1 or 4:1 may be better. For that reason, it's a good idea to find ways to increase the omega-3 fatty acid foods on your menu. This chapter will give you ideas how.

Fat in the Diet, Fat in the Body

Everybody knows that fats and oils make food taste good. They add richness, texture, and flavor. They aid in browning and emulsion

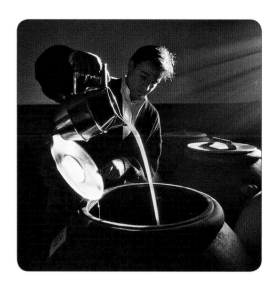

(making things creamy), and they make baked goods come out tender and flaky.

Fats do more than taste good, though. Because they take longer to digest than proteins and carbohydrates, fats help us feel full longer. They also stimulate production of a hormone that suppresses the appetite and signals us to stop eating. In terms of sheer survival mechanisms, stored fats represent the body's energy reserves—one pound of body fat provides enough energy for one and a half to two days of normal activity. The problem is, human beings often reserve more energy than we use, resulting in thicker waistlines.

A body's fat requirement varies throughout a person's lifetime. At birth, human breast milk provides a special combination of fatty acids (among other key nutrients), which is why many nutritionists and health professionals advise new mothers that "breast is best." As infants grow, fats help form cell membranes in all the organs. The retina and the central nervous system are mainly composed of fats. The body needs fats to produce growth hormones, sex hormones, and prostaglandins (hormonelike chemicals that regulate many body processes). Fat deposits protect vital organs and help regulate body temperature. Only when they are eaten with fats can the body can absorb some important fat-soluble vitamins, such as A, D, E, and K.

Body fat is not a simple function of the fat a person eats. The body is relatively efficient in storing dietary fat, but excess calories from carbohydrates and proteins are also converted to fat, leading to weight gain when energy consumed exceeds energy expended. A growing body establishes fat cells at certain key periods, such as infancy and adolescence. Once established, fat cells are permanent, though they may shrink with weight loss or expand with weight gain. Eating habits also begin early in life when children develop taste preferences and habits. Fats have their place in a healthy family's diet—but the right kinds of fats are key.

Those who eat an insufficient amount of fat in their diets can experience depression, heart disease, malnutrition, and other severe physical problems. On the other hand, those who maintain a diet high in certain kinds of fat face increased risks of heart disease, stroke, circulatory disorders, and cancer of the colon and rectum, prostate, breast, uterus, and ovaries.

Cholesterol and Trans Fats

Cholesterol is another fat essential for health. It is present throughout the body, especially in brain, nerve, liver, and blood cells. Of the two types of cholesterol—HDL (for high-density lipoproteins) and LDL (for low-density lipoproteins)—it has become common to speak of of HDL as "good" and LDL as "bad," but both are necessary—in the right proportion. HDLs are large molecules that circulate in the blood,

*Not only are fats essential to good health,
they taste good, too!*

scavenging unused cholesterol and recycling it back to the liver. Smoking, obesity, and a sedentary lifestyle can all lower one's HDL levels, leading to plaque deposits that block the arteries and limit blood flow (known as atherosclerosis). In the typical American diet, increasing vegetable fats and reducing animal fats will lead to a more balanced cholesterol count.

Another type of fat—trans fats, or trans fatty acids—forms naturally in the guts of some ruminant animals (cows and goats, for example) and is found in low amounts in many foods also high in saturated fats, such as milk, cheese, and meat. More significantly, trans fats are a key ingredient in many processed foods, in the form of partially hydrogenated vegetable oil.

Hydrogenation is an industrial process by which hydrogen is added to vegetable oil, transforming liquid oil into solid fat and improving the texture, stability, and shelf life of food made with it. This invention proved a real boon to manufacturers in the early to mid-twentieth century. Margarine, vegetable shortening, and all sorts of snack foods were developed containing partially hydrogenated vegetable oil. We have since learned, though, that of all the fats in the diet, trans fats have the most harmful effect on human health, particularly on blood cholesterol levels and risk of cardiovascular disease—more so than saturated fat or dietary cholesterol.

During the 1990s, studies seeking the causes for a rising incidence of heart disease in the United States identified trans fats as one of the culprits. Public health campaigns to eliminate trans fats from the American diet have since then proven effective, and many manufacturers now proudly claim "no trans fats" on their packaging. Trans fat content in our food has declined by 50 percent since 2005. Laws also limit the amount of trans fats that manufacturers and restaurant chains can use in the foods they offer, and health-conscious consumers avoid any items containing partially hydrogenated oil.

Know Your Fats

It is now well established scientifically that the type of fat a person consumes has a greater impact on that individual's general health than the amount of fat she or he ingests. Indeed, the heart-healthy Mediterranean diet, based on the culinary traditions of countries bordering the Mediterranean Sea, is actually quite high in unsaturated fats, such as those found in olive oil and nuts. The wisest diet choice is not to avoid fats altogether. Not only are fats essential to good health, they taste good, too! Instead, learn which kinds of fats and oils are most beneficial for your body and use that knowledge to shape your menu and adjust your eating habits.

CANOLA OIL

Extracted from the crushed seeds of the rape plant, rapeseed oil—also known as canola oil—was first used as a lamp fuel in Asia and Europe. The word "rape" comes from the Latin *rapum*, meaning turnip. The yellow-blossomed rape plant is related to the turnip, cabbage, mustard, and other members of the Brassicaceae family. Rapeseed oil was originally very high in erucic acid, which can damage cardiac muscle. Considered too toxic for human consumption, it was banned by the FDA in 1956. A new hybrid of rapeseed was later developed with a lower content of erucic acid, labeled Can.O., L-A for "Canadian Oilseed, Low Acid," hence the name "canola oil."

Once a specialty crop in Canada, canola is now a major U.S. cash crop, exported to Japan, Mexico, China, and Pakistan. Most U.S. canola is grown in North Dakota.

Choose and Use

Light yellow in color with a neutral flavor, canola oil is an inexpensive and versatile ingredient that may be used as a cooking or salad oil, when you want to highlight the taste of other ingredients. Canola's high smoking point (the temperature at which it breaks down and begins to burn) makes it a good choice for grilling, stir-frying, or deep-frying foods. This oil turns rancid when stored

GIVES YOU

Vitamin K
Vitamin E
Monounsaturated and
    polyunsaturated fats
Phytosterols (sitosterol,
    campesterol)

CONSIDER ✦ BIOFUEL

The global demand for vegetable oils like canola is expanding rapidly, due not only to increasing populations and individual preferences but also to the massive upsurge in growing it for biofuel. Canola's efficiency as a biofuel is unclear, however, and the deforestation that currently occurs to clear land to produce it leads to habitat loss.

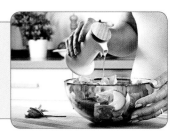

PREP TIP
✦
GREAT IN BAKING

Olive oil is lauded for its high mono-unsaturated fat content, particularly oleic acid. But mild-flavored canola oil has almost as much oleic acid, good news for people who don't care for the distinct taste of olive oil. Canola is a great choice for mellower vinaigrettes and marinades. With its healthier nutritional profile, it's also a terrific choice for baking in lieu or soybean or corn oil.

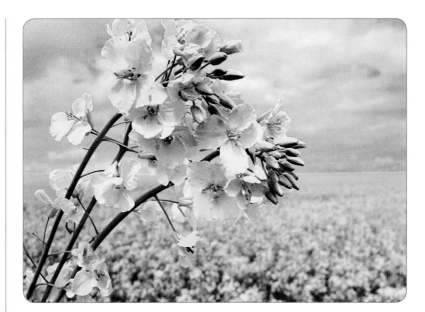

improperly, so keep it in a tightly sealed container away from heat and light. "Cold-pressed" canola oil has a longer shelf life.

For Your Health

Canola oil has the lowest saturated fat content of any oil commonly available in the United States, and it contains omega-3 and omega-6 fatty acids in healthy proportions. In fact, one tablespoon of canola oil contains 100 percent of the daily value of alpha-linolenic acid (ALA), an essential omega-3 fatty acid that the body cannot make and must get from the diet. Sixty percent of the fat in canola oil comes from monounsaturated fats such as oleic acid, which helps lower LDL, or "bad" cholesterol, and increase HDL, or "good" cholesterol, in the blood. Because of this, the FDA allows manufacturers to label canola oil as a food that reduces the risk of heart disease.

For Our Planet

In part because of consumer pressure, farm organizations are actively seeking ways to make rapeseed a sustainable crop. In 2012, the Cargill agricultural company supplied what they claimed to be the first verifiably sustainable rapeseed crop to Unilever, a multinational corporation that plans to source all of its raw materials sustainably by 2020. Unilever uses canola oil to make mayonnaises and margarines, among other food products.

✦ **TAKE AWAY**

Use this golden oil to accentuate flavors and lower your risk of heart disease.

CHOCOLATE

Chocolate is made from beans harvested from the large cacao pods that grow on a tropical tree native to South America. Both the Mayans and the Aztecs believed cocoa beans had magical properties and used them to brew a bitter drink called *xocolatl*, the probable origin of the word "chocolate." In 1502, Columbus brought cocoa pods back from the New World, and by the 17th century sweetened chocolate was a fashionable drink throughout Europe.

Cocoa beans are fermented, dried, roasted, and cracked, to separate the nib or central part of the cocoa bean, from the shell. The nibs are ground to extract a natural vegetable fat called cocoa butter, leaving a thick brown paste, which is further refined to produce cocoa powder and varieties of solid chocolate that include dark, semisweet, sweet, and milk chocolate.

Choose and Use

Supermarkets stock a mouth-watering array of domestic and imported chocolate containing varying percentages of cocoa solids and flavored with everything from mint to bacon—proof that the art of chocolate making is flourishing. Cocoa powder is used in beverages and baking (Dutch-processed has fewer flavonols, since the alkali process destroys some of the

---

FOOD SCIENCE ✦ WHITE CHOCOLATE

Unlike traditional brown-colored chocolate, whether milk, dark, or semi-sweet, white chocolate does not contain the dark-colored solids of the cacao bean. It does contain cocoa butter, however (as well as sugar and milk), which accounts for its mild chocolaty flavor and pale ivory color.

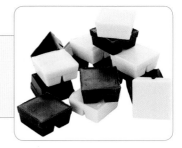

PAIRINGS
✦
FAIR TRADE CHOCOLATE

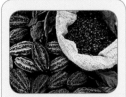

Cacao is often grown by farmers who do not receive just wages for their work, and reports have indicated child slavery is not uncommon. When satisfying your craving, look for the "Fair Trade Certified" label, which ensures your purchase supports farmers who receive a fair price, invest in their land, and do not employ child or slave labor.

GIVES YOU

DARK CHOCOLATE, 70-85 PERCENT COCOA SOLIDS:

Manganese
Copper
Iron
Magnesium
Dietary fiber
Phosphorus
Zinc
Potassium
Monounsaturated fats
Phytonutrients
  (flavonoids)

antioxidants). Solid chocolate may be eaten as is, or melted and incorporated into desserts. Chocolate has an incredible depth of flavor, since cacao features over 400 distinct smells (roses have 14). Tightly wrapped chocolate will keep for months in a cool, dry place.

For Your Health

The darker the chocolate, the greater its concentration of flavonol antioxidants, which can lower blood pressure and reduce the risk of heart disease. Consuming dark chocolate daily has been proven to reduce stress hormones in people with high anxiety levels. A good source of minerals such as manganese, copper, and iron, chocolate is also very high in saturated fats and when eaten in excess contributes extra calories and sugar to the diet. Choose dark rather than milk chocolate, and enjoy it in small quantities.

For Our Planet

To make sure your chocolate is sustainably sourced, purchase chocolate labeled "Rainforest Alliance Certified." This guarantees the cocoa is shade-grown, using practices that have a minimal impact on the rain forest and which conserve the habitat of native plant and animal species. This certification also ensures that cocoa farmers and laborers have decent working conditions.

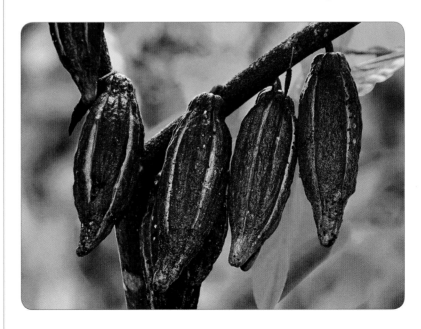

FLAXSEED: GROUND AND OIL

Humans have had an enduring relationship with the flax plant, which they named *Linum usitatissimum,* or "of maximum usefulness." For tens of thousands of years, flax has been cultivated as a source of food and textiles. Its strong fibers have been spun into sails for our ships, strings for our bows, and clothing and armor for our bodies. Graced with light blue, bell-shaped flowers, the flax plant is the source of linen fabric and produces golden or brown seeds used primarily today as a dietary supplement, and to produce linseed oil, an industrial lubricant.

Choose and Use

Flaxseed and oil can be found in natural food stores and in many supermarkets. Cooking does not diminish the omega-3 in flaxseed, so it may be baked into muffins and breads without losing this fatty acid. The seeds have a mild, nutty flavor. Grinding just before use, in a coffee or nut grinder, preserves their nutritional benefits. Sprinkle ground seeds on salads, yogurt, or breakfast cereals, or on ice cream or other desserts. Flaxseed can also be sprouted and used in salads and sandwiches. Some people experience bloating or flatulence when they first introduce this high-fiber food into their diet. Drinking more water should help such gastrointestinal symptoms abate over time.

Flaxseed oil is most often used as a dietary supplement. Practically flavorless, it may be added to protein shakes or other beverages or taken in capsule form. However, the whole seeds offer more complete nutrition, though the omega-3s it provides are not the long-chain EPA and DHA most critical for human health.

For Your Health

Flaxseed has a unique nutritional profile. The seeds and oil are remarkably rich sources of omega-3 fatty acids, which can help

GIVES YOU

GROUND FLAXSEED:
Monounsaturated and
    polyunsaturated fats
Manganese
Vitamin B1
Dietary fiber
Magnesium
Tryptophan
Phosphorus
Copper
Phytonutrients (lignans)

FLAXSEED OIL:
Monounsaturated and
    polyunsaturated fats
Vitamin E

✦ **TAKE AWAY**

Scatter the seeds over your favorite dishes for an added crunch loaded with antioxidants.

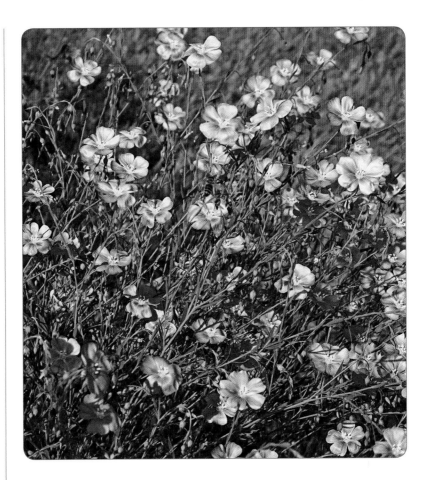

PREP TIP
✦
A NUTTY ADDITION

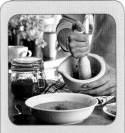

Flaxseeds have become a favorite among those looking to increase their intake of omega-3s. This small seed can be purchased raw or toasted and can be added to many different foods for texture with its mildly nutty flavor. Try as a topping for yogurt, sprinkle a handful on a salad, or add to cooked cereals to boost your intake of heart- and brain-healthy fats.

balance the omega-6 in Western diets, due primarily to the high corn content of many processed foods. Flaxseed is also the number-one source of phytonutrients called lignans, important antioxidants that may prevent precancerous cellular changes and reduce the growth of hormone-related cancers. Finally, flaxseed contains mucilage gums that support the health of the intestinal tract. Flaxseed oil lacks some of the nutrients found in the seeds and must be refrigerated, whether in capsule or liquid form, to preserve its benefits.

For Our Planet

Flax earns high marks for sustainability, in part because the entire plant can be used to make products such as linen cloth, twine, and linseed oil. After the oil is extracted, the remaining meal can be formed into nutritious bars called oilseed cakes and fed to cattle and chickens to create heart-healthier meat.

HEMP OIL

An ancient legend says that the Buddha, founder of Buddhism, survived for six years eating nothing but a single hemp seed each day. Hemp has a unique nutritional profile and has been consumed as a food since ancient times, but today this useful plant is transformed into insulation, auto parts, paper, and even stone.

Most industrial hemp is grown in China. In the United States, this versatile crop still suffers from guilt by association as a result of its relationship to the marijuana plant, and its cultivation is severely restricted. Hemp and pot both belong to the plant genus *Cannabis*, which contains molecular compounds called cannabinoids, including the psychoactive ingredient THC (tetrahydrocannabinol) and an antipsychoactive ingredient called CBD (cannabidiol). Unlike marijuana, hemp is very low in THC and high in CBD, and one cannot get high from smoking or ingesting it.

Choose and Use

Purchase small quantities of raw seeds in bulk or prepackaged, and sprinkle on granola, puddings, or other desserts, or blend into smoothies; toasting brings out their nutty taste, but eating the seeds raw provides the most nutritional benefits. Hemp oil is extracted from hemp seeds by cold-pressing, resulting in oil that ranges in color from off-yellow to dark green. Best used for cold and warm dishes where temperature is kept below the boiling point, hemp oil should not be used for frying. It adds a nice nutty flavor to foods and may be used in salads and baked goods, or taken by the spoonful as a dietary supplement. Store hemp oil in the fridge once the bottle is opened.

GIVES YOU

HEMP SEED (SHELLED):
Polyunsaturated fats
Phytosterols (beta sitosterol, campesterol)
Vitamin E
Protein
Magnesium
Zinc
Iron
Dietary fiber

HEMP OIL:
Polyunsaturated fats
Phytosterols (beta sitosterol, campesterol)
Vitamin E
Protein

For Your Health

One unique benefit of hemp resides in its particular ratio of omega-6 to omega-3 essential fatty acids (3:1), which exceeds the 4:1 ratio recommended for the body's health. Most people consume too few omega-3 fatty acids, and ingesting foods containing whole hemp seeds or hemp oil can help boost your intake. Hemp provides all of the essential amino acids that the body requires. The phytosterols in hemp also help lower LDL cholesterol by blocking the absorption of cholesterol into the intestines.

For Our Planet

Hemp is an environmentally friendly crop that requires few pesticides and no herbicides. It stabilizes and enriches the soil in which it grows. Sustainable hemp is currently grown on farms in Canada, Europe, and China.

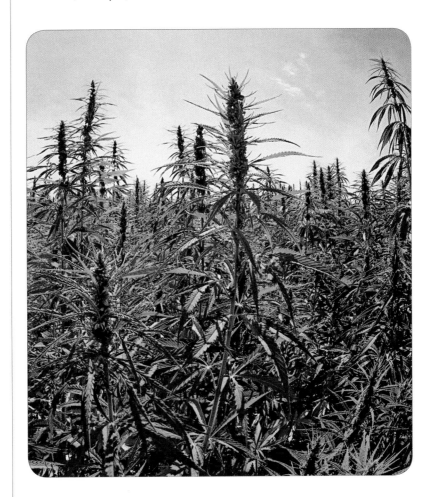

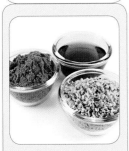

OLIVE OIL

One of the most ancient foods on Earth and a symbol of peace and wisdom, olives were cultivated before the invention of written language. Plucked straight from the tree, olives are inedible to humans and must be brined before they are fit for consumption. Originally the ripened fruit was pressed to extract oil for lamps and cooking, as well as cosmetic and ceremonial uses. Spanish missionaries planted the first olive trees in California, where most domestic olive oil is now produced. Imported olive oil may come from Greece, Italy, France, and Spain and varies widely in flavor and color, depending on the region of origin and the condition of the crop.

Choose and Use

Extra-virgin olive oil (EVOO), which derives from the first cold pressing of the olives, varies in color from straw yellow to bright green and has a flavor that ranges from peppery to fruity. Save the more expensive EVOO for use on salads and for drizzling over grilled vegetables; its low smoke point (the temperature at which it begins to burn and smoke) makes it less than ideal for high-heat cooking, though it can be used in faster-cooking dishes. Unlike flavor-filled extra-virgin and virgin olive oil, "pure" olive oil and "light" olive oil have a neutral taste and higher smoke point preferable to some palates and suitable for cooking and baking. Replacing the butter and cream in mashed potatoes with olive oil increases this healthy fat in your diet. Olive oil tastes best when used within two months of purchase but will last up to two years if stored in a cool, dark place. It turns cloudy and solidifies when refrigerated, but it will clarify and liquefy at room temperature.

GIVES YOU

Monounsaturated and
  polyunsaturated fats
Vitamin E
Vitamin K
Phytonutrients
Phytosterols
  (tyrosolesters)

PAIRINGS
✦
DRIZZLE AWAY

A cornerstone of Mediterranean cuisine, olive oil's flavor differs by variety, from mild and light to fruity or peppery. A staple in cooking, a drizzle adds a burst of richness and flavor to dishes likes soups, savory tarts, salads, and beyond. It's also great for dipping with a crusty loaf of bread—and more healthful than butter.

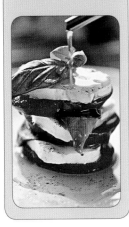

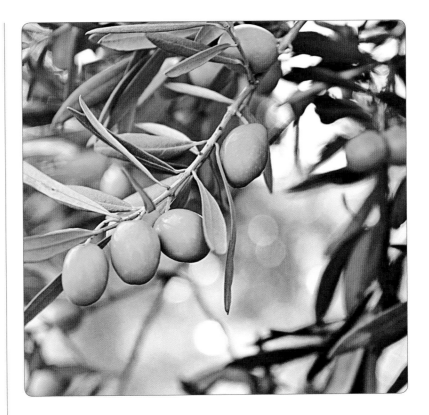

For Your Health

Olive oil is a staple of the Mediterranean diet, widely regarded as one of the healthiest in the world. Olive oil has been intensively studied, and research has linked it to weight loss, digestive and bone health, and improved cognitive function, especially in older adults. A review of the existing science, conducted at the University of Athens in 2011, concluded that a high intake of olive oil was associated with lowered odds of having any type of cancer. Nine different categories of polyphenols present in olive oil function in the body as both antioxidants and anti-inflammatory nutrients.

For Our Planet

Drought-tolerant olives require 50 to 75 percent less water than other crops, meaning fewer resources are used in their production. However, waste and residue are particularly high in olive oil production. In 2013, the development of software that calculates the carbon footprint of olive oil production processes will help olive oil businesses assess their environmental impact.

SAFFLOWER OIL

This ancient crop, related to the sunflower and native to the mountains of southwest Asia and Ethiopia, has been prized by various cultures as a medicinal plant and cultivated for its yellow, orange, and red thistle-like flowers, which have been used as a textile dye. Garlands made from safflower blossoms were found in the tomb of the pharaoh Tutankhamun. Now raised almost exclusively as an oilseed plant, most safflower is grown in India.

Choose and Use

This flavorless and colorless oil can be a nutritious yet silent partner in many dishes. Traditionally refined safflower oil is best used cold, whereas high-oleic oil has a high smoking point and may be used for frying foods. Expeller pressing is preferable to chemical processes used to extract oil from safflower seeds, which may leave traces of chemicals behind. As with all cooking oils, keep away from heat and light, and seal tightly to prevent oxidation.

GIVES YOU

Vitamin E
Monounsaturated and polyunsaturated fats
Phytosterols (campesterol, stigmasterol, beta-sitosterol)

FOOD SCIENCE ✦ PARTIAL HYDROGENATION

Like soybean oil, safflower oil is often used to make margarine by employing "partial hydrogenation." Through this process, the addition of hydrogen molecules to the oil creates a solid, more shelf-stable fat that mimics the look and mouthfeel of saturated fats like butter. The process also results in the creation of trans fats, however, a risk factor for high cholesterol and heart disease. Partially hydrogenated fats are commonly used in processed foods like cookies and crackers. While many foods have removed harmful trans fats, read the ingredients list to avoid purchasing foods with "partially hydrogenated vegetable oil."

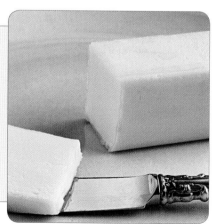

For Your Health

Nutritionally similar to sunflower oil, traditional safflower oil has more polyunsaturated fats than any other commonly used cooking oil. A variety high in oleic acid, often used in infant formulas, contains more monounsaturated fats. Some of the latest research into safflower oil has focused on its nutritional benefits for women. For instance, clinical studies in 2009 and 2011 demonstrated that postmenopausal women with type 2 diabetes who added safflower oil to their diets experienced a reduction in abdominal fat, increases in insulin sensitivity and "good" HDL cholesterol, and decreased inflammation. This oil contains heart-healthy phytosterols that may lower LDL cholesterol in the blood.

For Our Planet

Safflower grown in the United States is a high-yield crop that can survive with little or no irrigation, thanks to its deep taproot, and the application of insecticides and pesticides is often unnecessary. The lower water needs and the limited use of fossil fuel–intensive chemicals make this oil one of the most planet friendly.

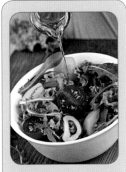

PREP TIP
✦
SIMPLE VINAIGRETTE

Safflower's orange flowers are a cheaper alternative to saffron. Its oil is neutral tasting and rich in monounsaturates, like olive oil. For those who prefer their salad dressings to feature the flavors of bright vinegars, fresh herbs, and spices rather than the oil, safflower is a good choice. An easy vinaigrette includes about one part vinegar to two or three parts oil seasoned with a bit of salt and freshly ground black pepper; garlic, shallot, or herbs provide additional flavor.

✦ **TAKE AWAY**

Reduce "bad" cholesterol by using safflower oil in your recipes.

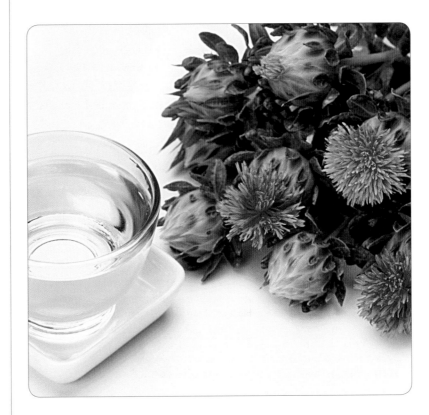

SUNFLOWER SEEDS AND OIL

One of the only crop species to originate in North America, the sunflower is well named; these plants swivel their golden heads to follow their namesake's passage across the sky each day. Sunflowers thrive in the bright heat of the wind-swept Great Plains, though more are commercially grown in the Dakotas than in the so-called Sunflower State of Kansas. The sunflower's broad face is packed with oily seeds, tucked inside hard shells. Many people enjoy snacking on the roasted kernels, but the seeds are also used for birdfeed and principally as a source of salad and cooking oil.

Choose and Use

Dried or roasted sunflower seeds are sold prepackaged or in bulk. They should look and smell fresh. Both shelled and unshelled are available, but shelling them yourself is a laborious process. Sunflower seeds are often heavily salted, so opt for the unsalted to avoid excess sodium intake. Sprinkle sunflower kernels on salads, or add to hot and cold cereals or baked goods. The seeds may also be ground and used in place of flour for coating meat or fish.

Light yellow to golden in color, sunflower oil has a mild flavor. Due to its relatively high smoke point (450° F) sunflower oil may be used for frying as well as in baked goods and as a neutral-tasting salad oil. Like other oils, it eventually turns rancid if exposed to oxygen, heat, and light.

For Your Health

Of seeds and nuts commonly eaten in the United States, sunflower seeds have the highest phytosterol content. Phytosterols reduce cholesterol levels in the blood, boost the immune system, and help protect against lung, stomach, ovarian, and breast cancer. The vitamin E in these seeds benefits the body in

GIVES YOU

SUNFLOWER SEEDS:
Vitamin E
Manganese
Copper
Tryptophan
Magnesium
Selenium
Vitamin B6
Phosphorus
Folate
Protein
Niacin
Pantothenic Acid
Iron
Potassium
Zinc
Phytosterols
  (beta-sitosterol,
  stigmasterol,
  campesterol)

SUNFLOWER OIL:
Vitamin E
Vitamin K
Monounsaturated and
  polyunsaturated fats

Oils like sunflower can be obtained from their seeds either by crushing them through an expeller press or through chemical extraction; either is safe to eat. Oil may also be "refined" or "unrefined." Unrefined oil is less heat stable and more flavorful, making it a good choice for vinaigrettes or marinades. Refined oil removes many nutrients but can be a safer choice when cooking at high temperatures, like frying.

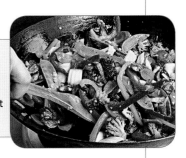

many ways, such as in building red blood cells and muscle tissue and protecting against heart disease.

Different types of sunflower oil have different fat profiles. Linoleic sunflower oil, the original and most commonly used variety, contains more polyunsaturated fats than high-oleic sunflower oil, which is higher in monounsaturated fats. A third variety, called NuSun, is a mid-oleic oil developed using standard plant-breeding techniques to provide the food industry with a heart-healthier frying oil.

For Our Planet
Sunflowers are drought-resistant, and herbicide use on commercially grown plants declined by 80 percent between 1996 and 2008 as a result of demand from eco-conscious consumers and companies pressuring for more sustainable farming practices. A major market for U.S. sunflowers, Europe enforces strict guidelines about sustainability.

PREP TIP
✦
GOOD FOR FRYING

Sunflower oil is a mild-flavored oil, making it a good choice when a mellow flavor is desired. It would work well in a simple marinade or salad dressing. Like canola, corn, and peanut oil, sunflower oil also has a very high smoke point, making it a good choice for frying food.

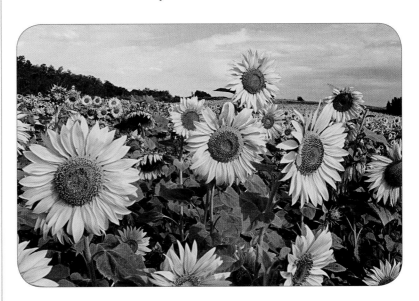

BEVERAGES

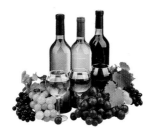

The history of beverages begins, naturally enough, with water. This mutable element varies hugely in form and character, It might issue from rivers, springs, or deep wells; fall from the sky as rain; or bubble up clouded with silt or fizzy with suspended gases. It has, until relatively recently, been more appropriately referred to as "waters." Humans, whose earliest ancestors were water-dwelling organisms, still possess bodies consisting of more than two-thirds water.

For millions of years—the vast majority of our evolutionary history—water was the only thing that human beings drank. Our billions of cells require water to function, and this clear, abundant, and calorie-free beverage is more essential to our daily survival than food. Once developing infants no longer require the nutrients present in breast milk, water provides everything we need to replenish the fluids our bodies lose through metabolism, perspiration, respiration, and elimination. So effectively does plain water address these physiological needs that it was not until the birth of agriculture 11,000 years ago that alternative beverages began to be developed.

Bottled versus Tap

At various times and places throughout history, people have lacked access to sources of clean water, as a result of both naturally occurring contaminants and human-created pollution. This problem originally led to the development of beverages that help purify water and thus provide a way to hydrate the body without putting health at risk. In the West, beer brewing and wine making developed, in part, as a way to decontaminate drinking water, as did the practice of brewing tea in the East. Boiling water to create a beverage from infused tea leaves kills waterborne contaminants, resulting in a beverage that is safe to drink. As an added boon, the caffeine present in this hot drink acts as a mild stimulant and provides other health benefits.

Much later, bottling water became another method of insuring its purity. Far from being a recent phenomenon, bottled water in the United States actually predates the American Revolution. Early consumers drank bottled water for health reasons, just as many people do today. By 1856, over 7 million bottles were produced annually at Saratoga Springs, one of the most popular bottling facilities and a natural source of mineral springs, which are purported to have therapeutic properties. In the early twentieth century, when chlorine was regularly added to municipal drinking supplies, bottled water fell from favor, since clean water was readily available from the tap.

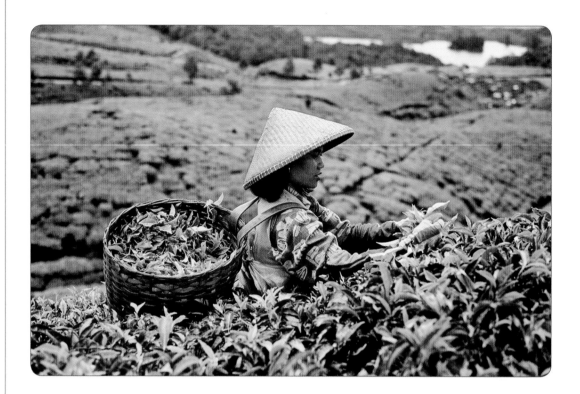

In the 1970s, concerns about the growing problem of water pollution led to renewed sales of bottled water. The French mineral water company Perrier launched a million-dollar marketing campaign that made its uniquely shaped green glass bottle a status beverage. In the United States, tap water costs just a fraction of a penny per glass, but since the 1980s bottled water has eclipsed it in popularity. Americans currently drink more bottled water than milk or beer, even though research has shown that bottled is no safer or better tasting than tap water, and may actually contain more contaminants. The economic and environmental costs of bottled water, in terms of waste, energy use, and production of greenhouse gases, have prompted local governments in the United States and Canada to consider banning its sale. Developing nations such as China, Pakistan, and India, where many people lack access to dependable sources of clean water, are now the world's second-largest consumers of bottled water.

Beer, Wine, and Spirits

Besides replenishing bodily fluids and purifying drinking water, beverages have evolved to fulfill a range of human purposes, from the sacred to the medicinal and recreational. Various types of alcoholic beverages have served all of these functions. Nearly every creature on Earth is attracted to the fermentation of yeast and sugar or starch, a natural process that results in ethyl alcohol. Alcoholic beverages have been consumed by virtually every culture in the world throughout most of their recorded history, in part as a health precaution in the absence of clean water sources. The ancient Egyptians brewed beer in their homes on an everyday basis. People in ancient Honduras drank a

Beverages have evolved to fulfill a range of human purposes, from the sacred to the medicinal and recreational.

fermentation of chocolate. Distilled spirits were first introduced during the 12th and 13th centuries. Prior to the Enlightenment, people in western Europe drank weak beer and wine throughout the day.

Imbibing alcoholic beverages to temporarily alter one's state of consciousness is one of the few universal features of human behavior. Over the course of our history, alcoholic beverages have served as a social lubricant and as a means of promoting relaxation. They have provided nutrition and increased the pleasures of eating. Intoxicating beverages have been ingested for their medicinal, antiseptic, and analgesic properties, as well. Alcohol, especially wine, is regarded by some cultures as a gift from God and afforded a prominent place in religion and worship. Alcohol can be misused, however, and chronic overconsumption produces long-term health problems. Certain cultures have periodically banned the consumption of alcohol for religious or public health reasons, such as during the Prohibition era in the United States (1920–1933). The religion of Islam expressly forbids the consumption of alcoholic beverages, as do some branches of Christianity, including Mormonism. However, current research has determined that alcohol in general—not just wine—is heart healthy, and moderate consumption is beneficial for most adults.

Sweet and Fizzy Drinks

An alternative to alcoholic or "hard" beverages, what came to be known as "soft" drinks were first marketed in the 17th century, specifically in France, where a mixture of water and lemon juice sweetened with honey was sold by street vendors who carried tanks on their backs. The invention of methods for artificial carbonation enabled the creation of beverages that imitated gaseous mineral waters that many considered therapeutic. This association of carbonated water with health led to the installation of soda fountains in drugstores, which used pressurized tanks of carbonic acid gas to create fizzy beverages. Pharmacists added tinctures of cocaine, caffeine, and tobacco to these energizing "health" drinks, along with different flavorings and sweeteners. By the time many of these additives were phased out, people had developed an unhealthy thirst for such sugary beverages, which were originally sweetened with glucose in the form of cane and beet sugar. Plentiful and cheap to produce, thanks to U.S. government corn subsidies, high-fructose corn syrup became the major component of most popular soft drinks by the 1990s.

Today, sweetened, carbonated beverages are thought to be a major culprit in the global obesity epidemic. Though research is ongoing, fructose does not seem to trigger the same appetite-suppressing signals as glucose does. Sugars of all kinds contribute excess calories and health risks. New laws seek to limit or ban sugary drinks in some schools.

BEER

Beer dates from at least 6,000 years ago, when the Sumerians began fermenting a low-alcohol beverage from barley. Originally, the drink was consumed as a nutritional supplement: an ancient inscription counsels every good mother to supply her school-age sons with two jars of beer to ensure their healthy development. Beer has long been a working man's drink, a grain beverage that almost anyone could make at home. The builders of the pyramids received some of their payment in unfiltered beer.

   Beer consists of four main ingredients: water, malt (germinated grain), hops, and yeast. Almost every culture worldwide has independently developed methods of brewing beer from local ingredients. In the United States, most beers range in alcohol content from 3.2 to 8 percent; anything over 5 percent must be labeled "ale."

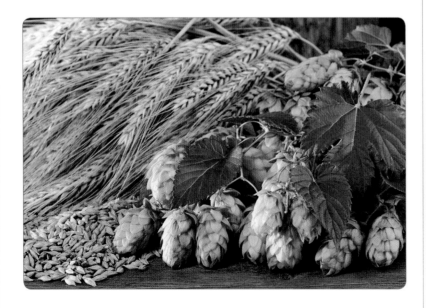

GIVES YOU

Niacin
Folate
Vitamin B6
Magnesium
Phosphorus
Potassium
Selenium

✦ TAKE AWAY

Choose from a wide variety of beers to find your favorite, but avoid overconsumption.

Choose and Use

Most supermarkets carry a wide assortment of domestic and imported beers, ranging from lighter beers such as lagers and pilsners, to darker styles such as porters and stouts. These have varying flavors, which pair well with different foods. Recently, craft beers from independent microbreweries have become popular. Unlike wines, most beers do not benefit from aging. Store bottled beer upright in a cool, dark place and refrigerate before serving. Once opened, bottled beer goes "flat," or loses its carbonation within a couple hours.

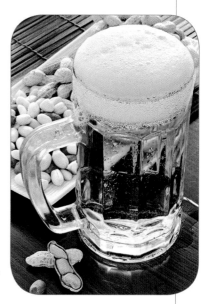

For Your Health

Most of the nutrients in grain are lost in the brewing process. Beer's proven benefits relate principally to its alcohol content, since moderate daily intake of alcohol has been determined to protect against heart disease, and to lower the risk of stroke and certain types of cancers, including those of the colon, ovary, and prostate. Studies also indicate that drinking beer may help prevent kidney stones, and that the silicon present in beer may increase bone density. However, overconsumption of this high-calorie beverage can contribute to abdominal obesity, aka the aptly named "beer belly," among other health problems. Notably, alcohol (of any kind) at higher intakes is a strong risk factor for breast cancer.

For Our Planet

Major beer producers use a huge amount of water in the brewing process. The carbon footprint of a pint of "suds" varies depending on whether it is bottled or draft, and where the beer is produced and consumed. Cans require far less energy to recycle than glass bottles. The footprint of an imported bottled beer may be three times larger than that of a locally brewed pint of beer on tap, so opting for a draft of local brew is a more sustainable choice.

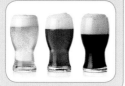

COFFEE

Coffee is a tropical evergreen shrub that grows in mountainous regions between the tropics of Cancer and Capricorn. Roasted coffee beans were first brewed into a beverage on the Arabian Peninsula around A.D. 1000. The practice spread throughout the Arab world in the 15th century as an alternative to drinking alcohol, prohibited under Islamic rule. Some historians argue that we have coffee to thank for the Enlightenment, the dramatic flourishing of Western thought that occurred during the 17th century. The French Revolution first percolated in a coffeehouse, and in these gathering places individuals from different backgrounds came together to socialize and exchange new ideas, under the stimulating influence of this naturally caffeinated beverage. Coffee drinking fueled commerce and became part of the rituals of business, and coffee is currently the second-largest traded commodity after crude oil.

Choose and Use

Beans labeled arabica are usually grown by organic and fair-trade coffee producers. A Fair Trade certification guarantees that the people who grow and pick your coffee beans have been paid a fair price, and that ethical labor practices have been followed. Fair-trade guidelines also require a limit on the use of pesticides and fertilizers in coffee production, and reduced impact on native plant and animal species. Avoid coffee labeled robusta, which is often of inferior quality and grown in environmentally damaging ways. You can purchase preground coffee or buy the beans and grind it yourself for maximum flavor. The finer the grind, the stronger the coffee; dense espresso, typically savored in small amounts, requires a very fine grind. Fresh beans yield the best flavor, so purchase in small amounts and store away from light in a cool, dry place—refrigeration or freezing does it no favors.

GIVES YOU

Riboflavin
Pantothenic acid
Potassium
Manganese
Magnesium
Phytonutrients
   (phenolic acids)

Choose Fair Trade, certified organic coffee to protect the farmers who grow it, and the planet too.

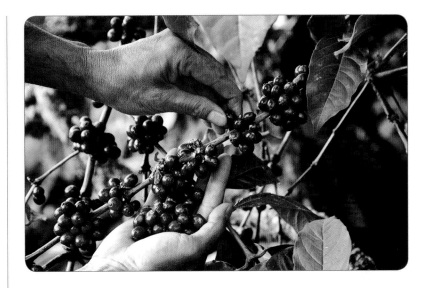

FOOD SCIENCE
✦
CAFFEINE

The myriad health benefits of coffee are due in part to its caffeine. Mildly addictive, the caffeine content varies depending on preparation as well as type and roast. Brewed coffee generally includes 150-200 mg in a 12-ounce serving, about the same amount of caffeine in a 2-ounce espresso shot; instant coffee contains about 100-150 mg.

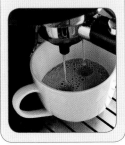

For Your Health

According to a 2005 study by researchers at the University of Scranton, Pennsylvania, coffee is the top source of powerful phenolic antioxidants in the U.S. diet, studies have shown that moderate coffee intake (two to four cups a day) may reduce the risk of liver cancer and gallbladder disease, improve alertness and concentration, and increase longevity. Caffeine itself is part of the healthful mix coffee provides, although decaf still includes the same range of antioxidants and phytonutrients and avoids potential insomnia and jitters that occur in some people. Good quality decaf tastes just as rich as caffeinated varieties. "Instant" coffees offer equivalent benefits, if not the same flavor, as fresh brewed. Many coffee-based drinks have added sugar and saturated fats, which considerably reduce the health benefits of this beverage.

For Our Planet

The world's thirst for coffee has led to monoculture plantations and severe environmental degradation in regions where this crop is grown. Swaths of rain forest land, essential to the biodiversity of the region and health of the planet, have been slashed and burned to clear land for more coffee plants. The fair trade movement offers economic incentives and training to encourage environmentally sustainable farming methods. Choosing Fair Trade Certified coffee helps support these efforts. Coffee that's certified "shade grown" by the Smithsonian Institution is the most sustainable.

MILK

Cave paintings depicting cows being milked offer proof that animal milk has been part of the human diet for thousands of years. People around the world consume milk from goats, camels, reindeer, llamas, sheep, and water buffalos, but cow's milk is the most popular, especially in the United States. European dairy cows were first brought to North America on Spanish ships during the 15th century. The inventions of two French scientists made the modern dairy industry possible: pasteurization, a high-heat process that kills harmful pathogens, and homogenization, which breaks up milk fats to keep them from separating and rising to the top as cream.

In 1993, the U.S. Food and Drug Administration (FDA) approved the practice of injecting dairy cows with an artificially produced growth hormone (recombinant bovine somatotropin, rBST and abbreviated BST, also known as rBGH), which increases milk production by 25 percent. Whether milk from BST-treated cows should be labeled, and whether BST adversely affects human health, is an ongoing controversy; organic dairy farms often choose to label their products "BST-free." Cow's milk is available in many varieties and can be made into a range of dairy products, including butter, yogurt, sour cream, and—most delicious of all— cheese, which first came about as a means of preserving milk during periods when animals were not lactating.

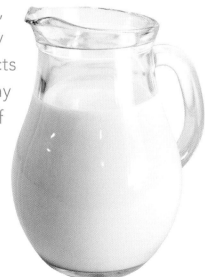

FOOD SCIENCE ✦ DAIRY ALTERNATIVES

While an excellent source of protein and calcium, the majority of the world's population is lactose intolerant. A wide array of non-dairy beverages is available, including soy, almond, rice, and coconut to name a few. Fortified alternatives often provide similar nutrition to cow's milk and have a lower environmental impact.

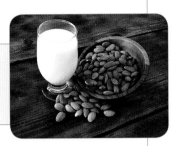

GIVES YOU

100 PERCENT
GRASS-FED COW'S MILK:
Iodine
Vitamin D
Calcium
Riboflavin
Phosphorus
Vitamin B12
Protein
Selenium
fatty acids
Magnesium
Phosphorus
Zinc
Potassium
Pantothenic acid
Vitamin A
Phytonutrients
   (carotenoids,
   isoflavones)

Choose and Use

The healthiest milk is from cows that have been pastured and grass-fed, so choose this whenever it is available. As a beverage, low-fat milk is most popular, but nonfat (skim) milk is a better choice for limiting saturated fat and saving a few calories. Used judiciously in cooking, whole milk, half-and-half,

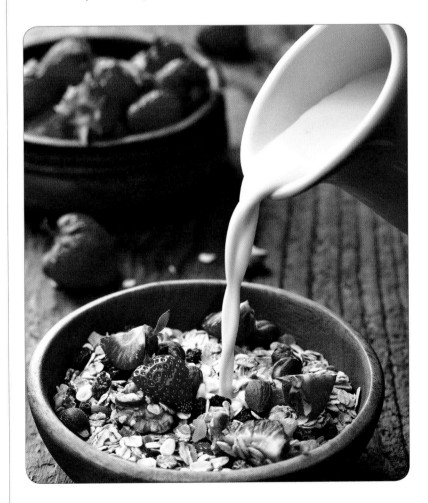

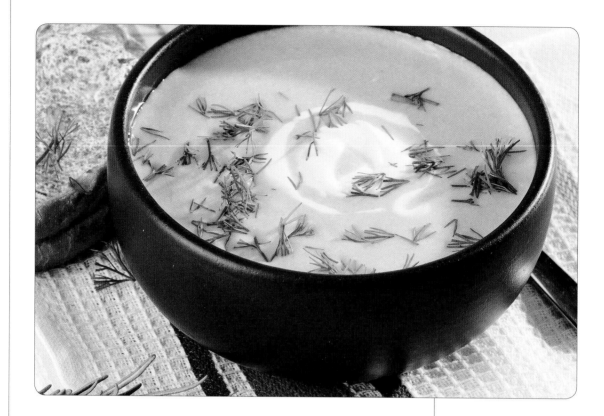

and cream add richness to soups and sauces. Ultrapasteurized boxed milk, popular in Europe and increasingly in the United States, can be stored without refrigeration. Foods rich in oxalate and phytates, which occur naturally in foods like spinach, berries, and grains, can inhibit calcium absorption somewhat, but there is no need to limit these foods if you are eating a varied diet with adequate calcium.

For Your Health

Fortified with vitamins A and D, U.S. cow's milk is a natural source of bone-strengthening calcium among a large set of vitamins, minerals, and phytonutrients. Conjugated linoleic acid (CLA) in milk has been associated with many health benefits, mostly in animal research, including immune system support and reduced body fat. Milk from grass-fed cows contains from two to five times as much CLA as milk from cows fed on hay and grain, as well as a higher content of omega-3 fatty acids. It also features a more balanced fat composition, with less of the saturated fatty acid often associated with heart disease.

✦ **TAKE AWAY**

Choose nonfat milk or dairy alternatives for a rich source of calcium and other nutrients.

FOOD SCIENCE
✦
RAW MILK

A growing interest in minimally processed foods has led to a surge in raw milk consumption. Raw milk is more likely to contain potentially fatal pathogens, and children are particularly vulnerable due to their developing immune systems. Do your health a favor by sticking to pasteurized milk.

For Our Planet

The 100,000 farms that constitute the U.S. dairy industry currently account for 2 percent of total greenhouse gas emissions due to methane-producing cows. In 2013, the U.S. Department of Agriculture and American dairy producers renewed an agreement to reduce emissions by 25 percent and increase the sustainability of the dairy industry in the years to come. Environmental scientists stress the importance of smaller herd sizes and the value of grass in making milk a more earth-friendly beverage.

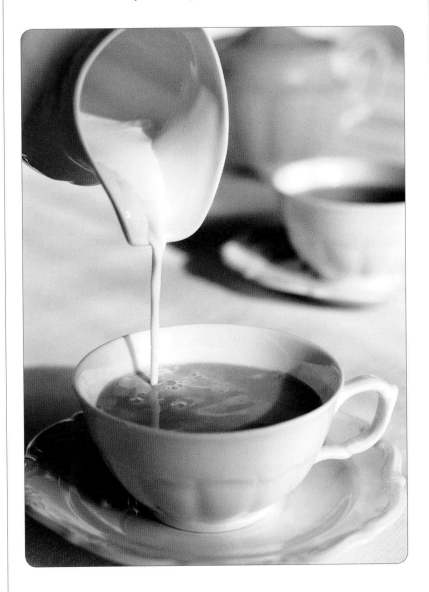

SPIRITS

The production of spirits, or distilled alcoholic beverages, depends upon fermentation. Organic (meaning, carbon-containing) materials containing carbohydrates naturally decompose, or ferment. When the ethyl alcohol produced by this process is heated, and the resulting vapor is condensed, the distilled condensation has a high alcohol content. The two ingredients essential to fermentation, carbohydrates and yeast, occur everywhere; as a result, civilizations all over the world have developed their own forms of alcoholic beverages.

The earliest spirits were made from grapes and honey, but eventually people used corn, rice, barley, and even potatoes to produce distilled "hard" alcohol. From the beginning, distilled spirits have served many purposes, from recreational to medical. Brandy made from distilled wine and rum from sugarcane molasses helped placate sailors during long sea voyages during the age of exploration from the 15th to the early 17th century. Grog, a mixture of rum, water, and lemon or lime juice, was a compulsory beverage for British sailors in the late 18th century. The vitamin C in the citrus helped reduce the incidence of scurvy. Today, spirits such as vodka (Russia), ouzo (Greece), tequila (Mexico), and scotch (Scotland) are all infused with deep cultural associations related to their countries of origin.

Choose and Use

Hard alcohol production is subject to many controls. Made from the blue agave plant, all tequila is imported from Mexico. Also strictly regulated, whiskey is made from fermented grain mash and aged in wooden casks. Different varieties of whisky, such as Scotch and bourbon, are produced in specific geographic locations (Scotland and Kentucky, respectively)

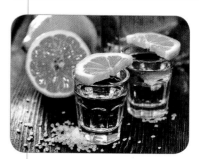

and are subject to different processes and ingredients. Gin and vodka are among the most popular types of clear spirits; vodka is neutral in flavor, whereas the taste of gin comes from juniper berries and can vary greatly depending on the herbs and other ingredients used in its production. Firmly capped and stored

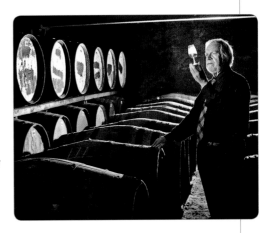

in a cool, dark place, spirits keep indefinitely. Hard liquor has a far higher alcohol content than beer or wine and should be enjoyed sparingly. Spirits may be savored on their own or mixed with other components in a cocktail. Rum and sweet liqueurs are also popular flavorings in desserts.

For Your Health

The health benefits of moderate drinking are well documented: alcohol can help prevent heart attacks and strokes and raise "good" high-density lipoprotein (HDL) cholesterol levels. Per ounce, distilled spirits have more calories than beer or wine, so moderation is key. Generally, equivalent alcohol doses are obtained from 1.5 ounces of liquor, 12 ounces of beer, and 5 ounces of wine. The number of calories in hard alcohol is correlated with its "proof" (200 proof is 100 percent alcohol)—the higher the proof, the more calories. Liquor is often blended with fruit juices and other types of alcohol, so the final calorie count for a single cocktail can be substantial. Mixing water, soda, or tonic water with spirits is a lower-calorie choice.

For Our Planet

The distillation process uses large amounts of water and energy, though some producers now convert waste products into fuel. On the whole, the alcoholic beverage industry sets fewer sustainability goals than other industries, but the sustainable spirit movement is gaining ground. Seek out microdistilleries in your area, and investigate producers that get high marks for sustainable practices.

GIVES YOU

Certain varieties of hard liquor contain trace amounts of vitamins and minerals. However, since these amounts are very small and alcohol should only be consumed in limited amounts, spirits offer virtually no known nutritional benefits beyond their alcohol content.

TEAS AND INFUSIONS: GREEN, BLACK, HERBAL

After water, tea is the second most popular drink in the world. Both green and black teas are made from the glossy leaves and leaf buds of a shrub called Camellia sinensis, related to the ornamental camellia and native to India and China. While botanically identical, black tea is prepared from fermented tea leaves and contains more caffeine and tannins than unfermented green tea.

Tea became a daily drink in China around the third century B.C., and several centuries later the Chinese introduced it to Japan. Made with boiled water, tea provided a sanitary beverage in places with dubious water quality. Preparing and drinking matcha, or powdered green tea, became a highly ritualized ceremony in Japanese culture. Trade relations with China introduced tea to the Europeans in the 17th century. This stimulating beverage has been credited with fueling the Industrial Revolution by keeping the laboring classes, who formerly drank weak beer throughout the day, more alert at their tasks.

PREP TIP ✦ STEEPING

In some parts of the world, drinking tea is a daily ritual. Critical to a splendid cup of tea or herbal infusion, steeping is an important step that differs by variety; whether the leaves were loose or prepackaged also matters. To steep the perfect cup, follow the instructions carefully. If you're planning on making iced tea, you'll want to brew a stronger pot to allow for the diluting effect when the ice melts.

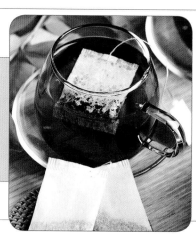

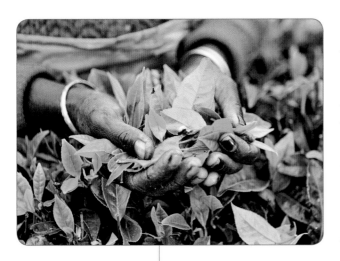

Choose and Use

Available loose or in bags, tea tastes good both hot and cold, served plain or with lemon and lightly sweetened with sugar or honey. Home-brewed teas are healthier than bottled, which often contain added calories and sugar and excess packaging. From delicate Darjeeling from India to England's Earl Grey, there are thousands of varieties; experiment to find a tea you love.

For Your Health

Green tea has a higher concentration of certain flavonoids than black tea. The most abundant is a catechin called epigallocatechin-3-gallate (EGCG), believed to be responsible for most of green tea's antioxidant and anticancer properties. These include the prevention of atherosclerosis and hypertension; protection against pediatric brain tumors, and geriatric cognitive decline, Alzheimer's, and Parkinson's disease; improved weight loss and bone density; and prevention of prostate, ovarian, and many other cancers. A 2006 study published in the Journal of the American Medical Association showed that drinking green tea lowers one's risk of death from all causes, especially cardiovascular disease. Results of this study were more pronounced in women than in men.

Black tea can reduce the risk of stroke, and its antibacterial qualities guard against cavities and gum disease. Flavonoids remain in decaffeinated teas, so feel free to switch to decaf later in the day. Herbal teas have been less studied, but health claims are likely in concert with their food source, potential benefits ranging from aiding digestion to promoting lactation.

For Our Planet

Tea farming raises a number of social and environmental issues. Acreage devoted to tea cultivation limits regional biodiversity and contributes to soil erosion and water pollution. Purchasing Fair Trade Certified and organically grown tea helps make this a more sustainable beverage. Compost your old tea bags and used leaves; loose tea requires less packaging than tea in bags.

GIVES YOU

HERBAL:
Health benefits depend upon the substance being infused, but they have lower concentrations of antioxidants than black or green tea. Most are caffeine-free, but beware that some commercially produced teas are black or green tea flavored with herbs and contain caffeine.

GREEN:
Phytonutrients
    (flavonoids,
    phenolic acids)
    catechins for both
Fluoride

BLACK:
Phytonutrients
    (flavonoids,
    phenolic acids)

WATER

Water is an essential nutrient, the basis of all life on Earth, and no civilization has survived without prioritizing this precious resource. On a planet covered with oceans, freshwater accounts for just 3 percent of the Earth's water supply, and two-thirds of it is frozen in glaciers or otherwise inaccessible. The available freshwater is unevenly distributed around the planet, and much is polluted or unsustainably managed. Agriculture soaks up 70 percent of the world's freshwater use, but 60 percent of this is wasted due to leaky and inefficient irrigation systems. At current rates of overconsumption, our freshwater reserves are being depleted twice as fast as the growing global population rate. By 2025, diminishing water supplies will likely impact two-thirds of the Earth's peoples and pit the needs of communities against industry, rich against poor, state against state, and nation against nation. We have yet to reach a global consensus about how to conserve and manage the world's water supply. However, people everywhere agree that water scarcity represents one of the greatest challenges of this century.

CONSIDER ✦ DESERT AGRICULTURE

Essential for human life, water is also fundamental to a country's economic stability given its critical role in food production. Many countries with arid regions or deserts face water shortages that threaten food security. An increase in severe weather due to climate change further strains this precious natural resource.

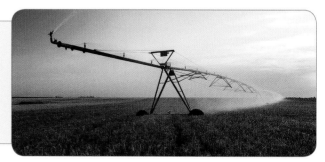

GIVES YOU

Drinking water collected from aquifers, lakes, and rivers contains a range of minerals, including calcium and magnesium, present in varying quantities, depending on the source and location. Water contains no protein, carbohydrates, fat, or fiber.

Choose and Use

Approximately half the bottled water sold in the United States comes from municipal water supplies. Those concerned about water quality should know that bottled water may actually contain more contaminants than tap water. Whereas 90 percent of U.S. tap water must meet strict Environmental Protection Agency (EPA) regulations for water quality, the bottled water industry is largely unmonitored. It takes about three liters of water to create one liter of bottled water: Fill up a BPA-free reusable bottle from your tap to conserve precious water resources and keep plastic bottles out of the landfill. Install a filter on your faucet if contaminants are a concern where you live. Approximately 15 percent of Americans rely on private wells for their drinking water, which are not subject to EPA standards.

Water from the tap should be your go-to beverage of choice to meet your nutritional needs, but there's little evidence to support the oft-repeated dictum to drink eight glasses of water a day. Among healthy individuals, it's best to listen to your body: when you're thirsty, drink. Downing a tall glass of water 30

✦ TAKE AWAY

Satisfy your thirst with tap water for a sustainable drink filled with nutrients.

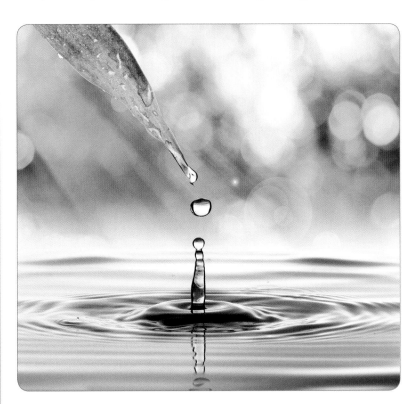

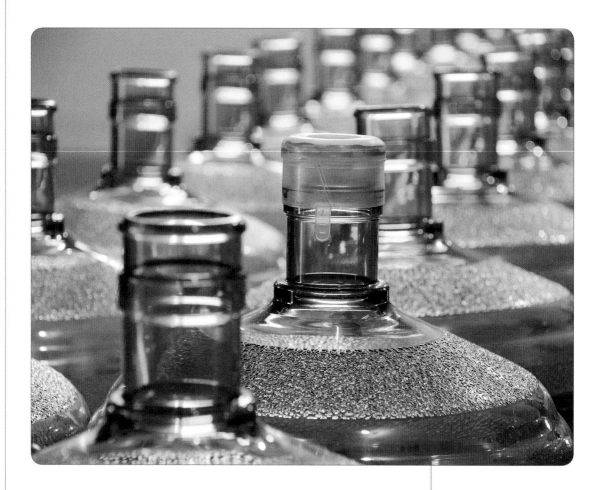

minutes before a meal can help with weight loss, since you will feel full and may eat less. However, drinking a lot of water during meals may interfere with the digestive process. About eighty percent of one's daily water requirements come from beverages like water, coffee, tea, and juice and the rest from food.

Sports drinks such as Gatorade have been developed to help athletes to quickly rehydrate and replace electrolytes and carbohydrates, as well as the potassium and sodium lost through sweating. Recently, coconut water has been touted as "nature's sports drink." This healthy and low-calorie beverage includes vitamins, minerals, and antioxidants and can help correct a potassium deficiency. However, those who exercise strenuously require the additional sodium that most traditional sports drinks contain. Markets sell many premixed flavorings for water, in liquid and powder form. Water may also be "enhanced" with various vitamins, minerals, and even caffeine, but many of these drinks contain additional calories. Pure, clean water is best enjoyed in its natural state, or with a wedge of lemon, a slice of cucumber, or a sprig of mint.

For Your Health

Water is essential to health. All our bodily functions depend upon water. Among its myriad benefits, it helps maintain blood pressure, improves mental performance, eliminates toxins from our bodies in conjunction with the liver, increases athletic performance, and aids in digestion. Water provides the most nutrients with the least amount of calories. Since the 1950s, fluoride has been added to drinking water in many U.S. municipalities to protect against tooth decay. Fluoridation is considered one of the top 10 public health achievements of the 20th century, although some claim that adding fluoride, a naturally occurring element in soil and water, is harmful to our health. Most developed nations do not fluoridate their water, and voters in some cities have rejected fluoridation.

For Our Planet

Bottling water uses energy and creates waste. Boxed water may soon replace bottled as a more environmentally friendly alternative, but filling up a reusable container with tap water is still the most sustainable option. In 2010, federal policies were established to help promote sustainability in the U.S. water infrastructure, requiring the government to partner with state and local agencies to ensure a clean, safe, and plentiful water supply.

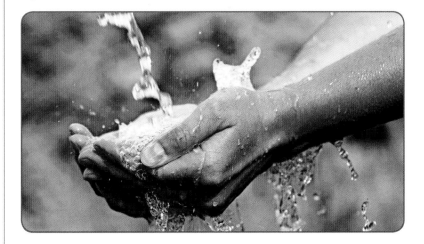

FOOD SCIENCE
✦
BOTTLED WATER

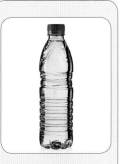

While convenient, drinking bottled water is not the greenest choice: it takes about 3 liters of water to create 1 liter of bottled water. Research has shown that most tap water is just as tasty as bottled so assuming your water is safe, using your tap is the top choice for the planet. It's best to bring your own reusable bottle that can be refilled when on the road.

WINE

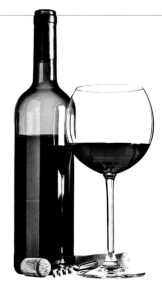

The roots of winemaking reach back many thousands of years into human history. A biblical story has Noah landing on Mt. Ararat after the flood and immediately planting grapevines. This alcoholic beverage may be even older than beer, as evidenced by stains inside vessels dating from the Neolithic period (8500–4000 B.C.). From early on, wine was employed in religious ceremonies, and better-tasting wines were reserved for the elite social classes.

The naturally fermented juice of grapes, wine is easier to make than beer but more difficult to store. A true art and science of winemaking had to wait until the mass production of glass bottles in the 19th century. Until recently, only a limited number of regions were known for winemaking. Today, vineyards producing excellent wines exist throughout the world.

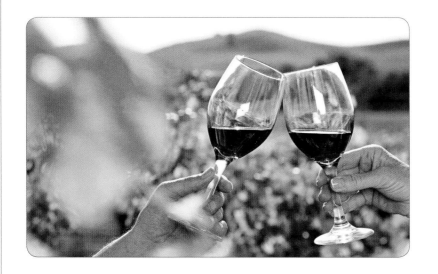

✦ TAKE AWAY

Enjoy wine in moderate amounts to help prevent heart disease.

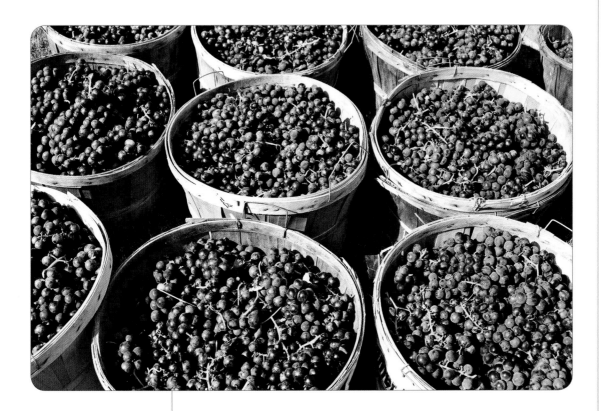

GIVES YOU

RED WINE:

Phytonutrients
 (stilbene, flavonoids,
 phenolic acid,
 resveratrol)
Manganese
Iron
Magnesium
Phosphorus
Potassium

Choose and Use

Most modern supermarkets stock a wide range of red, white,
rosé, sparkling, and dessert (sweet) wines. A wine merchant can
offer suggestions about which varieties best complement certain foods. The best advice, though, is be guided by your own
tastes. It is far better to enjoy yourself than to fret over choosing
the right combination of wine and food. Store unopened wine
in a cool, dark place. Bottled wine should be kept on its side
to prevent the cork from drying out. Some wines must be aged

FOOD SCIENCE ✦ FERMENTATION

Grape juice becomes wine through fermentation, in which added yeasts reacts
with sugars from the grapes to create alcohol (specifically, ethyl alcohol).
Temperature, speed, oxygen, and the container used for fermentation all
impact the nature and character of the wine. The same grape can produce
drastically different wines depending on how it's fermented, as anyone who's
compared a California chardonnay, produced in oak barrels, with a French
Chablis (also the chardonnay grape), produced in stainless steel casks.

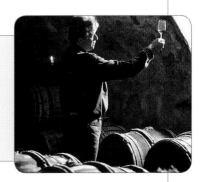

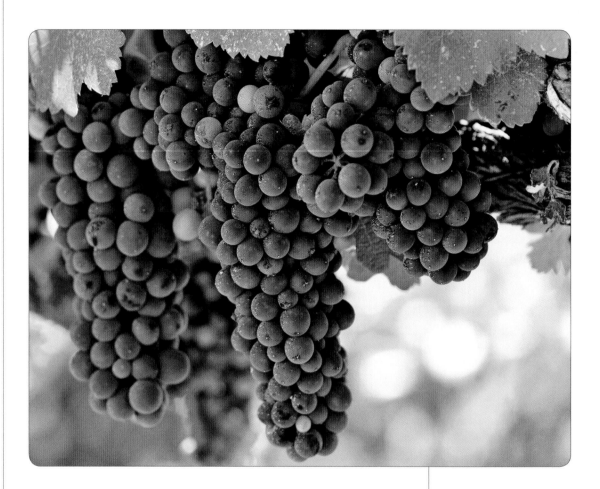

for a few years under proper conditions to achieve their full potential; however, many don't age well and are best consumed soon after purchase. Red wines are usually best served at cooler room temperatures (roughly 60 degrees). White wines should be refrigerated before serving and stored in the fridge after opening. Wines intended for use in cooking should be good enough to drink.

PREP TIP ✦ WINE PAIRING

Classic advice on pairing wine with food was overly simple: white wine with seafood or vegetables, red wine with beef, and either with poultry depending on preparation. There is considerable variation among red and white wines, however, and finding the best match to your particular dish can be a challenge. If you're not an expert, many agree to just drink what you enjoy.

Terroir comes from the French word terre, meaning "land" or "earth." Generally referring to climate, geography, and geology of a particular place, it's a term used to characterize differences among wines. Even within the same variety of grape, the smell, taste, and color of wine varies markedly due to terroir—as well as the style and specific ingredients of the winemaker.

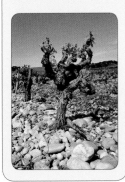

For Your Health

A polyphenol called resveratrol present in red wine may help repair blood vessels, prevent blood clots, and reduce "bad" low-density lipoprotein (LDL) cholesterol, although most research is in animal models consuming very high doses. Resveratrol resides in the grape skins, which give wine its red color. The skins also contain many of the bioflavonoids and phenols from which wine's health benefits derive, which is why purple grape juice shares some of its health properties. Research shows that moderate consumption of alcohol helps prevent heart disease; resveratrol may provide additional benefit, but wines of all varieties and colors are beneficial due to their alcohol content.

For Our Planet

Wine is shipped all over the world, but the largest component of its carbon footprint is packaging (predominantly glass bottles and corks), which accounts for 46 percent of wine's total carbon emissions. Wine grapes tend to grow in marginal-quality farmland, thus making good economic use of low-yield land. Grapevines are tough plants that don't necessarily require pesticides or fertilizers to thrive. In fact, vines grown in mediocre soil that lacks water produce smaller grapes. A higher skin-to-juice ratio is desirable for wine grapes, since most flavor components are concentrated in the skin. Composting the pressed skins and seeds back into the vineyard preserves the terroir—the unique character of a place that distinguishes the wine's flavor.

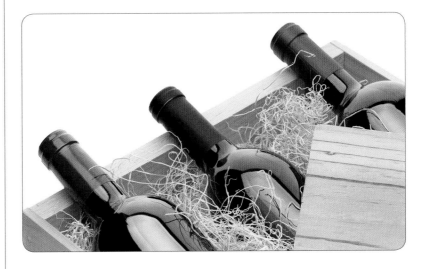

✦ TAKE AWAY

Wine, especially red, may offer more than a pleasing meal accompaniment.

SEASONINGS

A BRIEF HISTORY OF SPICES

Added to foods to intensify or improve their flavors, seasonings include herbs and spices as well as condiments. They have been considered important enough to wage wars over, and the human desire for them has proved stronger than our fear of the unknown. The demand for spices, in particular, has fueled great voyages of discovery, carved out intercontinental trade routes, and sparked armed conflicts. Spices have commanded astronomical prices, and they have been regarded as valuable enough to serve as currency at various times in history: cumin seeds were accepted as tithe, and people have paid their rent in peppercorns.

The story of spices typically begins in the Eastern Hemisphere, but in the Americas the Aztecs, Mayans, and Incas used seasonings as well. Besides enlivening bland or tainted foods, spices were valued in early cultures for their medicinal properties. They were used as antidotes for poisons and to cure disease and prevent illness. Ancient people invested certain spices with magical properties and used them in religious ceremonies to commemorate major life events such as births, marriages, and deaths.

The Role of Seasonings in Health

Today seasonings are still highly valued, less expensive, and available in supermarkets, specialty stores, or online. Used extensively to enhance the flavor of many processed foods, salt is an example of a seasoning that is cheap and plentiful today, but which was once one of the most valuable commodities on earth. Unlike other seasonings, salt is essential for human health, but our current craving for it far surpasses our body's daily requirement of this mineral. Introducing a wider range of herbs and spices into the foods we prepare may help wean our palates away from salt and help us limit our sodium intake. Many consumers think of herbs and spices as a means to add a bit of color, flavor, or heat to a dish without adding salt, fat, or calories; however, some seasonings have antioxidant levels that rival those of fruits and vegetables when regularly added to the diet. Current scientific research often bears out ancient beliefs and traditional medical practices, such as those in Ayurvedic and Chinese medicine, about the health benefits of herbs and spices.

The New American Palate

The increasing diversity of the North American population has led to a growing demand for a wider array of seasonings. Latinos now represent the largest-growing immigrant group, followed by Asians, bringing with them a taste for the flavors of home. The United States is the world's largest spice importer and consumer. Most supermarkets now devote an extensive amount of shelf space to "ethnic" ingredients from different world cultures, and seasonings once considered exotic have become commonplace. Half of the spices shipped to the U.S. come from India, Mexico, Indonesia, Canada, and China. Fresh herbs rarely travel well, but their seeds do. Herbs native to one global region become immigrants, too, taking root in new corners of the world, lending their flavors to local cuisines. Finally, a growing interest in healthy eating and "natural" methods of disease prevention have inspired many to learn about the nutritional benefits of seasonings.

BASIL

Highly fragrant basil is rich in bone-building vitamin K. The herb contains an array of volatile oils that help protect against unwanted bacterial growth, making this a beneficial additive to uncooked foods. The flavonoids present in basil help protect cell structures as well as chromosomes from radiation and oxygen-based damage. Best tasting when fresh, basil leaves should be added at the end of the cooking process to preserve their flavor. This summertime plant will flourish in a sunny windowsill garden, and growing your own means you can avoid buying it packaged in plastic. An abundance of basil can be made into traditional pesto, with the addition of ground pine nuts, garlic, Parmesan cheese and olive oil. During summer's bounty, make some extra and freeze to enjoy during winter months.

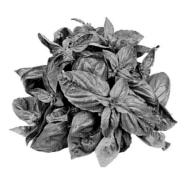

BLACK PEPPER

Found on every table in the country, pepper was once used as currency, and a man's wealth was measured by his supply of it. Black, green, and white peppercorns, which are ground to make pepper, are the fruit of the same tropical vine (though pink peppercorns are not) and reflect different stages of development and processing methods. Black pepper stimulates the taste buds and signals the stomach to secrete hydrochloric acid, which promotes digestion. It contains manganese, vitamin K, and iron, and works as a carminitive to help prevent the formation of intestinal gas. Green peppercorns are most likely to be found preserved in a pickle brine and are used in a quite different way from black or white pepper. The world's first sustainable black pepper was produced in Indonesia in 2013. The Rainforest Alliance Certified black peppercorns are grown in a manner that promotes biodiversity and reduces the use of pesticides and chemicals.

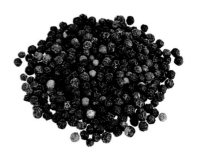

CAYENNE PEPPER

CILANTRO

Cayenne pepper is a spicy, orange-red powder made from a tropical chili pepper belonging to the Capsicum genus. Its warm color signals the presence of beta-carotene, an antioxidant that the body converts into vitamin A. Capsaicin, the volatile oil that gives cayenne pepper its heat, is widely used as a topical treatment for pain relief. Cayenne also has been shown to have cardiovascular benefits. Cultures where large quantities of chili peppers are consumed experience lower rates of heart attack and stroke. Cayenne has also proven effective in ulcer prevention. Surveys have shown that Chinese patients suffer from three times more gastric ulcers than Indians and Malaysians, who regularly consume chili peppers. Cayenne pepper also rapidly drains congested nasal passages by stimulating mucus membranes. International efforts to make spice production less damaging to biodiversity may soon result in sustainable cayenne pepper.

This ancient spice, mentioned in the Old Testament, is known by two names. Its fresh green leaves are called cilantro; the seeds of the plant (available whole or ground into powder) are known as coriander, and neither tastes like the other. Cilantro has a strong flavor (some say soapy) well suited to highly seasoned foods common in Indian and Mexican cuisine. Rich in beneficial phytonutrients, cilantro leaves are sometimes confused with those of Italian flat-leaf parsley. They belong to the same plant family but are not at all similar in flavor. When incorporated into uncooked foods, such as salsas, cilantro acts as a natural antibacterial to kill salmonella. Coriander seeds have a mild, aromatic character and are used in pickling and curry blends. Guidelines established by the Sustainable Spice Initiative (SSI) will soon be extended to coriander/cilantro, along with the other culinary spices recognized by the European Spice Association (ESA).

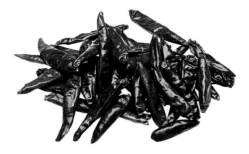

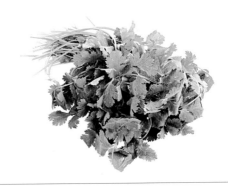

CINNAMON

Cinnamon is made from the inner bark of a tropical evergreen tree. Harvested when pliable, it is dried and ground to form the powdered spice sold in stores, or left in rolled tubes called quills and packaged as "sticks." Cinnamon's healing properties come from essential oils found in the bark and include preventing the growth of unwanted pathogens in food, limiting unwanted blood clotting, and reducing blood sugar levels in individuals with type 2 diabetes. The scent of cinnamon alone has been shown to boost brain functioning. Of more than one hundred varieties, the most commonly available types are Ceylon and Chinese cinnamon. Wonderful in many sweet baked goods, cinnamon is also often used in savory North African and Middle Eastern dishes, adding warmth and depth. Like bamboo, cinnamon is an inherently sustainable crop, which grows naturally without the aid of agrochemicals. The first Rainforest Alliance Certified cinnamon became available in 2013.

CUMIN

Native to Egypt, cumin was very popular in Europe during the Middle Ages and is used today in many Middle Eastern, Indian, and Mexican dishes. Available as both "seeds" and in powdered form, this aromatic spice is made from the fruit of a plant in the parsley family. The amber variety is most common, but white and black cumin seeds may also be found in specialty markets. Rich in iron, cumin blends well with curries and in chili. Traditionally, cumin seeds have long been recognized as a digestive aid, a belief supported by recent studies indicating that this spice stimulates digestive enzymes in the pancreas. Ground cumin will keep in a cool, dark place for six months. Whole seeds stay fresh twice as long. Sustainable Spice Initiative (SSI) guidelines will help ensure that this spice will be produced more sustainably in the future.

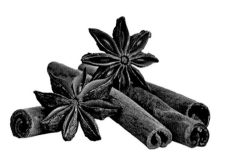

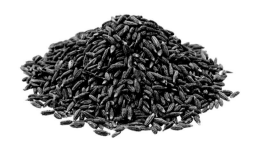

DILL

Mentioned in the Bible as well as in ancient Egyptian writings, dill has long been valued for its curative properties. Both the leaves and seeds are used as seasoning, though the seeds have a stronger flavor. Dill, especially the seed, is a good source of calcium, which helps prevent bone loss. Monoterpenes in this herb's oils make dill a "chemoprotective" food, which can help neutralize certain carcinogens. Flavonoids in this plant also provide beneficial components. Dill's wispy green leaves are frequent additions to Russian and Scandinavian foods. Fresh is superior to dried in flavor. Dill seeds can soothe the stomach after meals, so keep a small dish on the table. Organic dill is widely available, and this plant may be easily grown in a kitchen herb garden.

GINGER

Ginger root is the underground rhizome of the ginger plant. This versatile spice has an aromatic and spicy flavor well suited to both sweet and savory dishes. Ginger is especially popular in Asian dishes, where it is often paired with garlic. As a home health remedy, ginger has long been used to relieve the symptoms of motion sickness and nausea, but clinical studies have proven inconclusive. The root also contains anti-inflammatory compounds called gingerols, which can diminish the pain and swelling associated with arthritis. Fresh ginger must be refrigerated; unpeeled, it should keep for three weeks. The light brown skin is usually removed with a paring knife before grating or chopping the flesh. Powdered ginger root is often added to baked goods. Organizations such as Sustainable Harvest International are encouraging more farmers in countries such as Belize to produce sustainable, organically grown ginger.

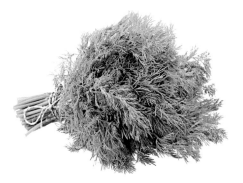

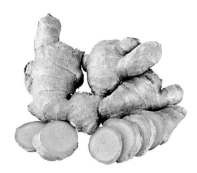

MINT

Mint is an ancient herb, long prized for its culinary and medicinal properties. Many varieties exist, including peppermint and spearmint, and its cooling, aromatic flavor may be used to enhance both sweet and savory dishes. Peppermint oil has been shown to soothe the digestive system, relieving indigestion and the symptoms of irritable bowel syndrome, although it may negatively affect people with heartburn or gastroesophageal reflux disease (GERD). A 2010 study of antioxidants in 3,100 foods, beverages, and seasonings placed peppermint at the top of the list of culinary herbs for its antioxidant content. Mint leaves are also infused into an aromatic herbal tea, a traditional beverage prepared to welcome guests in the Middle East. Fresh mint leaves have a vibrant green color. Refrigerated, they will keep for several days, wrapped in a dampened paper towel inside a loosely closed plastic bag. Mint will thrive in a kitchen garden; growing your own reduces packaging waste.

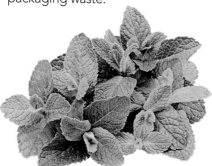

MUSTARD

The mustard plant is a member of the mighty *Brassicaceae* family, which includes broccoli, cabbage, and Brussels sprouts. Like its cruciferous relations, mustard contains certain beneficial phytonutrients called glucosinolates that may help guard against gastrointestinal (specifically, colorectal) and possibly lung cancers. Mustard seeds are sold whole, ground into powder, or processed with other ingredients and spices into a yellow or brown paste called "prepared mustard." Mustard seeds are available in colors ranging from white and yellow to brown and black, with varying degrees of spiciness. Mixing mustard powder with water prompts an enzymatic reaction that enhances the heat and pungent flavor of this popular spice, creating a homemade version of the familiar supermarket condiment. Guidelines established by the Sustainable Spice Initiative (SSI) will help make sustainable mustard seed available in the future.

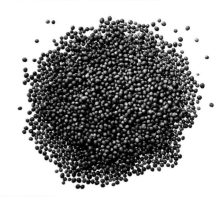

OREGANO

An aromatic herb with gray-green oval leaves often featured in Mediterranean cooking, oregano was little known in the United States until after World War I, when American GIs returning from Italy brought word of it back home with them. Derived from the Greek meaning "mountain joy," oregano is native to northern Europe, where this plant is sometimes called wild marjoram, to distinguish it from its cousin, sweet marjoram. The volatile oils thymol and carvacrol, both antibacterials, are present in oregano, and oregano oil can help fight MRSA (strains of antibiotic-resistant bacteria) and staph infections. Italian, Greek, or Mexican varieties of this herb taste delicious with tomato-based Italian dishes; many recipes call for dried, but fresh oregano offers greater health benefits though more must be used to impart the same flavor. Sonoran oregano, grown and harvested by the Seri Indians, is a sustainable crop.

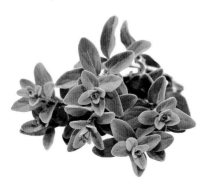

PARSLEY

Once relegated to mere garnish status on American plates, fresh parsley is rich in vitamins K, C, and A and lends its bright, grassy flavor to various foods. Originally used as a medicine in ancient cultures, the herb contains volatile oils and flavonoids, both highly beneficial to human health. The two most commonly available varieties are curly parsley and the milder flavored flat-leaf Italian type. Immerse stems in a jar of water and store in the fridge, loosely covered with a plastic bag; fresh parsley will keep for quite awhile this way, if you refresh the water every few days. Fresh is best; this herb loses its flavor quickly when dried. Plant parsley in a sunny windowbox, and you'll always have fresh leaves at hand.

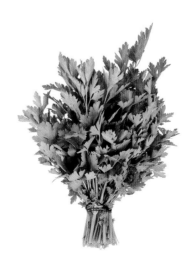

ROSEMARY

SAGE

This flowering evergreen shrub is native to the Mediterranean, where it has been prized since ancient times for both culinary and medicinal uses. Recent studies suggest that smelling rosemary improves long-term memory and brain function, which may explain why, in ancient Greece, students wore rosemary sprigs in their hair while studying for exams. As is true of many herbs, fresh rosemary is superior to dried. Most recipes use the plant's narrow, gray-green leaves, which are easily stripped from the stems. This herb's assertive flavor pairs well with lamb and other meats, as well as chicken and fish. You can grow your own rosemary, or choose organically grown using sustainable farming methods.

Long revered for its culinary and medicinal properties, the name of this herb derives from the Latin word *slavere*, meaning "to be saved." The lance-shaped, silvery green leaves of the sage plant are an excellent memory enhancer; a British study conducted in 2003 demonstrated that essential oil from sage may enhance memory in healthy young adults. The dried root of certain varieties of this herb contains active compounds similar to pharmaceuticals developed to treat Alzheimer's disease. Sage is also a source of beneficial flavonoids, phenolic acids, and enzymes with antioxidant and anti-inflammatory properties. Fresh sage leaves will keep for a few days in the refrigerator; dried sage leaves are also used to lend depth of flavor to soups and stews. Growing your own sage keeps those plastic herb packages out of the landfill.

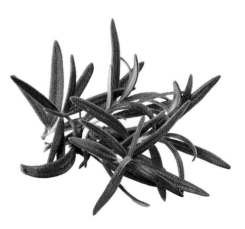

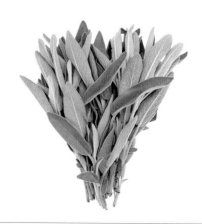

THYME

TURMERIC

Native to southern Europe and the Mediterranean, this delicate-looking herb has a penetrating flavor and was historically associated with bravery. Widely used in cooking, thyme also has a long history as a treatment for respiratory problems and is a good source of vitamin K for bone health. Thymol, the primary volatile oil in thyme, helps protect cellular membranes. The oils in thyme have been shown to limit microbial growth, so adding fresh thyme to a vinaigrette may help reduce any bacteria on salad greens. Fresh thyme and dried thyme are both widely available. Fresh thyme should be added to food toward the end of the cooking process, since heat causes a loss of flavor. Dried thyme can be added at the beginning. Thyme is a hardy plant that grows easily worldwide without the use of pesticides.

The root of a tropical plant related to ginger, this rhizome has multiple uses: as a textile dye, a spice, and a healing remedy. Ballpark mustard gets its bright yellow color from turmeric, and the spice lends its warm and bitter flavor to curry powder. Turmeric is an ancient spice native to Indonesia and southern India, used in traditional Ayurvedic and Chinese medicine. Turmeric's vivid color comes from curcumin, an antioxidant that may inhibit the growth of cancer cells by helping the body destroy mutated cancer cells. Many Indian recipes season cauliflower with powdered turmeric, a combination that may prevent prostate cancer and limit the spread of established cancers. The combination of turmeric and onions may afford protection against colorectal cancers. Sustainable turmeric cultivation can double a farmer's profit—an excellent incentive for sustainable production.

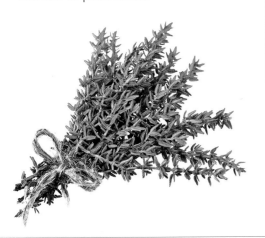

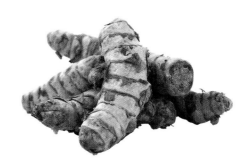

ABOUT THE AUTHORS

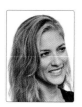

P. K. Newby, Sc.D., M.P.H.

Nutrition scientist, educator, food writer, and speaker, P. K. Newby has studied diet, chronic diseases, and sustainable eating for more than 15 years. She teaches in the Gastronomy, Culinary Arts, and Wine Studies program at Boston University and the program in Sustainability and Environmental Management at Harvard Extension School. She holds a doctorate from Harvard University's School of Public Health and master's degrees in public health and human nutrition from Columbia University. Newby shares sound science and fabulous cooking on her blog, *The Nutrition Doctor Is in the Kitchen: Where Science Is Sexy and Healthy Eating Is Spectacular.*

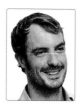

Barton Seaver

Chef, author, speaker, and National Geographic Fellow Barton Seaver is host of the National Geographic Web series Cook-Wise and is the director of the Healthy and Sustainable Food Program at the Center for Health and the Global Environment at the Harvard School of Public Health. A graduate of the Culinary Institute of America, he was named *Esquire* magazine's 2009 "Chef of the Year." In 2012 he was named by Secretary of State Hillary Clinton to the United States Culinary Ambassador Corps. He is the author of *For Cod & Country* and *Where There's Smoke: Simple, Sustainable, Delicious Grilling,* both published by Sterling Epicure.

CONTRIBUTING WRITERS

Monique Vescia
VEGETABLES | FATS AND OILS | BEVERAGES | SEASONINGS

Monique Vescia is a writer, dedicated home cook, and avid follower of foodie blogs. She has written on a range of subjects, including health, earth science, photography, and social networking. She lives in Seattle, one of the epicenters of the farm-to-table movement, with her husband and son, and raises bees in her backyard.

Katharine Greider
FRUITS | PROTEINS | WHOLE GRAINS

Katharine Greider is a freelance writer living in New York City. Her work has appeared in dozens of national and local publications. She is the author of two books, most recently *The Archaeology of Home: An Epic Set on a Thousand Square Feet of the Lower East Side* (PublicAffairs, 2011).

ILLUSTRATIONS CREDITS

Front Cover
Left (top to bottom): Joe Biafore/iStockphoto; 2009fotofriends/Shutterstock; blueeyes/Shutterstock; StevanZZ/Shutterstock; avs/Shutterstock; Right (top to bottom): Svetlana Lukienko/Shutterstock; Huguette Roe/Shutterstock; vkbhat/iStockphoto; Shulevskyy Volodymyr/Shutterstock; Suzanne Tucker/Shutterstock.

Back Cover
Left (top to bottom): Teodora George/Shutterstock; mpessaris/Shutterstock; GomezDavid/iStockphoto; mphillips007/iStockphoto; FotografiaBasica/iStockphoto; Right (top to bottom): jskiba/iStockphoto; Baloncici/iStockphoto; Valentyn Volkov/Shutterstock; Stieglitz/iStockphoto; Ragnarock/Shutterstock.

Front Matter
1, Carlos Gawronski/Getty Images; 2-3, ZERT/Getty Images; 4 (Asparagus), Debu55y/Shutterstock, (Squash), Olga Popova/Shutterstock, (Beets), Sasha Davas/Shutterstock, (Blackberries), alex7021/iStockphoto, (Apples), RusGri/Shutterstock, (Peaches), Dionisvera/Shutterstock, (Bananas), Maks Narodenko/Shutterstock; 5 (Lobster), Dani Vincek/Shutterstock, (Hazelnuts), Sukharevskyy Dmytro (nevodka)/Shutterstock, (Edamame/Soybeans), bonchan/Shutterstock, (Porridge), Volosina/Shutterstock, (Quinoa), marekuliasz/Shutterstock, (Flax Seeds), Picsfive/Shutterstock, (Chocolate), Andris Tkacenko/Shutterstock, (Coffee), Valentyn Volkov/Shutterstock, (Beer), Valentyn Volkov/Shutterstock, 6, Michael Piazza Photography; 7, Anthony Boccaccio/Getty Images; 8 (UP), Joe Biafore/iStockphoto; 8 (LO), Africa Studio/Shutterstock; 10, Thomas Barwick/Getty Images; 12, Bobkeenan Photography/Shutterstock; 14 (UP), Maks Narodenko/Shutterstock; 14 (LO), Bruce Block/Getty Images; 16, Michael Piazza Photography; 17, Premium UIG/Getty Images; 18 (UP), Roman Samokhin/Shutterstock; 18 (LO), Margouillat Photo/Shutterstock; 20, Bruce Block/iStockphoto; 22 (UP), Datacraft Co Ltd/Getty Images; 22 (LO), Valentyn Volkov/Shutterstock; 24 (UP), Andrii Gorulko/Shutterstock; 24 (LO), Aleksandra Pikalova/Shutterstock.

Chapter 1
26 (UP), Olga Popova/Shutterstock; 26 (CTR), Debu55y/Shutterstock; 26 (LO), Sasha Davas/Shutterstock; 27, MASAHIRO MORIGAKI/amanaimagesRF/Getty Images; 28, Cristian Baitg/iStockphoto; 29, Jeffrey Coolidge/The Image Bank/Getty Images; 30, Mark Thiessen, NGS; 31, Eric Broder Van Dyke/Shutterstock; 32 (LE), Olha Afanasieva/Shutterstock; 32 (RT), Lepas/Shutterstock; 33 (LE), Steve Cukrov/Shutterstock; 33 (RT), Kathryne Taylor/cookieandkate.com; 34 (LE), Luzia Ellert/Getty Images; 34 (RT), Debu55y/Shutterstock; 35 (UP), adlifemarketing/iStockphoto; 35 (LO), Philip Wilkins/Getty Images; 36 (UP), Valery121283/Shutterstock; 36 (LO), ElenaGaak/iStockphoto; 37 (UP), microgen/iStockphoto; 37 (LO), meltonmedia/iStockphoto; 38 (UP), pjohnson1/iStockphoto; 38 (LO), supermimicry/iStockphoto; 39 (UP), Profimedia.CZ a.s./Alamy; 39 (LO), Cathleen Abers-Kimball/iStockphoto; 40 (UP), SOMMAI/Shutterstock; 40 (LO), AnjelikaGr/Shutterstock; 41 (UP), feawt/Shutterstock; 41 (LO), Santanor/Shutterstock; 42, violetkaipa/Shutterstock; 43 (UP), B. and E. Dudzinscy/Shutterstock; 43 (LO), Suzifoo/iStockphoto; 44, KITSANANAN/Shutterstock; 45 (UP), littleny/Shutterstock; 45 (LO), BruceBlock/iStockphoto; 46, eye-blink/Shutterstock; 47 (UP), P.K. Newby; 47 (LO), boblin/iStockphoto; 48 (UP), Viktar Malyshchyts/Shutterstock; 48 (LO), siamionau pavel/Shutterstock; 49, Bo Valentino/Shutterstock; 50 (UP), monticello/Shutterstock; 50 (LO), Photo by Ian van Coller/Getty Images; 51 (UP), Feng Yu/Shutterstock; 52 (UP), Lilyana Vynogradova/Shutterstock; 52 (LO), monticello/Shutterstock; 52 (LO), Wittybear/iStockphoto; 53 (UP), kcline/iStockphoto; 53 (LO), AdShooter/iStockphoto; 54 (UP), Sergiy Telesh/Shutterstock; 54 (LO), Valentyn Volkov/Shutterstock; 55 (UP), Palo_ok/Shutterstock; 55 (LO), Cristina Negoita/Shutterstock; 56 (UP), Valentyn Volkov/Shutterstock; 56 (LO), Massimiliano Gallo/Shutterstock; 57 (UP), Denis and Yulia Pogostins/Shutterstock; 57 (LO), Elzbieta Sekowska/Shutterstock; 58 (UP), amst/Shutterstock; 58 (LO), Shumilina Maria/Shutterstock; 59 (UP), Foodpictures/Shutterstock; 60 (UP), Sce Hwai PHANG/Getty Images; 60 (LO), Elovich/Shutterstock; 60 (LO), Lidante/Shutterstock; 61 (UP), DonMcGillis/iStockphoto; 61 (LO), Hywit Dimyadi/Shutterstock; 62, loops7/iStockphoto; 63 (UP), missaigong/iStockphoto; 63 (LO), Lehner/iStockphoto; 64, Riverlim/iStockphoto; 65 (UP), siraphat/Shutterstock; 65 (LO), Lisa Charles Watson/Getty Images; 66 (UP), mashuk/

iStockphoto; 66 (LO), My Lit'l Eye/Shutterstock; 67 (UP), dlerick/iStockphoto; 67 (LO), Kathryne Taylor/cookieandkate.com; 68 (LE), vanillaechoes/Shutterstock; 68 (RT), xxmmxx/iStockphoto; 69 (UP), Kenneth Wiedemann/iStockphoto; 69 (LO), posteriori/iStockphoto; 70, Bob Ingelhart/Getty Images; 71 (UP), Susan Trigg/iStockphoto; 71 (LO), Creativeye99/iStockphoto; 72 (UP), Floortje/iStockphoto; 72 (LO), stuartpitkin/iStockphoto; 73 (UP), Timolina/Shutterstock; 73 (LO), FotografiaBasica/iStockphoto; 74 (UP), Nattika/Shutterstock; 74 (LO), Nickola_Che/Shutterstock; 75, Dana Gallagher/FoodPix/Getty Images; 76 (UP), Kristina Pchelintseva/Shutterstock; 76 (LO), AGfoto/Shutterstock; 77 (LO), Denise Taylor/Getty Images; 77 (UP), Andrew Scrivani/The Food Passionates/Corbis; 78 (UP), small_frog/iStockphoto; 78 (LO), WIN-Initiative/Getty Images; 79, sarsmis/Shutterstock; 80 (UP), JIANG HONGYAN/Shutterstock; 80 (LO), Foodpictures/Shutterstock; 81 (UP), Louis-Laurent Grandadam/Getty Images; 81 (LO), supermimicry/iStockphoto; 82 (LE), Masahiro Makino/Getty Images; 82 (RT), vig64/Shutterstock; 83 (UP), bonchan/Shutterstock; 83 (LO), Juraj Kovac/Shutterstock; 84 (UP), DNY59/iStockphoto; 84 (LO), Madlen/Shutterstock; 85 (UP), Temmuz Can Arsiray/iStockphoto; 85 (LO), keko64/Shutterstock; 86 (UP), imagestock/iStockphoto; 86 (LO), P.K. Newby; 87 (UP), BruceBlock/iStockphoto; 87 (LO), EasyBuy4u/iStockphoto; 88 (UP), Lehner/iStockphoto; 88 (LO), PicturePartners/iStockphoto; 89 (UP), Lena GabrilovichShutterstock; 89 (LO), Dream79/Shutterstock; 90 (UP), vasiliki/iStockphoto; 90 (CTR), Funwithfood/iStockphoto; 90 (LO), 4kodiak/iStockphoto; 91, svry/Shutterstock; 92 (UP), Nattika/Shutterstock; 92 (LO), nito/Shutterstock; 93 (UP), aquariagirl1970/Shutterstock; 93 (LO), Christian Draghici/Shutterstock; 94 (UP), Natalya Bidyukova/Shutterstock; 94 (LO), Anna Hoychuk/Shutterstock; 95 (UP), Peter Zijlstra/Shutterstock; 95 (LO), azure/Shutterstock; 96 (UP), Ju-Lee/iStockphoto; 96 (LO), Peter Zijlstra/Shutterstock; 97, Keith Szafranski/iStockphoto; 98, spectrumblue/Shutterstock; 99, PicturePartners/iStockphoto; 99 (LOLE), ElenaGaak/Shutterstock; 99 (LORT), Alan Richardson/Getty Images.

Chapter 2
100 (UPLE), alex7021/iStockphoto; 100 (UPRT), Dionisvera/Shutterstock; 100 (LOLE), RusGri/Shutterstock; 100 (LORT), Maks Narodenko/Shutterstock; 101, Jeffrey Coolidge/The Image Bank/Getty Images; 102, Maximilian Stock Ltd./Getty Images; 103, Rosemary Weller/Getty Images; 104 (UP), Maks Narodenko/Shutterstock; 104 (LO), perkmeup/iStockphoto; 105 (UP), Sea Wave/Shutterstock; 105 (LO), sampsyseeds/iStockphoto; 106 (UP), Goncharuk/Shutterstock; 106 (LO), Garry L./Shutterstock; 107 (UP), Dream79/Shutterstock; 107 (LO), Richard M Lee/Shutterstock; 108, Vasilevich Aliaksandr/Shutterstock; 109 (UP), Susan Schmitz/Shutterstock; 109 (LO), supermimicry/iStockphoto; 110 (UP), DebbiSmirnoff/iStockphoto; 110 (LO), Jodi Pudge/Getty Images; 111, BMJ/Shutterstock; 112 (UP), Valentyn Volkov/Shutterstock; 112 (LO), Lesya Dolyuk/Shutterstock; 113, Kativ/iStockphoto; 114 (UP), Viktar/iStockphoto; 114 (LO), vanillaechoes/Shutterstock; 115 (UP), rookman/iStockphoto; 115 (LO), pjohnson1/iStockphoto; 116 (UP), FineShine/Shutterstock; 116 (LO), ElenaGaak/iStockphoto; 117 (UP), Alina Vincent Photography, LLC/iStockphoto; 117 (LO), schankz/Shutterstock; 118 (UP), Madlen/Shutterstock; 118 (LO), Funwithfood/iStockphoto; 119, Truyen Vu/Shutterstock; 120 (UP), Aprilphoto/Shutterstock; 120 (LO), robynmac/iStockphoto; 121 (LE), f9photos/iStockphoto; 121 (RT), Andrew Hagen/Shutterstock; 122, Ivan Kruk/Shutterstock; 123, arka38/Shutterstock; 124 (UP), Antagain/iStockphoto; 124 (LO), GeorgeDolgikh/iStockphoto; 125 (UP), Barcin/iStockphoto; 125 (LO), Purestock/Getty Images; 126 (UP), Valentyn Volkov/Shutterstock; 126 (LO), antos777/iStockphoto; 127 (UP), DianePeacock/iStockphoto; 127 (LO), Photographer/Shutterstock; 128, YinYang/iStockphoto; 129 (UP), OGphoto/iStockphoto; 129 (LO), Karen Wunderman/iStockphoto; 130 (UP), Maks Narodenko/Shutterstock; 130 (LO), Albo003/Shutterstock; 131, AnjelikaGr/Shutterstock; 132 (UP), felinda/iStockphoto; 132 (LO), sayhmog/Shutterstock; 133, antpkr/Shutterstock; 133 (UP), leelakajonkij/iStockphoto; 134 (UP), YinYang/iStockphoto; 134 (LO), Sarsmis/iStockphoto; 135, Petko Danov/Getty Images; 136, Maks Narodenko/Shutterstock; 137 (UP), urbanlight/Shutterstock; 137 (LO), vanillaechoes/Shutterstock; 138, Frantysek/iStockphoto; 139 (UP), zmkstudio/Shutterstock; 139 (LO), sekulicn/iStockphoto; 140 (UP), Anna Kucherova/Shutterstock; 140 (LO), fabiofoto/iStockphoto; 141 (UP), studioVin/Shutterstock; 141 (LO), stonerobertc/iStockphoto; 142 (UP), SorenP/iStockphoto; 142 (LO), maxpro/Shutterstock; 143 (UP), nicolesy/iStockphoto; 143 (LO), Studio-Annika/iStockphoto; 144, Suslik1983/Shutterstock; 145 (UP),

ILLUSTRATIONS CREDITS

yuris/Shutterstock; 145 (LO), ElenaGaak/Shutterstock; 146 (UP), julichka/iStockphoto; 146 (CTR), Smileus/Shutterstock; 146 (LO), Synergee/iStockphoto; 147, NightAndDayImages/iStockphoto.

Chapter 3
148 (UP), Dani Vincek/Shutterstock; 148 (LOLE), Sukharevskyy Dmytro (nevodka)/Shutterstock; 148 (LORT), bonchan/Shutterstock; 149, Barcin/iStockphoto; 150, STUDIO BOX/Getty Images; 151, Susan Seubert/National Geographic Stock; 152 (UP), Garsya/Shutterstock; 152 (LO), grafvision/Shutterstock; 153 (UP), AnjelikaGr/Shutterstock; 153 (LO), Bon Appetit/Alamy; 154 (UP), Mehmet Hilmi Barcin/iStockphoto; 154 (LO), Jim Bowie/Shutterstock; 155, Jan S./Shutterstock; 156 (UP), Madlen/Shutterstock; 156 (LO), Mona Makela/Shutterstock; 157 (UP), Beth Galton/Getty Images; 157 (LO), Alex Koloskov/Shutterstock; 158 (UP), Creativeye99/iStockphoto; 158 (LO), Penny De Los Santos/age fotostock; 159, Allison Dinner/Getty Images; 160, lepas2004/iStockphoto; 161 (UP), Philippe Desnerck/Getty Images; 161 (LO), Aggie 11/Shutterstock; 162, Elena Schweitzer/Shutterstock; 163 (UP), Lilyana Vynogradova/Shutterstock; 163 (LO), marcomayer/iStockphoto; 164 (UP), Dream79/Shutterstock; 164 (LO), Luca Trovato/Getty Images; 165 (LE), Reza Estakhrian/Getty Images; 165 (RT), agitons/iStockphoto; 166, Dani Vincek/Shutterstock; 167 (UP), whitewish/iStockphoto; 167 (LO), MarkMirror/Shutterstock; 168, malerapaso/iStockphoto; 169 (UP), Omelchenko/Shutterstock; 169 (CTR), rusm/iStockphoto; 169 (LO), JOEYSTUDIO/Shutterstock; 170 (UP), Fanfo/Shutterstock; 170 (LO), Kubaeva/Shutterstock; 171 (UP), martellostudio/iStockphoto; 171 (LO), nycshooter/iStockphoto; 172 (UP), Nattika/Shutterstock; 172 (LO), cmnaumann/Shutterstock; 173, Topalov Djura/iStockphoto; 174 (UP), optimarc/Shutterstock; 174 (LO), cjp/iStockphoto; 175, martinturzak/iStockphoto; 176 (UP), Elena Elisseeva/Shutterstock; 176 (LO), paulprescott72/iStockphoto; 177, travellinglight/iStockphoto; 178 (UP), Alina Vincent Photography, LLC/iStockphoto; 178 (LO), Lepas/Shutterstock; 179 (UP), sauletas/Shutterstock; 179 (LO), funkybg/iStockphoto; 180 (UP), Kaan Ates/iStockphoto; 180 (LO), TwilightArtPictures/Shutterstock; 181 (UP), Lidante/Shutterstock; 181 (LO), magnetcreative/iStockphoto; 182 (UP), jeehyun/Shutterstock; 182 (LO), Karl Allgaeuer/Shutterstock; 183 (UP), sarsmis/Shutterstock; 183 (LO), ffolas/iStockphoto; 184 (UP), Robyn Mackenzie/Shutterstock; 184 (LO), agostinosangel/iStockphoto; 185 (UP), dionisvero/iStockphoto; 185 (LO), Foodpictures/Shutterstock; 186, Madlen/Shutterstock; 187 (UP), Elena Schweitzer/Shutterstock; 187 (LO), CGissemann/Shutterstock; 188 (UP), AlexStar/Shutterstock; 188 (LO), gmnicholas/iStockphoto; 189, Lauri Patterson/iStockphoto; 190, Maceofoto/Shutterstock; 191 (LE), Margouillat Photo/Shutterstock; 191 (RT), kcline/iStockphoto; 192, Africa Studio/Shutterstock; 193 (UP), Melica/Shutterstock; 193 (LO), isak55/Shutterstock; 194 (UP), SidorovichV/Shutterstock; 194 (LO), Cathy Britcliffe/iStockphoto; 195 (UP), lightfast/iStockphoto; 195 (LO), Zandebasenjis/iStockphoto; 196 (UP), Elena Schweitzer/Shutterstock; 196 (LO), 4kodiak/iStockphoto; 197, Viacheslav Nikolaenko/Shutterstock; 198 (UP), NinaM/Shutterstock; 198 (LO), Linelds/iStockphoto; 199, Myrmidon/Shutterstock; 200, Jacek Chabraszewski/Shutterstock; 201 (UP), MaraZe/Shutterstock; 201 (LO), taxzi/iStockphoto; 202 (UP), Pakhnyushcha/Shutterstock; 202 (LO), Ildi Papp/Shutterstock; 203 (UP), rtyree1/iStockphoto; 203 (LO), AKodisinghe/iStockphoto; 204 (UP), mexrix/Shutterstock; 204 (LO), Richard M Lee/Shutterstock; 205, grandriver/iStockphoto; 206, ElenaGaak/Shutterstock; 207 (LE), HLPhoto/Shutterstock; 207 (RT), Juriah Mosin/Shutterstock; 208 (UP), draconus/Shutterstock; 208 (LO), Ildi Papp/Shutterstock; 209 (UP), FotografiaBasica/iStockphoto; 209 (LO), Imcsike/Shutterstock; 210 (UP), PicturePartners/Shutterstock; 210 (LO), Picsfive/iStockphoto; 211 (UP), Suzifoo/iStockphoto; 211 (LO), Joerg Beuge/Shutterstock; 212, ermess/Shutterstock; 213 (UP), morganl/iStockphoto; 213 (LO), Sarsmis/iStockphoto; 214 (UP), kyoshino/iStockphoto; 214 (LO), Ekaterina Kamenetsky/Shutterstock; 215, Fotokostic/Shutterstock; 216, carlosdelacalle/Shutterstock; 217 (UP), Margouillat Photo/Shutterstock; 217 (LO), iinwibisono/iStockphoto; 218 (UP), maxuser/iStockphoto; 218 (LO), joesayhello/Shutterstock; 219, Brian J. Skerry/National Geographic/Getty Images; 220, Isantilli/Shutterstock; 221 (UP), Juanmonino/iStockphoto; 221 (LO), Paul Cowan/Shutterstock; 222, Chepko/iStockphoto; 223 (UP), vikif/iStockphoto; 223 (LO), adlifemarketing/iStockphoto; 224 (UP), syolacan/iStockphoto; 224 (LO), oksix/Shutterstock; 225 (UP), bazza1960/iStockphoto; 225 (LO), unkas_photo/iStockphoto; 226 (UP), studiogi/Shutterstock; 226 (LO), assalve/iStockphoto; 227 (UP), Uliana Bazar; 227 (LO), Gayvoronskaya_Yana/Shutterstock; 228,

B. and E. Dudzinscy/Shutterstock; 229 (UP), Olaf Speier/Shutterstock; 229 (LO), Martin Turzak/Shutterstock; 230, letty17/iStockphoto; 231 (UP), -lvinst-/iStockphoto; 231 (LO), ElenaGaak/Shutterstock.

Chapter 4
232 (LE), Volosina/Shutterstock; 232 (RT), marekuliasz/Shutterstock; 233, wasanajai/Shutterstock; 234, Creativeye99/iStockphoto; 235, Janine Lamontagne/Getty Images; 236 (UP), marekuliasz/iStockphoto; 236 (LO), joannawnuk/Shutterstock; 237, Simone van den Berg/Shutterstock; 238 (UP), Alasdair James/iStockphoto; 238 (CTR), svariophoto/iStockphoto; 238 (LO), robynmac/iStockphoto; 239, David Marsden/Getty Images; 240 (UP), Ivaylo Ivanov/Shutterstock; 240 (LO), robynmac/iStockphoto; 241, fotoflare/iStockphoto; 242 (UP), Seregam/Shutterstock; 242 (LO), Timolina/Shutterstock; 243 (UP), RossHelen/Shutterstock; 243 (LO), matka_Wariatka/iStockphoto; 244 (UP), Diana Taliun/Shutterstock; 244 (LO), Olga Miltsova/Shutterstock; 245 (UP), MKucova/iStockphoto; 245 (LOLE), Foodanddrink Photos/age fotostock; 245 (LORT), baibaz/iStockphoto; 246 (UP), bonchan/iStockphoto; 246 (LO), John Freeman/Getty Images; 247 (LE), Foodpictures/Shutterstock; 247 (RT), alexsvirid/Shutterstock; 248 (UP), Imageman/Shutterstock; 248 (LO), li jingwang/iStockphoto; 249 (UP), alle12/iStockphoto; 249 (LO), Ina Peters/iStockphoto; 250 (UP), Indigo Fish/Shutterstock; 250 (LO), lenazap/iStockphoto; 251, edoneil/iStockphoto.

Chapter 5
252 (LE), Picsfive/Shutterstock; 252 (RT), Andris Tkacenko/Shutterstock; 253, Africa Studio/Shutterstock; 254, Ira Block/NGS; 255, masaltof/iStockphoto; 256 (UP), iLight foto/Shutterstock; 256 (LO), Will Selarep/Getty Images; 257, Tobik/Shutterstock; 258 (UP), M. Unal Ozmen/Shutterstock; 258 (LO), Vizual Studio/Shutterstock; 259 (UP), eefauscan/iStockphoto; 259 (LO), Arie v.d. Wolde/Shutterstock; 260, Subbotina Anna/Shutterstock; 261 (LE), Ian O'Leary/Getty Images; 261 (RT), fotolinchen/iStockphoto; 262, xpixel/Shutterstock; 263 (UP), jurgajurga/Shutterstock; 263 (LO), Dave Reede/Getty Images; 264, Valentyn Volkov/Shutterstock; 265 (UP), mumininan/iStockphoto; 265 (LO), Tanya_F/iStockphoto; 266 (UP), Gary Ombler/Getty Images; 266 (LO), Roel Smart/Shutterstock; 267 (UP), etitarenko/iStockphoto; 267 (LO), Reika/Shutterstock; 268, bergamont/Shutterstock; 269 (UP), HughStonelan/iStockphoto; 269 (LO), Maxim Petrichuk/Shutterstock.

Chapter 6
270 (LE & RT), Valentyn Volkov/Shutterstock; 271, Africa Studio/Shutterstock; 272, Denis Waugh/Getty Images; 273, Africa Studio/Shutterstock; 274 (UP), Elena Elisseeva/Shutterstock; 274 (LO), prudkov/Shutterstock; 275, somchaij/Shutterstock; 276, Raja Islam/Getty Images; 277 (LE), Mariyana Misaleva/Shutterstock; 277 (RT), silver-john/Shutterstock; 278 (UP), Nitr/Shutterstock; 278 (LO), Vaclav Mach/Shutterstock; 279 (UP), Barnaby Chambers/Shutterstock; 279 (LO), Erdosain/iStockphoto; 280, NinaM/Shutterstock; 281 (UP), Ingetje Tadros/Getty Images; 281 (LO), StudioThreeDots/iStockphoto; 282, oriori/Shutterstock; 283 (UP), Lecic/Shutterstock; 283 (LO), Olga Miltsova/Shutterstock; 284, bitt24/Shutterstock; 285 (LE), Neustockimages/iStockphoto; 285 (RT), Pietus/Shutterstock; 286, gresei/Shutterstock; 287 (UP), Leon Harris/Getty Images; 287 (LO), HandmadePictures/Shutterstock; 288 (UP), demypic/iStockphoto; 288 (LO), al62/iStockphoto; 289 (UP), hadynyah/iStockphoto; 289 (LO), Elena Elisseeva/Shutterstock; 290 (UP), Christian Draghici/Shutterstock; 290 (LO), Image Source/Getty Images; 291 (UP), Kim D. French/Shutterstock; 291 (LO), c-vino/iStockphoto; 292, Brandon Bourdages/Shutterstock; 293 (LE), Belgium/iStockphoto; 293 (RT), Steve Cukrov/Shutterstock.

Back Matter
294 (LE), JIANG HONGYAN/Shutterstock; 294 (RT), Nata-Lia/Shutterstock; 296 (LE), Volosina/Shutterstock; 296 (RT), Alina Vincent Photography, LC/iStockphoto; 297 (LE), JIANG HONGYAN/Shutterstock; 297 (RT), YinYang/iStockphoto; 298 (LE), Nata-Lia/Shutterstock; 298 (RT), eye-blink/Shutterstock; 299 (LE), Volosina/Shutterstock; 299 (RT), Viktar Malyshchyts/Shutterstock; 300 (LE), Volosina/Shutterstock; 300 (RT), Chad Zuber/Shutterstock; 301 (LE), Scisetti Alfio/Shutterstock; 301 (RT), DenisNata/Shutterstock; 302 (LE), Nattika/Shutterstock; 302 (RT), Suzifoo/iStockphoto; 303 (LE), Volosina/Shutterstock; 303 (RT), Quang Ho/Shutterstock; 304 (LE and RT), Michael Piazza Photography; 318 Carlos Gawronski/Getty Images.

INDEX

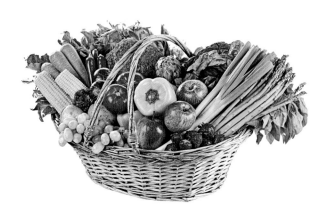

NATIONAL GEOGRAPHIC
FOODS FOR HEALTH

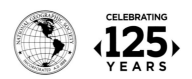

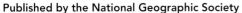

Published by the National Geographic Society

John M. Fahey, *Chairman of the Board and Chief Executive Officer*

Declan Moore, *Executive Vice President; President, Publishing and Travel*

Melina Gerosa Bellows, *Executive Vice President; Chief Creative Officer, Books, Kids, and Family*

Prepared by the Book Division

Hector Sierra, *Senior Vice President and General Manager*

Janet Goldstein, *Senior Vice President and Editorial Director*

Jonathan Halling, *Design Director, Books and Children's Publishing*

Marianne R. Koszorus, *Design Director, Books*

Susan Tyler Hitchcock, *Senior Editor*

R. Gary Colbert, *Production Director*

Jennifer A. Thornton, *Director of Managing Editorial*

Susan S. Blair, *Director of Photography*

Meredith C. Wilcox, *Director, Administration and Rights Clearance*

Staff for This Book

Gail Spilsbury, *Project Editor*

Sanaa Akkach, *Art Director*

Uliana Bazar, *Illustrations Editor*

Grassroots Graphics, *Design and Production*

Marshall Kiker, *Associate Managing Editor*

Lisa A. Walker, *Production Manager*

Galen Young, *Rights Clearance Specialist*

Kate Olsen, *Production Design Assistant*

Erin Greenhalgh, *Editorial Intern*

Susan Nguyen, *Editorial Intern*

Developed and produced by Print Matters, Inc. (www.printmattersinc.com)

Production Services

Phillip L. Schlosser, *Senior Vice President*

Chris Brown, *Vice President, NG Book Manufacturing*

George Bounelis, *Vice President, Production Services*

Nicole Elliott, *Manager*

Rachel Faulise, *Manager*

Robert L. Barr, *Manager*

The National Geographic Society is one of the world's largest nonprofit scientific and educational organizations. Its mission is to inspire people to care about the planet. Founded in 1888, the Society is member supported and offers a community for members to get closer to explorers, connect with other members, and help make a difference. The Society reaches more than 450 million people worldwide each month through *National Geographic* and other magazines; National Geographic Channel; television documentaries; music; radio; films; books; DVDs; maps; exhibitions; live events; school publishing programs; interactive media; and merchandise. National Geographic has funded more than 10,000 scientific research, conservation, and exploration projects and supports an education program promoting geographic literacy. For more information, visit www.nationalgeographic.com.

National Geographic Society
1145 17th Street N.W.
Washington, D.C. 20036-4688 U.S.A.

For information about special discounts for bulk purchases, please contact National Geographic Books Special Sales: ngspecsales@ngs.org

For rights or permissions inquiries, please contact National Geographic Books Subsidiary Rights: ngbookrights@ngs.org

Library of Congress Cataloging-in-Publication Data
National Geographic Foods for health: choose and use the very best foods for your family and our planet / contributions by Barton Seaver and P.K. Newby.
    p.cm.
  Includes index.
  ISBN 978-1-4262-1332-8 (hardcover : alk. paper) -- ISBN 978-1-4262-1333-5 (hardcover (deluxe) : alk. paper)
  1. Food. 2. Nutrition. 3. Functional foods. 4. Health promotion. 5. Consumer education.
  TX353.C6224 2013
  641.3--dc23
                                          2013026965

ISBN 978-1-4262-1332-8
ISBN 978-1-4262-1333-5 (deluxe)

Printed in the United States of America

13/RRDW-CML/1

STAY HEALTHY

with more books from National Geographic

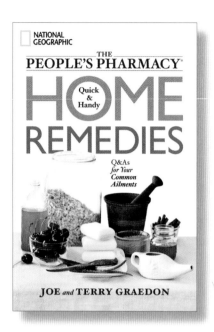

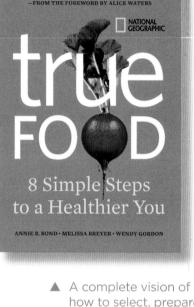

▲ Quick, easy, inviting, fun to read—this book offers as much information as a voluminous encyclopedia on home remedies.

▲ A complete vision of how to select, prepare, serve, store, and enjoy the planet's bounteous harvest.

Provides reliable and practical information about some of the most important medicinal herbs available.

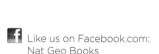

Like us on Facebook.com: Nat Geo Books

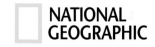

Follow us onTwitter.com: @NatGeoBooks

NATIONAL GEOGRAPHIC

AVAILABLE WHEREVER BOOKS ARE SOLD
nationalgeographic.com/books